BEARDS

BEARDS

THEIR

SOCIAL STANDING

RELIGIOUS INVOLVEMENTS

DECORATIVE POSSIBILITIES

AND

VALUE IN OFFENCE

AND DEFENCE

THROUGH THE AGES

BY

Reginald Reynolds

A HARVEST BOOK

HARCOURT BRACE JOVANOVICH

NEW YORK AND LONDON

Printed in the United States of America

Harvest edition published by arrangement with Doubleday & Company, Inc.

Library of Congress Cataloging in Publication Data

Reynolds, Reginald, 1905-
Beards

(A Harvest book ; HB 334)

Reprint of the 1950 ed. published by Allen & Unwin, London.
1. Beard. I. Title.
GT2320.R49   1976   391′.5   75-34138
ISBN 0-15-610845-3

First Harvest edition 1976

A   B   C   D   E   F   G   H   I   J

DEDICATION AD HOMINES

Non equidem Arma Virumque cano ast extollere Barbam
Intendo.   J. H. Schwabe

Beards and the Man I sing, who first his chin
Scraped with a flint, some woman's heart to win ;
I sing of controversies that ensued—
Deadly debates that led to deadlier feud—
Of beards political and beards religious
And legislation for the beard litigious,
Of Bluebeard and of Barbarossa (both
Lent local colour to the manly growth)
And Sacred Beards that dignify an oath.

Ye bearded swains, who scorn the razored cheek,
And trim your lawns with shears but once a week,
Thought you that Wisdom was with whiskers garbed ?
My chin is shaven, but my wit is barbed.
And ye, the martyrs of the daily moan,
Who reap each morning where ye have not sown,
Here is a mirror where your face is seen
Had not the razor carved the features clean—
The hoary Patriarch you might have been.

AUX DAMES

Votre sexe n'est là que pour la dépendance :
Du coté de la barbe est la toute puissance . . .
                                    L'Ecole des Femmes

ACKNOWLEDGMENTS

In these pages there will be found the names of some—there were, indeed, many others not named—who helped me with suggestions and criticisms. Among those mentioned is my old friend, Ben Vincent, who also greatly assisted me by reading the proofs. In this last (and most tiresome) task I was also much indebted to my good friends, P. J. Macmanus and Miss Marguerite Louis.

I take this opportunity, whilst expressing my deep gratitude to these scholars for their kindness, to mention also the names of Kenneth Fawdry and my nephew, Nicholas Hudson. Their corrections to the American proofs were of great value in preparing the present edition.

R. R.

CONTENTS

CHAPTER I

POGONOTROPHY IN SERENDIP

. . . And speak with such respect and honour
Both of the beard and the beard's owner.

HUDIBRAS

אָדָם בַּעַל זָקָן דַּק הוּא פִּקֵחַ עַבְדְּקָן הוּא כְּסִיל   BEN SIRACH

IT was the opinion of Mr. Pope, who spoke from personal experience, that a little learning is a dangerous thing ; though T. H. Huxley wondered who had enough to be out of danger. My own poor oddments, like the scrapings and clippings of a barber's shop, would perchance have been better used as Ezekiel was told to dispose of his hair and beard—*videlicet* : that one part should be burnt, one chopped up and the rest thrown to the wind. And were I not a confirmed Serendipitist such might have been their destiny.

Of this craft, feat or mystery of Serendipity, since some are ignorant (and therefore, by definition, too indolent to consult a dictionary) I will explain that it is the profession claimed by Autolycus and attributed to Mercury—that of a snapper-up of unconsidered trifles. The word itself was derived by Horace Walpole from the adventures of those princes of Serendip who, said he, were always making discoveries by accidents and sagacity of things they were not in quest of.

The Perils of Serendip

Now any good library is to a Serendipitist what a fly-paper is to a fly ; and the most dangerous of all such fly-papers to a fly of small learning, such as myself, is the Reading Room of the British Museum. You ask for some old pamphlet or broadsheet, and it is certain to arrive in a bound volume with some twenty others or more, that are all the more entertaining because they have nothing in common with your studies. Or again, you are reading a life of Pomponius Atticus, who does not interest you, when you find that he died of a *tenesmos*, which lays hold of your curiosity. A considerate footnote explains that this affliction is *a Violent Motion without the Power of going to Stool* ; and a new word with a sinister sound and a truly terrifying connotation is added to your vocabulary. It will explain almost any modern poet, except Mr. Betjeman, and can be swung on the head of any adverse critic of this book who has not himself written a volume on beards.

The God who keeps safe

Words alone are fatal to the Serendipitist. I have many drawers crammed with note-books and odd scraps of paper, where I have noted the gleanings of my dictionary digressions, the whole unassorted miscellany a magpie's nest of useless information. Here, for example, is a note on a Roman deity hight *Rediculus*, with his description as *the God who keeps safe*. The classical dictionary from which I obtained this vital information had added that Rediculus induced Hannibal to return home. Why should he be forgotten, while Scipio Africanus is so well remembered?

Being a Serendipitist I at once recall, and feel the itch to place upon record, such another deity of modern times. This itch is not the common malady of pamphleteers, concerning which it was written : *Prurigo scripturientium erat scabies temporum,* whereby scribblers itch when the times are scabby ; nor would I accuse myself by such excuses. For, as the Bishop of Hippo so well observed, we are the times ; such as we are, so are the times. Mine is an incurable disease, perhaps actually contracted in the Isle of Serendip (though I passed but one night at Colombo, and Sterne's sentimental journeys never took him so far, which did not save him from becoming a worse casualty than myself[1]). But I had almost forgotten the useful God whom my friend Verrier Elwin discovered among the aborigines of Central India. He is called *Sahibosum,* dresses in trousers and a solar *topee,* and is employed to deflect sahibs and memsahibs from the villages of the Saoras, by what my friend calls spiritual homeopathy. In my private Pantheon Sahibosum keeps company with Rediculus.

Had Rediculus a Beard ?

You may well ask by now when I am coming to the point ; but believe me, it is easy enough. Thus : *Had Rediculus a beard ?* I do

[1] I begin (he said) with writing the first sentence—and trusting to Almighty God for the second. He held it to be the most religious way to write a book, and so do I.

not know, and will refrain from the obvious inference. But I will lay heavy odds that he was so adorned, for such was the custom of Roman deities ; though my own patron, Mercury, is credited with the invention of shaving. As to Sahibosum, since he is Sahibo-morphic, I will assume that he is clean-shaven, as befits a modern deity ; but such are exceptions. For beards were unquestionably an attribute of the Gods in former times, also of patriarchs, prophets and Fathers of the Church—perhaps because (as Mr. Brophy suggests in his work on *The Human Face*) the mouth and jaws betray carnal appetites, whereas the eyes and brows convey dignity.

It was with some such general notions in my head that I was startled into my present studies by the most fatal shipwreck that ever marooned a luckless Odysseus on Horace Walpole's enchanted island. It fell about this way. I was guilelessly reading an article by Professor Rolleston in *Archæologia* (XLVII, 1883) when I found myself staring at this phrase, if I should not rather call it a rune or incantation :

THERE APPEARS TO BE SOME NECESSARY CORRE-LATION BETWEEN HIPPOPHAGY, POGONOTROPHY AND PERHAPS PAGANISM.

Pogonotrophy and Hippophagy.

You may imagine that, after I had read this seven times, I made as many circuits of the floor-space, looking (perhaps) not unlike Archimedes contemplating the memorable bath that brought enlightenment. Two courses lay open to me. To pursue the records of hippophagy, in search of eaters of horse-flesh who wore beards ; or to study the annals of pogonotrophy, in quest of bearded men who ate horse-flesh. I chose first what appeared to be the charted course of hippophagy, in company with Keysler, Grimm and the indispensable Walter Johnson, Archæologist of our British Byways.

In this voyage I examined the sacred horses of Kronos, Poseidon and Athene, and those of India, sacrificed in the *Asvamedhya*. I observed the horse sacrifices of Japan, and of the Mordvins in Eastern Russia. I traced these sacrifices home to the Midsummer festivals of the Celts, speculated upon the White Horses scoured from the chalk escarpments of Southern England and read of ancient Teutonic traditions that ascribed to giants and witches the habit of eating horse-flesh, on account of its magical properties. I found nowhere the suggestion that the horse, the sacrifice or the diet was related to the wearing of a beard, unless it were by implication, in the case of witches, who are well known to have black tufts on their chins. But these I will leave for later consideration.

Eating of horses a pagan practice

I did everything, even to frequenting the queues outside the establishment of a Belgian gentleman, who displayed a notice announcing that he sold horse-flesh exclusively for human consumption. I saw no abnormal percentage of beards among his clientèle, except upon the eager jaws of their little dogs. That the custom of eating horses was once tainted with paganism bore out one of the Professor's assertions clearly enough, and for this he himself provided evidence. Indeed, the pagan practice had crept into the Church itself, as is shown in the grace written by the monk Ekkehard in the eleventh century ; *Sit feralis equi caro dulcis sub cruce Christi*. Upon which Rolleston comments that Christian missionaries in Saxon times set their faces against this, *as also against the reprehensible practice of wearing beards*. But without short circuiting this connection, *post hoc, propter hoc* (like a Freudian psycho-analyst rationalising his own wish-fulfilments by tying up two ends of a strained hypothesis) I could still find no link between pagan beards and pagan horse-eaters.

However, as the Church was involved in both issues, I dug a little deeper. There was a letter written by Gregory III, who was Pope from A.D. 731-741, to St. Boniface, the apostle of Germany, forbidding the eating of wild horses ; but he did not mention beards. Another prohibition, also of the eighth century, was that decreed by the Council of Celchyth (no doubt my adopted Borough of Chelsea) deploring and condemning the eating of horse flesh by British Christians—*quod nullus Christianorum in orientalibus fecit*. I quote this for its memorable Latin, and also to show how complicated the quest had by now become. For, while the heresy to which Western Christians were addicted was clearly a passion for devouring their steeds, the East is here specifically absolved from the charge. And we shall soon see that, on the other hand, the heresy of pogonotrophy, the cultivation of the beard, is peculiarly Oriental (especially so far as priests are concerned) and has been less common among the Christians of the West. Ergo : the pogonotrophical paganism of the Orient does not appear to have any marked connection with Occidental hippophagy.

Horses, and how to eat them

Before I abandoned the Rolleston Riddle, for such (I must confess) it still remains, I had discovered enough to have written you a book on *Horses, And How to Eat Them*. This you shall be spared for the moment ; but I will put my mark upon the map of Serendip : HERE BE MEN WHO EAT HORSES. They are worth your attention, should you ever land there. You may consider, for example, the irregular and unconstitutional behaviour of Caligula in making his nag a Roman Consul, and the ingenious explanation, proposed by Walter Johnson, that it was by way of *homenaje* to his subjects in Gaul and Britain—a delicate tribute or compliment to their opinions on the sanctity of certain horses (for, as Mr. Wilde said, Each man kills the thing he loves). Or you may reflect upon the fact that, since John Fitzherbert wrote in 1534 (in his *Boke of Husbandry*) that *the horse, whan he dyethe, is but caryin*, most Englishmen have abhorred this meat, while their neighbours on the Continent of Europe have delighted in it. Like reformed drunkards, we English have become the very puritans of abstention—*But when will I be returning to Beards ?* Anon, anon, sir. Wiser men than I have held that full thoughts cause long parentheses. I tell you, it was in pursuit of this mare's nest that I first came by my subject, for I next gave my attention to whiskers, and found in them everything except the evidence of hippophagy ; from which agglomeration of by-products I thought fit to concoct a book.

Reverting to Beards

But since Professor Rolleston has failed to provide me with a useful text, I must look for another. Let us therefore consider an observation of E. B. Shuldham, M.D., in his monograph on *Clergyman's Sore Throat* (London, 1878), where he remarks that *the beard is an accident of sex, nay it is an accident of individual capacity for*

hair growing, but nature has been generous enough to give all her children
a nose. This is perilous ground for one of my habits. Remove
Tristram Shandy and say nothing of Slawkenbergius ; we must give
our undivided attention to the nature of a beard, before we are
led to debate with Coleridge whether the final cause of the human
nose be snuff, or no. Or worse, there is Martial, who held that
not all men have noses. *Non cuicunque datum est habere nasum*, as he
said in his first book of Epigrams ; which would invalidate Mr.
Shuldham's argument entirely, like the song of Quoodle, who
denied noses to the whole race of man. [1]

A Nose not indispensible

Let us then confine ourselves to that which we cut off from
vanity, rather to spite the face. Coleridge may say what he will ;
but his old salt might have held the wedding guest by his glittering
eye (and all the better had he been a Cyclops, with one only) even
in the absence of a nose. Indeed, it is not even specified that he
had one. But he certainly could not have prevailed without the
long grey beard. In the days of Coleridge a beard was a rarity
indeed, and this question of fashions in beards and beardlessness
must shortly claim discussion. But why this *accident of sex* ? What
purpose was it intended to serve ? On this subject I find the
greatest variety of opinion, and much hot controversy among
ancient authorities.

It was the view of Julius Cæsar Scaliger that human hairs were
not necessary, that some were useless and even hindered the *usus
vitæ*, the enjoyment of life ; of which he specified particularly : *ii
quos in superiore labro Mustaces Græci vocant,* those on the upper lip,
which the Greeks call moustaches. [2] He said, moreover, that

[1] For those who nevertheless insist upon pursuing this theme I recommend
the list of authorities given by Sterne, also Taliacotius (whom he curiously
omits) and Bishop Whately's *Notes on Noses,* which include a description of *the
anti-cogitative type.* I am considering the subject for a further study of my own.

[2] Even one of the defenders of the beard (Junius, *De Coma Commentarium*)
argued that the male face was not *entirely* covered with hair because this would
make man appear *sylvestris ac ferus* instead of *mansuetus* and *politicus.* Duckworth,
in his *Morphology and Anthropology,* mentions *the excessive hirsuteness of individuals
of feeble intellect,* which should encourage the yellow and black races ; but it is
a sobering thought for Europeans, Semites and others who suffer from pogoniasis.

excrements could have no end in themselves (*excrementa namque nullam habent finem ipsa*) and that such hairs grew merely that they might be shaved. To this I may add the opinion of Cicero, that the beard, although of a certain ornamental value, is of no use at all.

Virtues of the Beard

We have, on the other hand, the authority of Lactantius : *Jam Barbae ratio incredibilis est, quantum conferat ad dignoscendam corporum maturitatem.* He held that the beard helped to distinguish the mature body ; to which he added (and I think he *had something,* as the saying is) that it contributed to the differentiation of the sexes. He found it also an ornament of virility and strength. Not otherwise was the weighty opinion expressed by that bearded vegetarian, Clement of Alexandria, who thus interpreted the will of God :

> *Deus enim voluit feminam quidem esse glabram ac lævam, sola coma, sicut equum juba sponte naturæ exultantem : Virum autem cum sicut leones barba ornasset, virilem etiam fecit hirsuto pectore, quod quidem est roboris et imperii inditium.* (*Pædagogus* iii Cap. iii. *Adversus viros qui formam colunt.*)

From this and much more that Clement wrote on the subject,[1] which you will find in Migne's *Patrolologiæ*, Series Græca (viii, 578-592) it is clear that God intended woman to be smooth and silly, exalting naturally in her hair alone, like a horse in its mane. But man he adorned with a beard like a lion, making him tough, with a hairy chest, for such is the emblem of strength and empire.

Ideas likened to Beards

Here, indeed, we have it : the Beard is an aggressive portent of male domination. Did our Victorian forefathers trouble their minds over Women's Rights ? They did not. Their beards were

---

[1] He held the beard to be the male *signum* (*per quod vir apparet*), that it was older than Eve, and the sign of a better nature . . . So also Hoffman in his Commentary on Galen explained the beardlessness of women because *mores habent non aeque laudabiles.* Plotinus had a high opinion of the beard, and said that only God knew the number of hairs in it—a solemn thought.

the answer to all such flapdoodle and finookery. And even M. Voltaire, who lived in a shaven age, could say that ideas are like beards : *children and women never have them*. And some such sense of masculine superiority must surely have animated that author whom Isaac Disraeli quotes in his *Curiosities of Literature* (you will find it among the *Anecdotes of Fashion*). The writer, who spoke of education in the seventeenth century, felt strongly on the subject of *mustachios*. Of the young man who cultivated them he said that the time he employed in adjusting, dressing and curling them was no lost time ; *for the more he contemplates his mustachios the more his mind will cherish and be animated by masculine and courageous notions.*

Had Adam a Beard ?

Now since this hairy excrement is held by so many to be a vital distinction, indicating the superiority of the Sons of Adam to the Daughters of Eve, it is necessary that we should begin with the Garden of Eden. And here a great difficulty at once arises, because there is no agreement among the pogonologists as to whether Adam was created with a beard or without one. Jean Baptist Van Helmont (whose son appears to have become a Quaker, and no wonder) was of the scandalous opinion that Adam came into being without so much as a whisker, and that beards came (with other afflictions and diseases) after the fall of man, as Byron said :

> That ever since the fall, man for his sin
> Has had a beard entailed upon his chin.

The same opinion was maintained by Martinus Scriblerus, so I am informed, but I have failed to verify the reference among three writers of that pseudonym. It was against this monstrous heresy that Giuseppe Valeriano de Vanetti wrote his *Barbalogia ovvero ragionamento intorno alla Barba,* in 1759, to prove (as he said) that the father of the human race had a beard from the first instant of his creation, and that all men before the Deluge also had them.

Do Beards grow from excess of food ?

The opinion of Vanetti is, without doubt, more in conformity with orthodox theology. But that of Van Helmont so well

accords with the views of Jacob Boehme and of Swedenborg regarding the history of certain natural functions (of which I made
some mention in the xiith chapter of *Cleanliness and Godliness*) that
I should be rash to venture any judgment myself.   And this would
be a grave matter indeed, when faced with such a multitude of
conflicting explanations of the nature, origin and purpose of the
beard.   For Averroes held that all hair grew from an excess of
food, a view considered by the Abbé Fangé in his *Mémoires pour
servir a l'histoire de la Barbe de l'Homme* (Liége, 1774), wherein he
mentioned two theories to account for the relative absence of
beards among Red Indians, viz., that it was due to their smoking
of tobacco, or that it derived from their very simple diet.   For he
explains that from such aliments there might be less superfluity, of
which our own blood (being more *grossier*) furnishes a great
abundance, finding its way out of the body in the form of hair.
Père Fangé is properly cautious as to committing himself to such
a theory.[1]

Beards and Sins

But I cannot forbear from citing here the authority of a learned
scholar who wrote of the mystery of clerical clothing and said that
long hair

> is symbolic of the multitude of sins.   Hence clerics are directed to
> shave their beards; for cutting of the hair of the beard, *which is
> said to be nourished by the superfluous humours of the stomach*, denotes
> that we ought to cut away the vices and sins which are a super-
> fluous growth in us.   Hence we shave our beards that we may
> seem purified by innocency and humility and that we may be
> like the angels, who remain always in the bloom of youth.
> (From the *Rationale Divinorum Officiorum* of Gulielmus Durandus,
> 1459, Lib vi, cap 86.)

[1] I do not propose to discuss in this book the ethnological classification of
beards, but some interesting observations on Red Indian chins will be found in
Catlin's *North American Indians* (1841, vol. ii, 227).   C. S. Wake in the *Revue
d'Anthropologie* (Paris, 1880) wrote an interesting article on *La barbe considérée
comme caractère de race.*   For the effects of over-eating, compare *The Ancren Riwle*
(*Al Sodomes cweadschipe*, i.e.—wickedness—*com of idelnesse & of ful wombe*).

Have Angels Beards ?

Now, as to the shaving of priests, I shall have much more to say hereafter ; but in the matter of angels I must remark here that the same doubts exist which we have already recorded concerning Adam. For while angels are commonly depicted as clean-shaven (and, indeed, so smooth of cheek and fair of face that the term *angel* is commonly applied in our day to women, though every record concerning the species shows that angels are exclusively male, including Michael, Gabriel, the Prince of Darkness and those Sons of God who took wives of the daughters of men) in spite of this, I say, it must also be observed that certain old pictures, from Byzantium and other store-houses of ancient wisdom, show angels with beards.

To this it may be added that evil spirits, who are all fallen angels, are commonly represented with beards (see, for example, those shown by Francis Barrett in *The Magus, or Celestial Intelligencer,* London, 1801) ; but it may be argued, by those who hold that Adam produced a beard after the Fall, that these unfrocked angels grew them in similar circumstances. (Such, surely, were those sons of God in Genesis vi, 4, who toyed with the daughters of men.[1]) And why not, indeed, since the Creator himself is represented in art as sharing in the Fall of Man, Blake being among the few who gave him no clothes. But Blake also, on occasion, gave his angels beards, following the Byzantine tradition, or (rather) his own erratic genius. The matter is highly complicated, and while I am about it I will even put in a *caveat* against my own

[1] In the gnostic myth of Helen, a curious synthesis of Greek legend and Christian cosmogony, the story of the concupiscence of the angels is related to Helen of Troy—a story accepted by Epiphanius. Tertullian also (*De Cultu Feminarum*, i, 2) clearly assumes angels to be masculine, and mentions the crime of the sons of God as a reason why they are to be judged eventually by men (see I Corinthians, vi, 3). According to Bulwer's *Anthropometamorphosis* the reason for St. Paul's strictures in I Corinthians xi, as interpreted by Gulielmus Avernus, Bishop of Paris, was that *A Woman ought to have her Head covered, because of the Angels.* (Indeed, it is difficult otherwise to make sense of this chapter of Corinthians—see especially the tenth verse.) This makes it the more astonishing that Bulwer should add a conceit of his own, to the effect that male vanity may attract *succubi* in the same manner that women provoke *incubi,* ignoring the fact that there is no record of the Daughters of God among Lucifer's Party or on the Other Side.

naming of the fallen angels as *unfrocked* ; for (whether innocency wears a beard or no) it is certain that sin first wore clothes, the original garment of virtue consisting only of chastity. I admit to a personal prejudice, that I prefer my angels without beards, for these are ill sorted with wings. But this is among the unsolved riddles of the universe. And, for the matter of that, there are a few pictures that show Christ and the Apostles as clean shaven, though tradition has generally represented them as bearded ; but I decline to be involved in such controversies.[1]

Still other views on the meaning of beards and beardlessness will be found in *Erotomania, or a Treatise discoursing of the Essence, Causes, Symptoms, Prognosticks and Cure of Love, or Erotique Melancholy,* a work by Jacques Ferrand, published in 1640. I quote what is relevant to our present studies :

And agen, those that have little, dry, hollow eyes, with a long, thin wrinkled visage, are lewd, crafty, slaunderous, envious, covetous, treacherous, sacrilegious rascally fellowes : Especially if they are wont to looke very stedfastly on any thing, and use to bite their lips when they are thinking of their businesse : But above all, if they have but little beard.

> Poco barba, & men Colore :
> Sotto 'l ciel non e peggiore.
> Saies the *Italian.*

He that has but little beard on his face, and lesse colour ; there cannot possibly bee found a worse complexion than his.[2] And such a one is that Villaine *Melitus Pitheus,* the false accuser of *Socrates,* described to be in *Plato.*

Of Erotique Melancholy

Nevertheless, should M. Ferrand be thought to imply, by his contempt for those who have but little beard, that an excess of

[1] There is also the problem of the Devil's beard. According to a Moslem story quoted by T. S. Gowing (*The Philosophy of Beards*) Satan has only one long hair on his chin. I cannot commit myself either way on this subject. The Devil, as Luther said, can take many forms.

[2] Compare the saying of the Rabbi ben Sirach at the head of this chapter, for a different opinion.

hair is a sign of virtue, I will do him the justice to cite what he says a few pages later, which is to this effect :

> We conclude then, that a man may know by Physiognomy, not onely those that are actually possest with this Malady of Love or Erotique Melancholy ; but also those that are Inclined, or subject unto it.   For if I see a man that is Hot, Hairy, high-coloured, with a black thick curled head of haire, great veines, & a big voice I dare be bold to say, that this man hath a hot and dry Liver, and his Generative parts are also of the same Temper ; and that consequently he is inclined to lustfull desires.[1]

Beards for the British

Certain authors insist upon the *utility* of the beard, and find here its principal function.   Of these I will quote first one who wrote in 1860 a tract entitled *Shaving, A Breach of the Sabbath and A Hindrance to the Spread of the Gospel.*   I know no more of him except his own assurance that he was a Cambridge M.A. and that he signed himself ΘΕΟΛΟΓΟΣ.   This is what Theologos says regarding nature's own protector (as he calls it) for the most delicate part of the whole body :

> There it hangs, full and flowing, across the throat and down upon the breast, with the obvious intention of softening the keenness of the advancing blast . . . What can be more merciful than such a provision in the humid climate of Britain !

Why, to be sure, Providence played an odd trick, to have given all men beards because the English had need of them.   But let Theologos continue :

> How clearly is it the property of *man*, exposed in his outdoor toil, in contradistinction to the *woman* whose province it is to be a keeper of home.

Madame, I did not say it, and you must hold me guiltless.   *Not I, but Theologos said it,* as Erasmus almost pleaded.   He will not have you fit to live in England, unless you will remain within doors, and all because you wear no beard.   *Were it* (says he) *in any*

[1] It may have been with this in mind that a certain Martin Pohl published, in 1671, a *Disputatio physica de quæstione an Esau fuerit monstrum.*

other position its benefit and purpose might be doubted, but situated where it is no physiologist will dare to deny its intention. Us only cruel Providence has armed ; and women must be defenceless.

Why Women have no beards

There was also a certain Mr. T. S. Gowing, who wrote a small book on *The Philosophy of Beards,* being the published version of a lecture delivered about the time of the Crimean War. He was of the same opinion as Theologos regarding the purpose of the beard, and quoted no less an authority than Edwin Chadwick for the beard as a protection against iron and stone dust, for those whose occupations exposed their lungs to such dangers. Having referred also to articles in *The Builder* and in Dickens' *Household Words,* to the same effect, Mr. Gowing then set himself to answer the conundrum which we have already discovered. Why, he asks, if Beards be so necessary for men, have women no provision of the kind ? Let Mr. Gowing state his case :

The reason I take to be this, that they are women, and were consequently never intended to be exposed to the hardships and difficulties men are called upon to undergo. Woman was made a help-meet for man, and it was designed that man should, in return, protect her to the utmost of his power from those external circumstances which it is his duty boldly to encounter.

So, Madame, you are answered ; a bushy chin is the emblem of man's power to protect as well as the banner of his right to dominate. *Floreat Barba ;* and we will deal with bearded women in their turn. But here I must admit that the learned French doctor, Jean Rioland the younger, was dissatisfied with the explanation that beards are given to us for protection precisely for this reason, *that women most need such protection* and are not provided with it. To him I must ascribe yet another explanation, that Nature intended the beard as a warning of puberty in order that sexual segregation may take place when the *lanugo* begins to sprout.

Of Male Majesty

The case for male pride has been most ably summarised by Père Fangé. Cette barbe, says he, qui lui orne le menton, & qui le rend tantôt terrible & tantôt simplement respectable ; cette Barbe, bien considérée, découvre aux femmes les intentions de la nature, & *leur apprend à s'humilier, à se soumettre, à obéir* . . . Lacking the assurance that might accompany a beard, I dare not English this. Even M. Fangé adds hastily, and very wisely : *Je ne prétends pas examiner si ces raisons sont bien plausibles.*

For myself I am more inclined to accept the view of which there is a hint even in the writings of such pogonophiles as Mr. Gowing, who more than once suggests that he finds unshaven features distasteful to his eye. Such was the opinion boldly expressed by Théophile Gautier, who argued that—since few faces were good enough to appear without one—*Dieu avait créé ce magnifique cache-sottises, la barbe.* Is it not for a like reason, above all others, that we clothe our bodies, and prefer to see the limbs of others decently draped ? Therefore let those only who can be proud of their bodies, display them, and only those who believe their faces to be worth showing remove Nature's face-cloak. And beards shall be a form of *purdah* for males who lack chins or have mouths that are weak or ugly. That is a reasonable apologia for one who shaves. The painter Liotard is said to have lost the love of his wife when he removed the beard in which he had wooed and won her. Happy the shaven husband whose wife, having seen his features before marriage, could still sign the contract open-eyed and undeceived. He may live to be called a pig, but not to be reproached with having been purchased in a poke.

Summary of Findings

From these exhaustive researches we may now summarise the results. We have discovered that some have considered the beard to be without use or purpose ; that others held it to be an emblem of dignity. Some have held it to be a sign of sexual conquest, as though Nature had wished to say : *In hoc signo vinces.* Others have seen in it the result of over-eating, or the symbol of our sins. Some believe it to be a natural protection, because it is given to man in his strength, while others have disputed this because it is denied to woman in her weakness. Some hold that Adam was created with a beard, some have held otherwise. Some have seen their angels bearded, most have beheld them smooth of cheek, though indubitably male.   One writer finds that lack of beard is proof of a lewd and crafty disposition, but the same fellow finds in excess of hair the evidence of lust.   But we have found four truths that cannot be denied, viz. :

(1) That not all are given beards, though all (*pace* Martial, Chesterton and others) appear to be born with noses.

(2) That these beards appear to originate from an accident of sex, though some women have produced them.

(3) That they may be worn to conceal a sorry countenance, though not prohibited to persons with well-cast features.

(4) That there is no discernible evidence for the view that bearded men are more addicted than others to the eating of horse flesh.

Now I would not have the reader imagine that I am one of those pernickety fellows who cavil upon small points, or upon how many angels, bearded or otherwise, could stand upon one.   I am not such as Pagenstecher had in mind, when he wrote in *De Barba Prognosticum* (a work to which I am heavily indebted) *Quæris, an intra domus januam stanti extra domum mingere permissum sit ?* I am a simple man and desire only to simplify.   I will not so much as trouble you with definitions, for (as Pagenstecher also observes) *Barbæ definitionem non putamus necessitatis.* But I will divide my subject into heads or chapters, like Jean Pierre Camus, the bearded Bishop of Bellai, who divided his beard in this manner at the beginning of each sermon, that he might count off the chief headings as he dealt with them.   And this splitting of beards is not to split hairs, but rather to number them.   So the first head shall be of Antick Beards, as here follows.

CHAPTER II

OF ANTICK BEARDS

How Homer could write with so long a beard, I don't know.
TRISTRAM SHANDY

Non tamen ludicrum erit si adjunxerim exemplum Alexandri Macedonis,
qui barbam militibus radi jussit ne hostile prædæ ansam darent.
J. F. W. Pagenstecher

THE genealogy of human decay is so simple and direct that it is
not difficult to prove the true pattern of civilisation to have existed
beyond the horizon of history.

Of Change and Decay

The late Sir Walter Raleigh—himself a mere bookman, while
his illustrious namesake beaconed from the abode of the buc-
caneers—lamented the decline of the Scholar-Gentleman ; whose
disappearance I (in a yet baser age) regret principally because it may
lose me a profitable public. Sir Walter said it was time to remember our ancestry ; but Cobbett had been saying much the
same thing seventy years earlier, when he located his Golden Age
about the time of Edward III. For him England was already a
land of domestic misery and of foreign impotence, which (said he) *amidst
all her boasted improvements and refinements, tremblingly awaits her fall.*

Thirty years earlier Wordsworth was invoking Milton in a land
which was even then a fen of stagnant waters, where altar, sword
and pen had forfeited their English dower, because something had
to rhyme with *hall and bower.* But the Age of Chivalry had already
disappeared a dozen years previously, the funeral sermon being
preached by Edmund Burke. Not only England, but the glory
of Europe had then been extinguished for ever ; and the age of
sophists, economists and calculators had already been proclaimed.
Crabbe, anticipating this by another seven years, had noted the
decline of patriotism, poetry and gallantry :

> *No shepherds now, in smooth, alternate verse*
> *Their country's beauty or their nymphs' rehearse . . .*

As to rural life, Goldsmith had read its requiem in *The Deserted Village*, the year being 1770. He could speak of a time (*ere England's grief began*) when health, plenty and innocence were universal and labour was light. But times, he said, were altered . . . and about the same time Smollett's Squire Bramble was doubting whether the world could always have been as contemptible as it then appeared to him, for he thought the morals of mankind had, within the past thirty years, contracted an extraordinary degree of depravity.

Skip over another century, and here is Isaak Walton enjoying old-fashioned poetry, which he found *much better than the strong lines that are now in fashion*. An early seventeenth century song compares unfavourably the young courtier of King James's days with the old courtier of the Queen's. The king himself complained of the times, attributing to long peace and wealth *a general sluggishness, which makes us wallow in all sorts of delights*. He found the clergy negligent and lazy, the nobility and gentry prodigal ; for all of which he damned the increase in luxuries, and namely tobacco.

But continue the course, and you will find Bishop Latimer, preaching in the reign of Edward VI, and deploring an age when pity and compassion had so declined since the days of open-handed charity. Sir Thomas Mallory, some eighty years before, had lamented the decline of Love. *Soon hot, soon cold,* said he, *this is no stability. But the old love was not so.* In the time when *Cursor Mundi* was written they must have been saying the same thing :

> *He praises all thing that is gone*
> *Of present thing he praises none.*

Orderic Vitalis, whose observations on beards in the twelfth century (indeed, I have not forgotten them) we shall consider presently, saw nothing but change and decay even in *his* time.

The Golden Age

Rome and Greece looked back to the Golden Age, lamented by Hesiod. Laotzu could write in the sixth century B.C. that China had once, long ago, been ruled with wisdom, only some of which tradition had passed on to his own decadent generation, which adhered to codes because it had forgotten how to live. The writer of Genesis vi, 4, some three centuries earlier, spoke of the mighty men which were of old, men of renown—and indeed, the information provided indicates a very low death rate among the patriarchs and no infantile mortality at all, apart from an occasional massacre. But the men servants and the maid servants, the sheep and the oxen, the asses and the camels, the gold and the silver, the wine and the oil, and even a life of 969 years must all have seemed small beer to those whose family album began with the Garden of Eden.

From all this I conclude that, to find the best beards and how best to deal with them we must examine the earliest chins of which we have any record.

The First Beards were false

Now it is not for me to discuss the question of priority among the ancient civilisations of the world. I recall that an Egyptologist was once announcing to his colleagues that he had found pieces of wire in his excavations, from which he surmised that the early Egyptians knew the use of telegraphy ; but one of his hearers capped his conclusions by observing that, since no such wires had been found among the remains of the Assyrians, these people must have enjoyed *wireless* telegraphy. And much that has been argued on such matters appears to me to be equally conclusive. Indeed, I am not sure that I could not undertake to prove that telegrams were sent in Saxon times, also ; for the word *Telligrapha* is found often enough in their writings, though Du Cange disappoints me as to its meaning. And was there not a Divinity called Telephos ? However, I will take an example from the student of theology who (being asked in an examination to give lists of the major and minor prophets of Israel) wrote after some thought : *Far be it from me to distinguish between these great and holy men, but I will give a list of the kings of Israel.* Therefore I will not be so rash as to say that Egyptian beards were the oldest in the world, but I will say and maintain that the first beards of Egypt were false ones (except, of course, that of the Sphynx), Nature having subsequently imitated Art, just as she is even now in labour to keep up with Salvador Dali.

These false beards of the Egyptians were tied to their chins only for ceremonial occasions. They were sometimes made of metal, and even the queens of Egypt came eventually to wear such beards, theirs being of gold, like the beards of the Pharaohs. On special occasions, such as a funeral procession to the Pyramids, these false beards were worn and the mourners must have made an imposing spectacle.

Egyptian loathing of Hair

As to the assertion in the Talmud that the Pharaoh who ruled in Egypt at the time of the Exodus had a beard which was an ell long, I am convinced that if such a beard was worn at all it was mere postiche, assumed in order to compete on equal terms with Moses and Aaron, and for no other reason. We have even the assurance of Herodotus as to the horror with which the Egyptians regarded the bearded Greeks of his time, so that no Egyptian (of either sex, said he) would kiss so repulsive a face. Indeed, the priests among these people shaved their whole bodies three times in a week such was their loathing of hair ; and in this all persons of note imitated them, for the purpose of cleanliness, as Herodotus makes mention. Nor is it the only curious resemblance between these people and those of ancient Peru that the Incas made laws against the wearing of. beards ; and when the Spaniards first appeared—such fellows as those who stood silent upon a peak that was not in Darien, but which could not be squeezed into iambic pentameter (for which reason its name was forgotten, while Chapman's is remembered by those who never read his works)—these strangers were called the *Bearded Ones*. So did the smooth Egyptians see the *Barbarians*, the long-bearded Greeks, the pointed beards of the Bedouin Arabs, the round beards of the Syrians, forever trampled upon by the victorious arms of shaven Egypt in Egyptian art. According to Cheyne and Black's *Encyclopædia Biblica* the negligent Rameses VII is caricatured in his tomb at Thebes, wearing an unshorn beard. These same authorities speak of false beards made of plaited hair, though this use of hair was certainly not universal. They note the difference between the common beard and that of the king (longer and square at the bottom) or of a god, which was longer still and curled at the end.

No more need be said on the subject of Egyptian beards. But when we turn to Assyria and Babylon there is lyrical matter in the ornamental variety to be observed, chiselled in sculpture by artists who, with light hand, traced the parallel waves of royal and military whiskers. Here, indeed, we may find the first *bona fide* beards ; for if those of Egypt were false, those of China, were they never so ancient, could not have been compared with such magnificent growths. And though Mr. John Brophy assures me that some Chinese attribute their hairlessness to their long centuries of highly refined civilisation (which he thinks might account for the normal beardlessness of women), it has always been an axiom among those who share Esau's birthright that hairiness is a sign of virility and manly dignity.[1]

The Beard of Assurbanipal

Look well, then, at the beards of Assyria. Observe the square-cut ornament, cross-laced and surely held in position by a bag of fine silk or some such stuff, to make it stand out like a stone cornice upon the chin of Assurbanipal. There he stands in his cylindrical hat, with an ice-cream cornet in his hand, sharing a ponderous milk-float with a charioteer, bearded like himself. But the third figure beneath the royal parasol wears no beard. Nor do three of the four pedestrians behind the chariot. These are smooth of cheek, full-faced and glandular, like the overfed cherubs who support celestial scrolls in our eighteenth century engravings. These are *castrati*, whose voices scandalise their breeches (as the author of *Anthropometamorphosis* said of the Choirs at Florence) or would have done, were they not clad in dressing gowns. Were all then, bearded, save the eunuchs ? Georges Perrot and Charles Chipiez thought otherwise, finding in the beard the prerogative of kings and the military caste.

Thus, in addition to the Court Eunuchs, who had beardlessness thrust upon them, these authorities would have us believe that

[1] Abraham Rees (article on *Beards* in his *Cyclopædia*) took another view. Le Compte, he said, observes that the Chinese affect long beards extravagantly, but that nature has balked them and only given them very little ones.

the lower orders generally, holding no licence to kill, were not permitted to honour their chins with the emblem of the killer. Like the moustache before the Crimean War, the beard marked the soldier, but his was not the elongated mass that adorned the king. Perhaps such a beard as that would have incommoded a fighter in his professional duties ; or it may have been a matter of rank (for size and length increase, according to Assyrian sculpture, in keeping with the wearer's dignity of function). Whatever the cause, the fighting man of Assyria wore his beard short—a fashion common among soldiers of other races and later ages. But all who had a beard to curl used the irons on it. Dyes they used too and, on occasion, gold dust to give it lustre.

Curled and immaculate as the beards of her kings was that of the winged bull of Nineveh, with its human face, standing guard in its top-hat over the Assyrian capital when Jonah arrived with his cargo of curses. I was misled by Herman Melville into supposing that the prophet circumnavigated Africa in three days, but on a careful reading of the text I can find no reason to suppose that the Great Fish landed Jonah at the citadel of Idolatry, cruising from the Mediterranean to the Persian Gulf and up the Tigris. I drop the theory with reluctance, the more so as I have been fascinated by the description of Jonah's voyage *apud* Sidonius Apollinaris :

> . . . *resonant dum viscera monstri*
> *Introrsum psallente cibo* . . .

—the bowels of the monster resounded with the psalms of his food (a pretty fancy).

But this will not help us. I am relieved to learn from Burchardus de Bellevaux that Isaiah vii, 20, where the Assyrians shave everybody and everything (also Isaiah xv, depicting the baldness of Moab) should not be taken literally *quia in solo misterio dicebantur.* The earliest Babylonians, imitators perhaps of Egypt, are believed to have been clean shaven ; but they too came to wear beards that tempted sculptors to ecstatic exaggeration. Weighed in the balances and found wanting, their empire passed to the Medes and Persians, whose laws changed not and whose beards were plaited with golden threads.

Of Hittite Beards and Lion-killing

And the Hittites—those unfortunate people whose crime it
was that they defended themselves against the unprovoked
aggression of the children of Israel—why does the *Jewish Encyclopedia*, in its article on Beards, state that they were clean shaven ?
Old Abraham claimed their land among the *lebensraum* promised
to his seed by the tribal divinity—a claim renewed by Moses,
who added (not having at that time received the tenth commandment, though the Code of Mount Sinai does not appear to have
altered his predatory habits) that it was a land flowing with milk
and honey—a fact which he repeated as often as he had occasion
to mention his unsuspecting victims. Eventually they were, as
the chronicler expresses it, *cut off*. But not their beards. The
basalt reliefs at Carchemish show some, it is true, who are
shaven, but others well bearded, as the encyclopedist should have
known. Indeed, he could have seen a very fine sculpture of two
Hittites, with admirable square laced beards, lethargically killing
a lion—one holding its stern in the air by its tail, while both
plunge their weapons into the dumb beast *in locis posterioribus*, as
William of Malmesbury said when describing the murder of
Edmund Ironside. A *tour de force*, indeed. But as to the *Jewish
Encyclopedia*, it has provided me with one of the most remarkable
Serendipitations I have ever chanced upon, which is to be found
in an erratum slip to Vol. XII (1906) where the reader is advised
to delete the words *committed suicide at Frankfurt-on-the-Main*, on
page 102, col. b, *the subject of this article having been regrettably
confused with another person of the same name*. So how could one
hope that such scholars would know a Hittite beard when they
saw one ?

Well, these same Hittites having been treated much as their
conquerors fared later (Thou shalt make no covenant with them,
said Moses, nor shew mercy unto them), the Israelites made
themselves free of their possessions, as it is written in the Book
of Joshua, *a land for which ye did not labour, and cities which ye built
not*, with vineyards and oliveyards which they had not planted.
(The whole story has been repeated in our own time.) And not
much more is heard of the Hittites apart from the unfortunate
Uriah, whose ancestors must have contrived better in escaping the

massacres of Moses than he, in his misplaced loyalty, when pursued by King David's treachery. As for the Israelites themselves, they counted shaving or even clipping the beard among the sins of the Gentiles which made them fit for cat's meat. For the ancient Hebrews as vigorously maintained the sacredness of God's handiwork upon their chins (*neque in rotundum attondebitis comam, nec radetis Barbam*) as they fanatically insisted upon improving the Divine Image in certain other particulars, that is to say, by such trimming as they held to be impious if applied to the corners of the beard. The particular prejudice reflected in Leviticus xix, 27, which some early writers have attributed to Egyptian customs, is now clearly seen to have had reference to the habits of neighbouring peoples about the time of the Captivity.

The Shaving of Joseph

Indeed, the first Israelites in Egypt appear to have conformed to the customs of the country ; for Joseph (who had clearly either been deprived of a razor in his prison, or merely neglected the growth from despair, or perhaps to repel the advances of Mrs. Potiphar) had a shave when released from his dungeon and brought before Pharaoh. But the obelisk of Shalmaneser II shows the children of Israel cherishing the long beards that became traditional among them.

So, while the shaving of Joseph indicated the termination of his misery, that of Job was a sign of mourning. Was this, as Sir James Fraser suggests (in his *Folk-lore in the Old Testament*), a form of self-mutilation such as the uncircumcised practised, with their misplaced slashings and other forms of ritualistic masochism ? If so, the prohibition, *Ye shall not round the corners of your heads, neither shalt thou mar the corners of thy beard*, may concern the extravagance practised in their mourning by Lesser Breeds without the Law, rather than any fashion in corner-marring popular among these Gentiles in their normal toilet. Indeed, as Sir James points out, the writer returns to the matter in Leviticus xxi, 1-5, with a milder prohibition that appears, in making certain concessions, to point to some such explanation. The law-giver compromises—it is only to the priests that he now addresses himself.[1] They are only to defile themselves in mourning for their nearest of kin, but *they shall not make baldness upon their head, neither shall they shave off the corners of their beard.* The making of baldness, according to Robertson Smith, referred to the use by the Hebrews (continued, in spite of this prohibition, in many recorded instances) of the tonsure in mourning—a custom which Herodotus (iii, 8) ascribed to the Arabs of his time, in honour of their God Orotal, the Arab Bacchus.

Leprosy of the Beard in misterio

There is also some mention in Leviticus xiii, 29-30, of a man or woman having *a plague upon the hair or the beard.* This the priest is to examine, and if he find it deeper than the skin the person is to be pronounced unclean—*it is a dry scall, even a leprosy upon the head or beard.* In such cases all hair is to be shaved off (xiv, 8-9) including even the sacred beard. On this point I must quote the authority of a French abbot, Burchardus de Bellevaux, whose *Apologia de Barbis,* a twelfth century MS, has been available since 1935 in the limited edition edited by Ernst Philip Goldschmidt. Where, says Burchardus, there is mention of a leprous beard in Leviticus, this is said *in misterio* and not *in re* —it is to be taken allegorically—*nemo enim unquam vidit barbam leprosam.* No one, forsooth (says he) ever saw a leprous beard.

David, to simulate madness (while enjoying the very kind hospitality of Achish, king of Gath, which he later rewarded in

[1] The laws which were evidently not too rigidly kept by the Jewish laity were enforced far more strictly among the priests, as this passage makes clear. It is curious that a shaven clergy, i.e., that of Rome—still seeks to identify itself with these Levites, to whom the razor was anathema (and to whom the idea of Peter and the Apostles as priests would have been repugnant had it not been too ludicrous to contemplate). Father Seghers, in an article often quoted in later chapters, even speaks of the shaven priest as a *young Levite,* in a passage which describes the mystical significance of removing all hair from the face. He might as reasonably have discussed the shape of a square circle. Levi was one of the sons of Jacob who participated in the revolting massacre mentioned on page 76 ; and why anybody, Jew or Gentile, should wish to be associated with him I cannot imagine, for even his father on his deathbed could not find a good word to say about him. As an ancestor I think he should be kept secret, if possible, and as a prototype he should be studied merely as an example of what to avoid.

his habitual manner) *let his spittle fall down upon his beard*—it being
assumed that no man in his senses would so defile the ornament
of his face (or was it an imitation of frothing at the mouth?)
It took in the King of Gath, who agreed that David was mad
indeed (I Samuel xxi, 13-14). Poor credulous Achish : he har-
boured David in spite of his alien birth and his apparent lunacy,
trusting him in spite of his own advisors, the Lords of the
Philistines, and believed all David's stories of his sallies against
his own countrymen, when in fact the young brigand had been
looting and exterminating the neighbouring peoples *which were of
old the inhabitants of the land*, leaving no one alive to contradict his
bulletins (I Samuel xxvii). David this credulous king dismissed
eventually with a first-class reference : *Thou hast been upright*, the
simple Philistine said (and we are not told if David's ruddy
countenance showed a deeper red) *for I have not found evil in thee,
since the day of thy coming unto me* . . . It is sad that the Philistines
left no history, for the little that we know of them from their
worst enemies show them as good fellows, whose fault was that
they lived on the fertile plains and held the sea-coast, which
Ahab's ancestors coveted—though it took some 3,000 years to
annex that vineyard from the present descendants of their
hereditary foes.

An offence against Israelite Beards

To offend against an Israelitish beard appears to have merited
the most frightful reprisals. The war in which Uriah the Hittite
met his end, sent deliberately to his death that David might enjoy
his wife, was fought on account of an insult to the Hebrew ambassadors who had been sent to Hanum, King of the Ammonites.
As Coverdale gives it, *Then toke Hanum the Servantes of David and
shove of the one halve of their beardes*. In the war waged against
Hanum, to avenge this insult, the Ammonites were defeated
after a battle and a protracted siege of the royal city of Rabbah.
David had spent the time amicably with Mrs. Uriah ; and a long
siege it must have been, for she had time to bear him two sons
(one of them being Solomon ; from which we must suppose
that the end justifies the means, such credit attaches to David's
progeny through this démarche). David's reference in Psalm Li,

7, to being purged with hyssop after this affair might be taken to infer that he contracted leprosy from it. But I take it the leprosy was *in misterio*, and not *in re*.

The King was summoned to Rabbah by the faithful Joab, who was unwilling to take the credit for the victory he had earned. Little did he know that David's dying instructions to the babe he had begotten during that war would include a king's gratitude to the general who had framed Uriah's death ; for David was to say of Joab *let not his hoar head go down to the grave in peace*. (Solomon saw to that, in due course—glad enough, no doubt, to wipe out the tool of his father's infamy without whose aid his mother might have remained an honest woman and he himself would never have been born.) So David arrived just in time to lead his army into the defeated city and to collect the loot. As to the inhabitants of Rabbah and the other Ammonite cities, the story is told in II Samuel, XXXI. They were treated to various refinements of cruelty—some sawn in pieces, some ripped up with harrows, some chopped up with axes and others thrown into brick-kilns. If any Ammonites survived, they knew better than to interfere with an Israelite beard.

The shaving of half the beard has been common enough as an insult. Yet John Bulwer affirmed, on the evidence of Captain John Smith, Admiral of New England, in his *History of Virginia*, that the Red Indians in those parts were wont to shave half their beards—merely as art for art's sake—or rather to cause their squaws to do so with two shells. Bulwer, who was both gullible and imaginative, supplied a wood-cut on page 201 of his *Anthropometamorphosis* (1653), showing an Indian with such a beard as I am sure no Indian could ever have grown, cut in this style—a single mustachio with one half of a square beard. Apart from a story about Chopin I know of no other case of such a style being adopted from choice, unless I accept an instance where a four-teenth century romance describes a man as wearing such a cut in order to play the fool.[1] This is in the metrical romance, *The Lyfe of Ipomydon*, published by Wynken de Worde about 1500 (it is available in vol. ii of Weber's collection, 1810). Here we have it :

[1] There is also the case of Demosthenes, who is said to have shaved off half his beard in order to induce himself to stay at home.

And also he shove halfe his chynne :
He semyd a fole, that queynte syre,
Both by hede and by atyre.

But to return to the Jews. Except in the case of Joseph, to which we have referred, all shaving was with them a mark of mourning, as it is written in the Epistle of Jeremy to the first captives of Babylon : *And in their temples the priests sit on seats, having their clothes rent, and their heads and beards shaven, and nothing upon their heads* (Baruch vi, 31).

Of Aaron's Beard

This Jewish predilection for beards is indeed as ancient as it is famous. The beard of Aaron is renowned principally for an incident which I find personally a little revolting—*the precious ointment upon the head, that ran down upon the beard, even Aaron's beard : that went to the skirts of his garments.* That of Moses is familiar in the statue by Michelangelo (whose authority I would not presume to dispute) being of a preposterous length, and looped round his fingers [1] : without such a beard how could he—or Aaron—have conjured so successfully ? The very word by which the Hebrew language distinguished the Elders of the People was ZAKEN or long-bearded, and an old Hebrew saying has it that the adornment of a man's face is his beard. This the orthodox Jew has since Biblical times worn long, though a wall-painting at Benihassan shows some Semitic people—who may well be Israelites—wearing their beards neatly trimmed to an oblong, and continued across the cheekbones by well-cut lines of side-whiskers. Why J. A. Repton (in his monograph on the Beard and the Moustachio) speaks of Aaron's beard as *forked*, I cannot imagine. There is nothing in Exodus on which to plant this assumption.

Joab (himself, as we have observed, ever faithful in his treachery) made use of what must have been a Hebrew courtesy when he decided to liquidate a rival. *And Joab took Amasa by the beard with his right hand to kiss him. But Amasa took no heed to the sword that was in Joab's hand. So he smote him therewith in the fifth rib . . . and he died.*

[1] A corbel in Wimborne Minster, carved in King Alfred's time, shows Moses with a *plaited* beard—an even pleasanter fancy.

These heroes were sinister, so to speak. It was that little trick and such another that David remembered against his old friend when he had seemingly forgotten his own peccadilloes. He felt this was a stage worse than the pranks they had played together ; and (in view of his strong feeling about beards) I am inclined to think it was Joab's use of Amasa's whiskers that really upset the King of Israel.

David beards a lion

Such things could be done in fair fight ; and David himself by his own report, once killed a lion just that way, when he was a mere boy—catching it by the beard and sticking it as easily as killing a sheep. The lion seems to have gone hunting in company with a bear, according to David's rather tall story in I Samuel xvii, 34-36. David claimed to have killed both ; but it is not clear which he seized by the beard, except that a lion, if it stood still, would give some sort of a hold in the way of whiskers. But David claimed actually to have dispatched both beasts, and for all I know he used on them the strategy which was later used so effectively by the Persians that Alexander the Great made his whole army shave.[1] *Persicos odi puer apparatus*, said Horace, perhaps with this beard-grabbing technique in mind : *Boy, I dislike these Persian gadgets*. But we should still be in the Holy Land—I will not say in Palestine, for that word is the same as Philistine, and signifies the place where the Israelites never lived until our own time.

The Beard of Mephibosheth

Of Mephibosheth we read that he came to meet David, after the defeat of Absalom, having neither dressed his feet nor trimmed his beard (though some say that, the word being *safam*, for *beard* we should read *moustache*). This Mephibosheth, whose name one ancient authority derives from *Memfiboste* (*de ore ig-nominia*, says he) was a mascot, in a manner of speaking, of David's charity to the descendants of Saul. David had murdered

[1] So Plutarch says in his Life of Theseus. But medals show Alexander's father, Philip of Macedon, and his two predecessors (Amyntas and Archelaus) as beardless ; so the story is somewhat suspect.

the young soldier who claimed to have taken Saul's life, though the deed was done as an act of mercy to a dying man about to fall into the hands of his enemies. But such gratuitous magnanimity did not prevent the king from handing over seven of Saul's innocent descendants to be hanged by the Gibeonites. That order was hardly given before we find him burying the bones of Saul with every appearance of solicitude, for it is always easier to be generous to the dead, in whom David found *nil nisi bonum* and even included the seven victims aforesaid in his pious regard for the bodies of those who could no longer wield a spear. Mephibosheth of the unkempt beard was allowed to live, doubtless because he was lame in both legs (a poor thing, quite disqualified as a rival in the days when kings sometimes had to fight their own battles instead of exhorting others to be courageous from the safest spot to be found).

The Beard as a Symbol

In spite of Leviticus, beard marring appears to have long continued as a sign of grief. Ezra plucked his out by the roots, and Ezekiel elaborately disposed of his shavings *in misterio*, as a token of what should befall his countrymen. As a symbol the beard was much in use among the prophets, Isaiah likening the king of Assyria to a razor which God would use to shave the Israelites—*it shall also consume the beard*, he said, in the peroration of his threat. So also he says of Moab that on all their heads should be baldness, *et omnis Barba radetur*—a promise also made by Jeremiah with respect to the Moabites. In Jeremiah xli, 5, we meet eighty men in mourning, whose beards are shaven—they come to an unhappy end, like most people of whom Jeremiah wrote. (His forebodings reached far, and included names worthy of some speculation : *Dedan and Tema and Buz, and all that are in the utmost corners*, reads the Authorised Version ; but the R.V. says *and all that have the corners of their hair polled*.)

Aubrey Beardsley (who should have known better, and doubtless did) represented his Salome holding a beardless head on the celebrated charger, though I doubt if the Baptist used a razor in the wilderness, or was provided with one in the *oubliettes* of Herod Antipas. The Jews of his time clung tenaciously to their beards, as symbols of nationality in a country that had been over-run by shaven Greeks and was now ruled by smooth-cheeked Romans. Herod's father (a criminal known for some reason as Herod the Great) can hardly have been approved in the best Jewish circles, for his beard was dyed ; but the Herods were mere *Uitlanders* and I will leave their new-fangled habits, for we are concerned here with beards of more ancient vintage. So next we will consider those of India.

The Beard in Ancient India

When I visited the Indian Exhibition held at the Royal Academy, 1947-48, I was delighted to find that the first exhibit in the catalogue was the bust of a bearded man, found at Mohenjo-daro and supposed to have belonged to the period 2400-2000 B.C. —a wide enough margin. The buried city of Mohenjo-daro, peopled by a race of whose origin nothing is known, shares with Harappa the distinction of belonging to a lost civilisation, the oldest in India of which anything is known. The sanitary arrangements of these people having entertained me (and, I hope, my readers) when I wrote *Cleanliness and Godliness*, I will say no more of them here except that evidently some at least of the men among them were bearded. There was nothing that I can re-member in the least remarkable about the beard of the figure exhi-bited : it was not of exceptional length, it was not ornately plaited and it showed no sign of being a false one. It was merely a beard—*fungus menti vulgaris*.

The culture of later civilisations in India bears the mark of the razor. A head of the second century B.C., from Sarnath in the United Provinces, shows a smooth chin but long curled *mustachios* —always the sign of the dandy. On the right uses of the razor the sacred books of India are most explicit. It appears that, *in the beginning, Savitar, the knowing one, shaved the beard of King Varuna ;* like Mercury, who began on his old Dad (though Poppa Jupiter never allowed himself to be portrayed without his beard and evidently soon grew a new one). So you will find it in the *Sankhayana-Griha-Sutra*. The other *Griha-Sutras* amplify the theme. *Paraskara* says that this Savitar, or Savitri, shaved both King Varuna and King Soma. Two things seem to obsess the writers : the fee to be paid to the barber and the need to urge him to spare his customer's life.

The Barber's Fee

To the barber the vessels of grain, says one authority. Another—the *Griha-Sutra* of Gobhila, says that the fee for shaving head and beard in the sixteenth year is an ox and a cow for a Brahmin, a pair of horses for a Kshatriya or two sheep for a Vaishya. The charge seems to be somewhat steep, and my suspicion that the goods did not really go to the barber is strengthened by Hiranyakesin, who allocates boiled rice and butter to the barber and a cow to the young man's *guru*, his spiritual advisor. That seems more likely. The same writer speaks of the razor as having been used to shave the gods, those of India being commonly clean-shaven.

Great Danger of Shaving

As to the fear of the operation proving fatal, one of the *Griha-Sutras* (*Asvalayana*) in its account of the Ceremonial shaving in the sixteenth year, known as the *Godanakarman*, gives this mantra : *Purify his head and face, but do not take away his life.* In *Paraskara* the tonsure of the child when twelve months old is to be performed *with the razor, the wounding, the well-shaped.* But again the words are added : *Do not take away his life.* And the *Arthava-Veda* provides this invocation : *When thou, the barber, sheareth with thy well-whetted razor our hair and beard, do not, whilst cleansing our faces, rob us of our life.*

From all this we may gather that Ceremonial shaving was an expensive business in India and regarded as entailing a certain risk. Razors were known to the Aryans before they invaded India (and, indeed, some even claim that barbers' tools of a sort can be identified among implements of the Neolithic Age). Certainly the Aryans of India always used the razor extensively, as Hindus do to this day. But in specified categories the wearing of the beard has been considered proper. The *Anugita* says that the *Brahmakarin* is to live as a mendicant ascetic, preserving his hair and moustache ; but whether the beard is included is not entirely clear. I do not think any more need be said about

Indian beards at present, though a mass of further material exists of the same *genre* in the Hindu Scriptures.

Chinese beards, as I have already suggested, are hardly worth mentioning, except to say that Confucius is always represented wearing one, which has varied in accordance with the imagination of the artist. Therefore I will confine my final observations upon Antick Beards to those of the Greeks and the Romans. [1]

A speculation as to the Amazons

Herodotus assumed that the shaven Scythians of his time were all smitten with a disease which made them resemble women, as a punishment for plundering the temple of Aphrodite at Ascalon. Such was the unfamiliarity of a shaven face among the ancient Greeks (though the art of ancient Crete shows that razors were used there, and they were mentioned by Homer). Why should not these beardless Scythians have been the true originators of the legend of the Amazons, since they looked to the Greeks like women but fought like men ? (The Amazons, we must remember, amputated their breasts and were famed for their archery—two further points in the legend which the appearance and habits of the Scythians might have sustained.)

Among the many offensive utterances attributed to Diogenes on the subject of beards was his reply to one who came to him shaven : *Nihil tibi ad propositam quaestionem repondebo*, he said (or so his namesake Diogenes Laertius renders him) *nisi prius vestem deponas et ostendas num vir vel mulier sis.* He would have no converse with him till he unrobed and showed whether he were man or woman. And again, the old dog roughly asked a shaven stranger (for though he would order a king out of his daylight he could not himself keep long to his own business) *Numquid naturam accusas, quia te virum, non autem mulierem fecerit ?* He would know whether this fellow quarrelled with nature for making him a man, not a woman.

---

[1] Some of the information that follows is culled from the invaluable Messrs. Daremberg and Saglio, where the reader may find further facts regarding classical beards (v, *Barba*).

The Beard of Diogenes

> Such was Diogenes, wearing himself a beard
> *that hung in candles*
> *Right from his chin down to his sandals.*

Small wonder that he went through the streets of Corinth at high noon, peering at the shaven chins of strangers with the aid of a light, to see if he could find a man amongst them. The beard that rebuked great Alexander (and no wonder, for there indeed was an enemy of whiskers, a tyrant of the razor), such a man would at least have known how to deal with the dictators of slave labour in modern Britain. *What is your profession,* asks the clerk at the Labour Exchange of the bearded cynic hailed before him by a couple of narks. The only trade I know, replies the sage, is that of governing men, therefore give me to an employer who needs a master. Such at least was his answer when sold into slavery ; and I wish my countrymen had shown as much spirit when the heirs of Wilberforce were themselves trucked by the pediculous Hitlers of Whitehall.

Of Beards and Solar Deities

Ignacz Goldziher, in *Der Mythos bei den Hebräern und seine geschichtliche Entwickelung,* claims that man's solar deities have been traditionally represented as long bearded—giving as examples the Viracochaya of the Peruvians (themselves enemies of the beard among mortals) the Quetzalcoatl of the Toltecs, and the Coxcox of the Chichimecs. But he does not explain why the most famous of all sun gods, Apollo, was commonly represented as beardless, and that in a bearded age. Did it escape his attention that his long-bearded American gods lived among people who could themselves show little in the way of whiskers, even if they had let them grow ? There would have been nothing remarkable in a beardless God among such people. But the smooth-cheeked Apollo of the Greeks signified Eternal Youth among men who could grow a good beard and in an age when they commonly did. He was (as Lucian of Samosata has it) a youth in the flower of his age. Yet Lucian himself had seen at Hierapolis a Syrian Apollo—or so he considered him—bearded and robed, the same which Macrobius saw, speaking of the pointed beard and the cloak, bordered with serpents. As to the beard, Lucian tells us that the Hierapolitans considered it a mark of ignorance to assign imperfect forms to the gods, and that these people looked upon youth as imperfection. Doubtless the mature years of this bearded deity account, in turn, for the cloak, provided by decency for so venerable a figure.

John Garstang in his notes to *The Syrian Goddess* remarks that *the beard presents no difficulty, for in early art the Greek Apollo was frequently represented with this feature,* as may be seen in L. R. Farnell's *Cults of the Greek States* (Vol. IV, chap. vii) where the *Ideal Types of Apollo* are discussed. He was however more commonly seen without a beard, as also was Saturn, according to Tertullian.

The Golden Beard of Æsculapius

But it was of the familiar youthful Apollo that Dionysius of Syracuse was thinking when he excused himself for stealing the golden beard of Æsculapius by saying that it was not fitting for the son to wear this ornament, when the father had none (so Cicero tells the story) ; though one sculptor at least, perhaps mindful of this very point, carved Æsculapius beardless, that he might share eternal youth with his adolescent parent. So is Bacchus commonly represented, though the bearded Bacchus is not unknown, as though even he could be grave as well as gay.

But as to the tyrant of Syracuse, Caxton says in his own bold Black Letter that *for fere and doubte of the barbours he made hys doughters to lerne shave ;* but such was his small confidence even in the children of his loins that *he would not they shold use ony yron to be occupied by them.* They were to burn off his whiskers (some say with hot nutshells, an operation having need of more skill than common barbering requires) or, as William says, *to brenne and senge his heeris ;* as you will find in the second chapter of the third tractate on *the Game and Playe of the Chesse.* From such a character there is no truth to be had, and I conjecture that Dionysius stole the golden beard from plain villainy, without any mitigating circumstances.

Other golden beards were known in Greek statuary, notably that of Zeus, in emulation of whom the Emperor Caligula would sometimes affect the same fashion, as Suetonius tells us, wearing a false beard of gold upon his shorn chin. The heroes of Homer entwined their beards with gold ribbon, like the kings of Persia.

Did the Spartans wear Beards ?

Of the Spartans various things are said. Some will have it that they shaved the chin, as Alexander later caused his soldiers to do, in order to give no handle to the enemy ; and for the same reason they are said to have let their hair grow long behind, as Valeriano Bolzani tells us (*Pro Sacerdotum Barbis*—I use the words of his translator in 1533) that *theyr enmies might take theyr hands ful, and draw them backe ageyne : and so for feare of that they shulde not intende to flee.*[1] But Plutarch (in a passage which I shall quote in its proper place) says that the Spartans were compelled to shave the upper lip, from which one would infer that the chin was unshorn. There is, indeed, evidence in support of this view in a story of the Spartan King Nicander, which will also be found in Plutarch (Life of Theseus). Here we are given Nicander's reply to the question, *quare Lacedæmonii barbam alerent*. The answer, typical laconic pomposity, is of small importance compared with the question— for why should anyone ask why Spartans cherished or nourished their beards if, in fact, it was clear they did nothing of the kind ?

The Dedication of the First Beard

By ancient custom the first down on adolescent chins was dedicated in some temple. Thus, according to Plutarch, it was the custom of youths to dedicate this *lanugo* to Apollo at Delphi— a tactless reminder to the God, as he was there represented. For those who would have young men give their first beards to the Gods did not do so in scorn of what they removed from their faces but (as Valeriano's translator has it) *as a deere and thankfulle gyfte, thynkinge that nothynge mighte be offered more meeten for that age.*[2]

---

[1] Lycurgus, according to Plutarch, said that long hair made good-looking men more beautiful and ill-looking men more terrible. This in the life of Lysander. In the same passage Plutarch says the Argives *after their great defeat shaved themselves for sorrow.*

[2] See Appendix E.

This custom was attributed originally to Theseus who (I quote from the same source) *to the intent he might professe his valyantnes by that same mannely state,* shaved not at all himself. But a vase found at Anzi shows this hero clean-shaven (like many of the statues of the classic period) ; and, as the occasion represented on the vase is the fight with the Centaurs, Theseus must have been old enough to have shown a very fine beard if it were not to be assumed—as it evidently is—that he had removed it with a razor. So here is another contradiction.

But we may safely assume that most Greeks were bearded until Alexander set a new military fashion ; and we shall often observe how military fashions have shaped those among civilians. So in due course the Athenian barber's shop became a familiar resort of the local Areopagites (such as *spent their time in nothing else, but either to tell or to hear some new thing*). And there we will leave them, to consider the Romans.

The antiquarian Varro (Lib ii, cap ii) testifies regarding the beards of ancient Rome from the evidence of ancient statues, *quod pleræque habent capillum et barbam magnam,* which he accepted as proof that there were then no barbers in Rome. And Pliny (for what his opinion is worth) considered that shaving had been adopted later among the Romans than among other peoples. According to both these authorities barbers were first brought from Sicily by Ticinius Mena, *ab urbe condita* 454, that is to say B.C. 299 ; though Pliny claimed that the first Roman to remove his beard entirely was Scipio Africanus. But Livy gives a much earlier date for the introduction of the razor, which he fathers upon the elder Tarquin. At one time (according to Lardner's *Cyclopædia,* which gives no authority) it is said that Romans were not allowed to shave after the age of forty-nine.

A Tree of Beards

As with the Greeks, and those Syrian youths at Hierapolis, it was customary in Imperial Rome (as Marquardt makes mention), and doubtless in earlier times also, for the adolescent to dedicate his first beard to the Gods. Nero's first shavings were enshrined on the Capitol, in a casket of gold, adorned with pearls, as recorded by Suetonius and by Dion Casius. So also

Suetonius speaks of the ceremonial first shaving of Caligula ; and that of Augustus is on record. And the grammarian, Sextus Pompeius Festus, speaks of a *capillaris arbor*, a tree of hair, whereon the youths of Rome hung their first beards. Such ceremonies, adopted by the Christian Church, later found their place in the Roman *Barbatoria*, the Greek *Pogonocuria*. (See Appendix E.)

In Christian times we learn something from St. Augustine of a deity, *Fortuna Barbata*, whose votaries sought by propitiation of their patroness to grow worthy beards. In his great work *De Civitate Dei* the saint speaks of the many who have honoured Fortuna Barbata that never had good beards and of those with beards who scorned the Goddess and mocked at her vain, beardless worshippers. Two-faced Janus showed both a beard and a smooth visage—*vultu uno barbato, altero imberbi*—perhaps (as Goldziher suggests) because he was a solar deity, bearded with strength like Samson, in the heat of noon, but shorn by night of his whiskers and therefore of his strength.

The Beard is mightier than the Sword

Formidable indeed were the beards of those Roman senators before whom (seated in majesty, as Livy tells us) the invading Gauls stood in silent awe. Not, indeed, until an inquisitive barbarian stroked one of these senatorial beards, doubtless to see whether he had to do with flesh or with stone, was the spell shattered by the sudden anger of the Bearded One,[1] followed by the massacre of the Conscript Fathers. But of the first impact of those patrician whiskers upon the barbarians Valeriano Bolzani has well said *Illi quos Romanorum gladiorum vis non edomuerat, Barbarum iam erant reverentia mitigati*—or (as his contemporary translator has it) *they that the Romaynes sworde coude not tame, were appeased by the reverence of their berdes*. To which this author adds that these senators preferred to lose their lives with their beards rather than to have the majesty of their mouths defiled.

In these early days grief was expressed by cutting off the

---

[1] Or, as I find it in an early translation of Polydore Vergil (Camden Society, 1846) *M. Papirius did smite one of the Frenchemen on the hedd with a sticke, for that unreverentlie he stroked his bearde.*

beard or by tearing it out in handfuls ; for if life had ceased to be worth living or could only be continued in shame and dishonour, of what significance was a beard, the token of manly pride and well-being ? But in a later age, when to shave was the fashion, the growing of a beard became for many the evidence of mourning, as though the wearer had valued life so little that he could not even be at pains to remove this noxious growth upon his face.[1]

Of the Beard Philosophic

Pliny speaks of the *respect and fear* inspired by the beard of Euphrates, a Syrian philosopher, and Strabo says much the same of the bearded Gymnosophists. The Beard Philosophic, whereby every man who could grow as long a beard as Socrates deemed himself as good a philosopher, survived into the shaven age. Of such beards the younger Pliny wrote when he praised that of the philosopher Euphrates ; for (as my translation of Valeriano puts the matter, a work I come to love more as we proceed) *a philosopher without a bearde was very lyttell estemed.* As well a plumber with no tools or a wind-jammer without sails. Small wonder that, in later days, when the celebrated grammarian Francesco Filelfo had a dispute with the Greek *savant* Timotheus, who was evidently short of cash (or perhaps over-confident) the Greek wagered his beard against the Frenchman's hard cash. So Paolo Giovio, the Italian historian, tells the story. The Greek thought his beard was worth all and more. And so did Francesco when he won the wager ; for he took the beard, refusing all offers to redeem it with a resolution worthy of Shylock, though what use it was to him only malice can explain. As Junius tells us (*De Coma*, cap. ii) he shaved the Greek *inexorabile superbia.* (I cannot discover other examples of betting for beards ; but Edmund Campion, in his *Historie of Ireland*, said that the Irish in the sixteenth century wagered their hair and—the rest is not repeatable.) Erasmus, in his *Moriae Encomium* has a curious reference to Stoic beards, implying that the philosopher might just manage to behave humanly without laying aside his whiskers.

[1] Slaves in Rome once shaved as a badge of servitude, but were forbidden to do so by Roman law in Juvenal's time, for the same reason.

Wit is not to be measured by Whiskers

That the Beard Philosophic could be a mere disguise, and a poor one at that, is recorded by Aulus Gellius, as I find him quoted in a footnote to the work of Musonius Rufus (*Reliquiæ*, Leipzig,—1905). Here is the source of the famous saying of Herod Atticus, *I see the beard and the cloak, but I do not see the philosopher.* [1] This Musonius Rufus was himself a Stoic Philosopher and a militant pogonotrophist, often quoted by later authors. But, as an epigram in our own tongue has it (from the *Musarum Deliciæ* of Mennis and Smith) :

> *Thy beard is long, better it would thee fit*
> *To have a shorter beard and longer wit.*

So many Romans felt. Thus Horace, addressing a friend who affected the Stoic philosophy and wore the uniform on his chin, invoked the blessing of the Gods and Goddesses in this wise, in his second book of satires (iii) :

> *. . . Di te, Damasippe, Deæque*
> *Verum ob consilium, donent Tonsore . . .*

May they send him, says he, a barber. And indeed, such was the prejudice against beards at one time among the Romans that when Marcus Livius returned from his place of exile, with a beard which he had acquired (perhaps as a mark of grief, or it might have been from mere neglect) he was compelled by the

[1] There is no end to stories relating to the Beard Philosophic, showing how little human nature has changed. Horace's *lascivi pueri* molested the bearded Stoics (Satires I, 1), Apulius commented rudely on them, and *Video barbam et pallium, Philosophum non video* might serve today, *mutatis mutandis*. So also Lactantius (*De Falsa Sapientia*, cap. XXIV) noted the fraudulence of beards—*quod mysterium eius barba tantum celebratur et pallio*. Such ridicule of the beard was *in modo* rather than *in re*. Ronsard rendered some classical lines in a well-known quatrain :

> Si la grande barbe au menton
> Faisoit philosophe paroître
> Un bouc barbassé pourroit être
> Par ce moyen quelque Platon.

Homer may have had a long beard—but so had Zoilus. Mockery of beards is common in the Roman satirists, e.g., Martial's shaggy farmer with a kiss like a he-goat (*Epigrams* xii, 59).

Censors to remove it before he was suffered to take his seat
in the Senate.

The First Beard Imperial

Julius Cæsar shaved, as Suetonius tells. He was (says Suetonius)
not only shaved, but plucked—for depilators were by then in
common use among the Roman fops, of whom Cæsar was a
fashionable leader as a young man. (He was soon, however,
afflicted with baldness, and as concerned about the lack of hair
on his head as he was with the growth of it elsewhere.) Pagenstecher (*De Barba Prognosticum*) quotes some curious verses which
imply that Cæsar made every effort to grow a beard :

> *Nec dare cessabat medicata liquimina mento*
> *Sedulus, et votis sollicitare Deos.*

But this is contrary to all known facts. Cæsar only once grew
a beard, and that once as an expression of his grief, like the Saxons
and the Franks upon certain notable occasions. Suetonius tells
us (*D. Julius Cæsar*, LXVII, in his *Twelve Cæsars*) that upon one
occasion Julius let his beard grow until he had avenged a defeat of
his soldiers. (In similar circumstances Augustus expressed his
chagrin in the same way.) But there is a coin showing Cæsar with
side-whiskers.

Of the revival of beards (Hadrian was the first Roman Emperor
to wear one, and Julian the Apostate the most notorious, by reason
of the publicity he gave to the fact) we will speak later. There
was even a revival of short beards from the middle of the first
century until about A.D. 140. Christians during these changes
evidently followed whatever was the custom of the place and time
in which they lived, though shaving was on occasion denounced
by Churchmen as ungodly, as will be seen from the strong language
quoted from the writings of Clement of Alexandria. In the
Annales Ecclesiastici of Cardinal Baronius (Tom I, Annus 57, XCIII)
I find it admitted that the first Christians wore the beard *quod sit
virorum insigne*. The Cardinal even quotes Clement of Alexandria
to show how the Church felt about the matter *de communi usu
barbæ* ; but he will not have it that this held good for the priests.
Of this matter, and the great controversies to which it gave rise,
we will speak in a later chapter.

CHAPTER III

OF BARBERS AND BARBARIANS

*The chief of Namosi in Fiji always ate a man by
way of precaution when he had had his hair cut.*
Sir James Frazer

THE old ruffian who heads my chapter will be discovered in
Taboo and the Perils of the Soul (London 1914, p. 264), where a
great deal of information will be found with regard to barbering.
As, for example, the numerous *taboos* affecting barbers and all who
cut hair, an operation considered so grave in some parts of New
Zealand that the most sacred day of the year was assigned to it.
Or there are the numerous dangers that attend the shorn head,
from the subsequent fate of the shearings. If birds take them to
build their nests the head that lost them will ache. Should
mice so use the shearings, idiocy may result, so say the Huzuls of
the Carpathians. Small wonder that the Todas of Southern India
conceal their hair clippings so that they may not be found by
crows. (Bats ? Bats are not specified.) But, though it has nothing
to do with my subject, I like best the consideration shown by
these same Todas in burying the parings of their nails *lest they
should be eaten by buffaloes,* wrote Sir James, *with whom, it is believed,
they would not agree.*[1]

The Perils of Barbering further considered

It will easily be imagined, then, that the cutting or shaving of
the beard is not to be undertaken lightheartedly ; and the sacred
books of Hindustan have already made this more than clear. It
has been suggested to me that Moslem apprehension centred
around the sacred hairs on the top of the head, whereby a True
Believer is to be lifted into the Prophet's Paradise after his death.
But these fears are too universal, and concern the beard as much
as any other hairs, so I leave the meaning of it all to wiser men
than myself.

[1] Compare Marco Polo's account (Pinkerton vii, 163-4) of certain Brahmins
who, when they ease themselves, disperse the matter *lest it should breed worms
which might die for lack of food.*

Notable Casualties

How dangerous the operation could actually be was demonstrated by the late Mr. Sweeney Todd, of Fleet Street, and long before him by the Roman Emperor Commodus, who would commandeer a barber's shop to beguile a dull afternoon and amuse himself by cutting off the noses of his customers. There was also the *Assassin Perruquier* of Paris. Of him R. W. Procter wrote in *The Barber's Shop* that he despatched his customers with a neat stroke and gave their bodies to a neighbouring pastrycook *whose shop in the Rue de la Harpe became famous for its savoury patties*. And another Parisian practitioner was Joseph Orcher, of the Faubourg St. Antoine, to whom the Marquis de Courzi went for his last and fatal shave, leaving the barber in possession of his corpse and of a thousand louis d'or that he had collected from a tenant farmer. Perhaps there was wisdom in the precautions of long standing custom in so many parts of the world, including those we have observed in the case of the Tyrant of Syracuse. Shaving is no frivolous matter.

Even more clearly there may have been, in the days before Mr. Gillette and his confrères made it more easy for the amateur to shave himself, yet another reason for wearing a beard, apart from those reasons which we have examined. In most places un-influenced by the religion of Egypt or by Græco-Roman foppery the beard was normal wear, in ancient times. Fosbroke, in his *Encyclopædia of Antiquities*, describes the beards of the Parthians and inland sovereigns as bushy, being finically dressed and curled. Of Rome's neighbours he remarks that the Etruscans showed their own habits in the images of their anthropomorphic gods, who (for the most part) wore the short curled beard, like that of the Greek heroes. That of the Etruscan Mercury he noted as crooked, and turned up in front, like the Pantaloons of Italy.

Though the Goths and the Franks at their first appearance in history seem to have worn the moustache only, the later Franks came to regard the beard as a privilege of nobility ; and according to Dulaure's *Pogonologie* there was a time, in Gaul, when only Frankish nobles and priests were permitted to go bearded. The same has been asserted of Burgundy.

Beards laced with Gold.   The Ride of the Beardless One

St. John Chrysostom tells us of the threads of gold wherewith the kings of Persia laced their beards—a custom to be imitated later by some long-haired, long-bearded Merovingians in France. Among the Persians of the seventeenth century some similar decoration was in use, according to André Favyn, who wrote that *le Sophy de Perse, & quelques Rois des Indes portent leur barbe poudree de limaille d'or.*   And just as it is considered a source of mirth among us for a man to be bearded,[1] insomuch as the wearing of a false beard is a jest in itself, so among the ancient Persians there was nothing more ludicrous than a man unbearded.   Hence it is, as Frazer shows in his work concerning *The Scapegoat,* that the scape-goats of Persia were the strangest goats in the world, being bald of face.   Such a one, a beardless and (writes Sir James) if possible, a one-eyed buffoon, being set naked on an ass, would ride through the streets of every Persian city at the beginning of the year, according to the old Babylonian calendar.   His was the *Ride of the Beardless One,* an Oriental Saturnalia in which shame and de-formity were honoured, and heavy tribute paid to this representa-tive of our Abbot of Misrule, attended by a royal retinue, or at least that of the local Governor.

Whether Sir James was right in identifying with this ancient ceremony of the Persians (and of the Babylonians before them) the Jewish feast of *Purim,* I have no means of judging.   But as such a supposition would clear the reputation of the Jews from the responsibility of a revolting and vindictive massacre (though it was but one of many, and for once not entirely unprovoked according to their own account) I prefer myself to think that Mordecai was a one-eyed, beardless buffoon, chosen from the captive Israelites to play this rôle in a Feast of Fools.   In which case national pride and an Oriental capacity for hyperbole may well have metamorphosed the Roman holiday of a half-wit into a sanguinary triumph worthy of Moses or Genghis Khan.   As to what an Israelite was doing without a beard, I cannot imagine, unless Mordecai was a eunuch or a freak ;   or, again, king Ahasuerus may have had the man's whiskers removed on purpose for the occasion.

[1] In Hollywood beavers are known as *Airedales.*

Shaving as a Punishment

The Abbé Fangé provides many examples of the loss of the beard as a punishment, inflicted (he says) among certain peoples of India in ancient times—in evidence of which he cites Alexander of Alexandria—and by the Arabs in his own time, of whom he wrote that there was not one of them who would not sooner lose his head than his beard. In Crete and Candia he found the same punishment to be greatly dreaded, according to the *Cosmographie Universelle* of André Thevet ; and he could even produce from the *Acta Sanctorum* the case of a crime discovered by divine intervention, which resulted in the removal of the beards of two sacriligious thieves as a penalty. The miraculous discovery of the crime was credited to the account of the appropriate saints and the beards displayed as a warning to others, their removal being evidently considered a sufficiently terrible threat to a weak or wavering conscience. Of the same *genre* is the penalty which Père Fangé notes in Plutarch's account of Agesilaus, whereby a Spartan convicted of cowardice in time of war was compelled to wear half of his moustache only, the other half having been removed—though (unless Plutarch intended to contradict himself) the delinquent would already have had his upper lip shaven by the custom of the country, and must have been compelled in practice, to grow one half while keeping the other in check.

The dedication of the first beard, as already noticed in the case of the Romans and described by Lucian (*De Dea Syria*) was common among the barbarians of the earliest times and is, in fact, an ancient and universal rite of which much has been written, notably by Robertson Smith in his ninth lecture on *The Religion of the Semites*. The Arabs appear in all ages to have cherished as sacred the few hairs which fall (or which they can be persuaded to remove) from their heads ; and the pilgrim to Hierapolis in the second century A.D. shaved not only his head and his beard but his eye-brows as a votive offering (upon which Robertson Smith comments that the laws of the Incas also demanded the sacrifice of hair from the eyebrows). We have even the word of Lucian for the custom—by no means unique in history—of offering to women the choice of losing their hair or their chastity, which he says was the case at Byblos, when they mourned there for Adonis.

But for the young man who must dedicate his beard there was no such alternative.

The Makoko and the Missionaries

I never knew the Makoko of the Anzikos. He is but a name to me, and yet a name immortalised in *The Golden Bough* (iii, 271) where it is recorded that he begged the missionaries to give him half their beards as a rain charm. Who these bearded missionaries were I do not know, but in view of the reference quoted (*Die Deutsche Expedition an der Loango-Küste*, i, 231 sq.) I see them as bearded Lutherans, their gravity shocked no less than their godliness. The sense of futility and frustration which these worthy men must have experienced can only be paralleled by the fruit of long and patient education of the Gonds, in Central India, whom my friend Verrier Elwin undertook to teach the rudiments of public health. *They now know*, he recorded, not without some trace of bitterness, *that syphilis comes from being bitten by a mosquito.* Some such diffused light had dawned upon the Makoko of the Anzikos when he reached out into immortality : the labours of the missionaries had at least convinced him of their true worth. He knew that it resided in their beards, and that half—merely half (such was the virtue of those evangelical whiskers)—would suffice to induce rain-fall. [1] Could one ask or expect more of any Prophets ? The Makoko has strayed out of his own dim world and I have enlisted him among the ancients, his spiritual peers. For beards have often been used among peoples since the beginning of time for purposes of weather wizardry, like those first

[1] Beardless races (or those poorly endowed) vary between horror of the beard—of which I shall later give examples—and great reverence for it. Mungo Park notes that West Africans had a great idea of the dignity of the beard, but few Africans can produce good ones themselves. It was even for years a subject of dispute among learned men as to whether Negroes grew hair or wool (see, for example, the treatise by a certain P. A. Browne, published in Philadelphia, 1850, on *The classification of mankind by the hair and wool of their heads*, which contains an answer to the heterodox opinion then held by another writer that *the covering of the head of the negro is hair, properly so termed, and not wool*). There is further information in *Taboo and the Perils of the Soul* concerning the value of the beard in inducing rainfall. Fraser says that the Masai of the El Kiboron have this secret, and that for this reason their head chief and sorcerers do not pluck out their whiskers as others do in those parts.

fruits of the chin which the adolescents of Delos sacrificed to Calais and Zetes, Sons of the North Wind, of whom Callimachus sang.

That the devotion to their beards of the peoples of the Eastern Mediterranean has not had an uninterrupted history is clear from many known facts. The denunciations of effeminacy by John Chrysostom, no less than the Levantine levity encountered by the bearded Emperor Julian in the fourth century show us something of the habits commonly practised in those times. So also Mohammet, in his days, spoke of the idolators as shaven. And at Byzantium, at one time, though shaving was forbidden under grave penalties, it was commonly practised ; as was also the case at Rhodes, or so Valeriano informs me. For the beardless period in Persia and the Levant Alexander the Great appears to have been largely responsible. Doubtless the conquering Greeks introduced their new fashion among the conquered. But Semiramis, the warrior queen of Assyria (desiring to be treated as a man, but unable to produce one visible essential) is said by some to have introduced shaving at an even earlier age among her people—making the appearance of men conform to her own, since she could not make hers conformable to theirs—a story which I regard with scepticism.

Of Teutonic Nazarites

Of our German ancestors we learn from Tacitus that it was customary for a young man to make a vow in order to show his individual daring, whereby he would undertake to leave both hair and beard uncut until he had killed an enemy. Which custom, confined to such personal bravado in other tribes, had become general among the Chatti, who inhabited the hills of the Hercynian Forest. Of such metal were those Saxons of whom St. Gregory of Tours tells us in his *Historia Ecclesiastica Francorum,* where in the fifth book (Cap. XV) he records the defeat of a Saxon army of which the survivors swore never to cut their hair nor their beards until they were avenged ; a determination which did not save them from a second, and even more disastrous defeat, so that the beard trimming problem was solved finally for many of them. (A comparable story is told by William Ellis in the fourth volume of his *Polynesian Researches*—1834, vol. IV, 387—where he speaks of some islanders who were forbidden to trim their beards for a period of thirty years.)[1]

Of the ancient kings of France André Favyn wrote in his *Histoire de Navarre* (Paris, 1612) that those of the first three dynasties wore their beards long, the first kings having *leur barbe nouee & boutonnee d'or*, though I think this was true only of the Carlovingians. The first to shave, said Favyn, was Louis the Young, at the request of Peter Lombard, himself a *renegado* of a long-bearded race. But Clovis took his beard so seriously that it was by touching the sacred hairs that the king of the Visigoths, Alaric the Second, was invited to become his God-father,[2] *ut Alaricus Barbam tangeret Clodovei, effectus patrinus,* as one chronicler has it (though it may well be that the beard was to be cut off altogether, as other writers imply ; for the cutting of the hairs and their presentation to one whose protection was sought was common enough among our ancestors, as Père Fangé shows in his seventh chapter).[3] Pogonolatry, or swearing by the beard seems to have been not uncommon among the Northern barbarians whom the missionaries of Rome and of Ireland were slowly converting to a semblance of Christianity ; but touching the beard came later to imply an insult—hence in 1603 Ulmus (*Physiologia Barbæ Humanæ*) has the rubric : *Barba alterius tangere indecorum est, et causa.*

Thirty thousand bearded Gods

Such oaths may be compared with those of the pagan Romans, who would swear by the beard of Jupiter (according to Juvenal) or, indeed, by any beard of the many Gods available. The Etruscan Lars had but nine by which to swear ; but the devout Roman had a good selection of bearded deities, *all which beards, as Varro tells*

---

[1] Compare page 50. Sir Walter Scott in his autobiography recorded that his great-grandfather wore his beard uncut in mourning for the Stuarts.

[2] The offer was rejected and the Frankish ambassadors insulted. In the war which followed the Franks (following the Teutonic custom mentioned above) swore not to shave till they had avenged the insult—which they did.

[3] There was, for example, an Archduke of Austria (I think Frederick the Quarrelsome) who cut off his beard and sent it to the King of Hungary—an odd present to receive.

me (I quote from *Tristram Shandy*) *upon his word and honour, when mustered up together, made no less than thirty thousand beards upon the Pagan establishment ; every beard of which claimed the rights and privileges of being stroked and sworn by.* I will pass over, for the moment, the well-known invocation of Islam. This swearing by the beard is a venerable means of perjury once practised by the Greeks too, and perhaps by men of yet earlier civilisations. (Among the Greeks the touching of the beard in begging a favour is also noted by Pliny, who tells us : *Antiquis Graciæ in supplicando mentum attingere mos erat.*) But the oath by the beard is not so safe as it sounds for those who value such superfluities, as a peasant once found when he swore by his beard in the presence of the holy relics of St. Maur. His beard, which he was holding in his hand, fell off like the tail of a lizard, and could by no means be persuaded to grow again, as you will find in the third tome for the month of March in the *Acta Sanctorum,* in the fourth chapter of the fifth book of the miracles of St. Benedict.

Of insult, injury and punishment

As an insult the cutting of the beard continued among the Franks, so long as Frenchmen wore them. Prince Dagobert—later crowned as king of France, the first of that name—revenged himself upon Duke Sadregisile, his tutor, by de-bearding him. Such was the treatment, also, of Charlemagne's ambassadors at the Danish Court, according to an old romance *La Jeunesse d'Ogier le Danois ;* and the Emperor is supposed to have taken it as ill as King David himself received the news of Hanum's insult, for he made it the occasion of war—though not (I am glad to say) of any revenge on the same scale of frightfulness. There was an old law of the Alemanni which ran : *Si Barbam alicujus tonderit non volentis, cum sex solidis componat,* that is to say that the fine for shaving a man against his will was fixed at six gold coins. And in later years the Emperor Frederick Barbarossa, who had clearly a vested interest, fixed the fine for this offence at twenty pounds, with ten pounds damages to the victim.[1] Fines were, in fact, frequently mentioned, among old Teutonic laws, for forcible shaving as an injury and insult.

[1] Frederick I *in constitutione de pace tenanda* 2, F. 77.

King Alfred among his laws (Doom XXXV) ordained fit fines for anyone who, to insult a *ceorlish* man (that is to say, a freeman of the lowest rank), should shave his head like a *homola*. As to this word *homola*, the editor of the *Ancient Laws and Institutes of England* (1840) found some difficulty in explaining it, but considered that, though its derivation could not be traced, the reference was evidently to the shaven head (and chin ?) of the slave or criminal. To treat even the least of free-men in this manner merited a fine of ten shillings :

> *If, without binding him* (the Doom continues) *he shave him like a priest, let him make bōt with XXX shillings. If he shave off his beard let him make bōt with XX shillings. If he bind him, and then shave him like a priest, let him make bōt with LX shillings.*

A vulgar Anglo-Saxon prejudice

It was of our own bearded ancestors that Fosbroke wrote in 1825 (before the beard had returned to its place on Victorian chins) that *the vulgar idea of a man without a beard having the aspect of a catamite is an old Anglo-Saxon prejudice, mentioned by Alcuin.*

According to Fangé many lawyers in the Middle Ages maintained that such compulsory pogonotomy was equal to the severance of a limb, meriting the same punishment. Among the Visigoths and the Burgundians, in the early days of their conquests, the beard was the prerogative of the ruling race, and to be shaven marked a man as a mere native, a Celt-Iberian aborigine. So, in later days, the Turks shaved their slaves.

Of the shaving of the beard as a form of punishment Bulwer in his *Anthropometamorphosis* said that even in his day (1650) according to Thevet's *Cosmographie*,

> In the Isle of Candy it is a kind of punishment to cut a man's Beard. Paradine writeth, that certaine young Gentlemen who followed the Earle of Savoy, were so served for forcing a Damosell and the Father made Declarations that he was well satisfied. The Beglerbegs and Bossas of the Sultan wore very long Beards ; If the Sultan were displeased with any man he caused his beard to be cut for a punishment and shame.

No Beard Laws among the Welsh

I cannot discover that the Britons had any specified punishment for such offences, but if Cæsar's description of them is to be credited there may have been a simple explanation. The Gwentian Code belongs to a much later date (that of Howel the Good, son of Cadell, who styled himself king of the Cymru in the tenth century). Here the worth of a person's component parts are given cash-values, down to the value of a finger-nail, assessed at thirty pence. *Holl aelodeu dyn pan gyuriuer y gyt wyth punt aphedwar ugein punt atalant* is the summing up (Book ii, vi, x). All the members of a person, when reckoned together are four score and eight pounds in value. There is even, in the Demetian Code of the same era, the precise value of a cat that is killed or stolen, which will be found in Book ii, Chapter xxxiii, *Of Cats*. The head of the cat is to be put downwards upon a clean, even floor and its tail lifted up. Wheat is then to be poured about it *until the tip of its tail be covered, and that is to be its worth*. There is also, in the same code (ii, xviii, xxix) a meticulous regulation to control marriage. (Whoever shall leave his wife, and shall repent leaving her, she having been given to another husband ; if the first husband overtake her with one foot in the bed and the other out, the first husband, by law, is to have her . . .)

Assessment of hair pulled from the roots

In a word, there is Serendipity enough to drive a man mad, but not a word that I can find about fining a man for pulling another's whiskers—only a fine (*Dull Dyved*, ii, xvii, xviii) of a penny for every hair pulled by the root from his head and of twenty-four pence for the front hair. But the Venedotian Code (*Dull Guynedd*, iii, xxiii, xxvi) says that the worth of hair plucked from the roots is a penny for every finger used in plucking it out, two pence for the thumb and two pence for the hair. That way of reckoning must have made the pastime very much more costly. As to beards, however, there is still no mention ; and those who recall the tiresome wars of Cæsar will remember the probable reason, the British habit of shaving the chin. They retained long moustaches in those days, *which was ever attributed to their Barbarisme*, says John Bulwer in his *Anthropometamorphosis*. And for all I know they may have been as barbarously unbarbed and mustachioed in the days of Hywell Dda. Fosbroke certainly says they were so in the twelfth century.

Fashions change ; and what was considered fair play by the Persians (when Alexander out-witted them by barbering his phallanges) had become foul play by the time Rotharis was giving laws to the Lombards. Men, he decided, were not to pull one another's hair, nor—an even greater temptation in a people named and famed for length of beard—was a man to tug at another man (*hominem liberum,* which meant slaves excepted, of course) *per Barbam.* The penalty, as usual in Teutonic laws, was a fine ; there was even a smaller fine for pulling the hair or beard of certain slaves in specified circumstances.

The unreasonable Irish

It is hard to visualise a world where men had to be restrained by law from pulling one another by the hair or beard ; but even in the sixteenth century an English resident in Ireland thought it strange that the Irish should object to such a practice. My compatriot of Glastonbury, William Good, who became a Jesuit in 1562 and subsequently taught and preached as a missionary at Limerick, wrote of the Irish *having a long head of haire with curled Gleebes, which they highly value and take it hainously if one twitch or pull them.* So runs the passage, as quoted in Camden's *Britannia.* Even English Catholics in those days wrote scurvily of the Irish, and their Spanish allies were no kinder, if Bacon may be credited for the words he ascribed to a Spanish Captain. (The reference will be found in his *Considerations Touching a Warre with Spaine.*) The Spanish General Don Juan d'Aquila, who surrendered to the English at Kinsale, is reported to have said that when the Devil upon the mount did shew Christ all the kingdoms of the earth, and the glory of them, he did not doubt but the Devil left out Ireland, and kept it for himself. D'Aquila was fortunate in surviving to make this observation, if he did ; for the Elizabethan English had a way of massacring Spaniards who surrendered, as he would have soon discovered had he been dealing with Raleigh. But I fear the reported words reflected a prejudice common enough, that must make us wary of all reports that concern Ireland for many a century.

As to John Bulwer, who wrote a century later than William Good, he found the Irish *a Nation estranged from any humane excellency* (which is the way we English have always talked about those we have robbed or are about to rob) ; and he said of them that they :

Scarce acknowledge any other use of their Haire then to wipe their hands ... for which cause they nourish long fealt locks ... which they are wont to use instead of Napkins to wipe their greasie Fingers.

A Royal Prank

But in exhibiting the scurvy writings of my countrymen against the Irish I am forgetting beards. Bad King John, who visited Ireland as a young prince in 1185, pulled at the long beards of the Irish chieftains, a royal sport which they held for a deadly injury, though the prince doubtless saw no more harm in such buffoonery than did William Good of Glastonbury when recording the strange prejudices of the Irish in later years. I shall have more to say later regarding the persecution of the Irish on account of their long hair and beards, but I cannot forbear from recalling here a curious and confusing passage in Spenser's *View of the Present State of Ireland* (1596) :

And first, I will, for the better creditt of the rest, shewe you one of theyr Statutes, amongest which it is enacted that noe man shall weare his bearde but onely on the upper lipp like muschachoes, shavinge all the rest of his chinn. And this was the auncient manner of the Spaynyardes, as yet it is of all Mahometans to cutt of all theyr beardes close, save only theyr muschachoes, which they weare long. And the cause of this use was that they being bredd in a hote country, founde much haire on theyr faces and other partes to be noysome unto them ; for which cause they did cutt it most away, like as contrarily all other nations, brought up in cold countryes, doe use to nourish theyr haire, to kepe them warme, which was the cause that the Scythians and Scottes weare Glibbes (as I shewed you) to keepe theyr heades warm, and long beardes to defend theyr faces from cold.

Whatever statute Spenser had in mind, there is plenty of evidence that the Irish did not adhere to it. Though the clean-shaven chin with the long moustache on the upper lip is not unknown among early representations of the Gaelic *Galloglach* (notably in the well-known Dürer of 1521), Irish beards are even more frequent and sometimes of great length—that of Hugh O'Neill, as portrayed in his old age (the picture is now in the Victoria and Albert Museum) being very creditable. But Spenser's wildest statement concerns the habits of Moslems, and this seems a suitable occasion to say something of the beards of Islam.

The Beard of the Prophet

That Prophet by whose beard so many millions still take their oaths, wore it dyed red, and set great store by it. His followers were ordered to clip their beards and moustaches in such a way as to distinguish themselves from the Jews, but apart from such trimming the beard was held to be sacred, and even the clippings from it were commonly preserved for burial with their owner. For whilst the clipping of the beard distinguished the Moslem from the Jew, the wearing of a beard was said to have been ordained by the Prophet to distinguish his followers from the idolators, who evidently shaved ; and this we may infer regarding many peoples of Asia Minor, before the time of Mahomet, from various sources. Hence in the *Mishkatu 'L Masabih* (XX, iv) Mahomet is represented as saying, *Do the opposite of the Polytheists and let your beards grow.* But the Moslems afterwards admitted shaving as a badge of servitude—a custom noticed in the Memoirs of Alexander Gardner as common in Central Asia. And of the manumission of a slave they were wont to say that he was *suffered to let his beard grow.* Among the Wahabis shaving of the beard was once a punishment for grave offences.

Of Oaths valued by the inch

It therefore came about, among the Turks, that a man was respected according to the length of his beard ; so that in hiring witnesses, a practice once common among them and (for all that I know) still obtaining, a man's testimony being valued by the inch, he could hope to earn a good living in the courts if his whiskers were sufficiently creditable. As to the general esteem in which the beard is held among Islamic peoples,[1] François Pyrard de Laval, in his observations on the Maldives claimed that :

They curiously keepe the shavings of their haire and nailes, without losing or letting fall any, and are carefull to interre it in their Churchyards.

Some Moslems, when burying these relics, break each hair to release the guardian angels. Such customs have been common enough among many peoples of various religions, as we have already noticed. With respect to the Moslems of his time Monsieur Fangé (*Mémoires*, pp. 187-188) not only asserted that they kept all hair combings in a handkerchief for burial, but supplied the following information regarding insults to the beard :

Un homme qui cracherait (says he) sur la Barbe d'un autre, ou qui, crachant à terre, lui diroit, *c'est pour ta barbe*, ou celui qui, lachant un vent, diroit, je peterai sur ta Barbe, seroit rigoureuse-puni en justice, comme un sacrilège, un profanateur de la Barbe, & un impie, qui méprise les Anges, qui en sont les protecteurs & les gardiens.

A mishap to Mohamet's moustache

Indeed, two stories, which are quoted by Père Fangé from the writings of the Chevalier d'Arvieux, make it very clear that—in each method of insult described by him—the intention need not be present ; for the merest mischance, if the Chevalier can be credited, has endangered a man's life in one instance—that of a French cook who inadvertently spat on the beard of a Turkish peasant (*On ne parloit pas moins que de faire bruler le Cuisinier*, wrote d'Arvieux, *ou de l'empaler*). As to the other offence of which he speaks, it nearly caused an international crisis, for which the reader is best referred to the *Mémoires* of Laurent d'Arvieux, Tom iii, page 206 *et seq*. The same Chevalier is given by

[1] I may add here that this was one of the Islamic principles adopted by the Sikhs, who to this day wear their beards at great length, but rolled up under the chin.

Monsieur Fangé as the authority for a formidable story of the
Prophet himself, tracing the origin of the clipping of the moustache, practised by Moslems, to a mishap which befel Mohamet
in a jakes.

Cullinary Instructions for Christian Cannibals

Everyone who, in youth, read *The Talisman* and Scott's appendix
to the introduction will remember that gruesome feast in which
Richard Cœur de Lion is cheerfully credited with cannibalism by
an admiring panegyrist. The doggerel which Scott quotes is of
no small interest as a reflection of the Age of Chivalry, which was
apparently a period in which the highest praise of a popular hero
was not considered inconsistent with the belief that he roasted
and ate his prisoners of war—indeed, the incident is recorded *ad
majorem Ricardi Gloriam*. John Repton, in his monograph on the
Beard and Moustachio, claims that the shaving of the Saracen
heads which were to be served up at the banquet was probably
an act of malice (and not merely, as I had myself imagined, a
utilitarian measure like filleting a fish). The removal of the
beard, once sacred to its now dead and defeated owner, would be a
final consumation of revenge almost as sacramental as making a
meal of him.

Hence we are told that *the Sarezynes off most renown* are to be slain
pryvyly and their names inscribed upon parchment scrolls. This
is just to rub in the joke for the benefit of the Sultan's ambassadors—perhaps friends or near relatives of the gentry in the
table d'hote—for these emissaries are to be entertained at the
macabre banquet. But Richard's orders to the kitchen are even
more specific. The hair is to be removed *off hed, off berd, and eke
off lyppe,* and each head to be served on a platter *the teeth grennand*.
This bare-faced grin is evidently important, as shown by the king's
minute stage directions. The admiring bard tells us of the not
unnatural dismay of the Arab ambassadors, to whom Richard
explains (after eating the head before him as fast as it could be
carved) that his army will not starve :

> *While we may wenden to fight*
> *And slay the Saracens downright,*

Wash the flesh, and roast the head
With one Saracen I may well feed
Well a nine or a ten
Of my good Christian men.

And finally, after a eulogy of Saracen flesh, the king makes an alarming promise to the emissaries of Saladin that :

To England will we nought gone
Till they be eaten every one.

The epic has been published in various collections of Metrical Romances (e.g., in that of Henry Weber, Edinburgh, 1810, vol. ii) where the reader will find the passages of which the spelling has been modernised in these extracts. On the whole I find myself that the original spelling adds to the horror fascination. As, for example, when the ambassadors :

sat stylle and pokyd othir
They said : This is the develys brothir
That sles our men and thus hem eetes.

The Beard as proof of credit

In his *Anthropometamorphosis* Bulwer, in spite of stating that in his time the Turks shaved all but their mustachios, in the same chapter gives a more accurate account of them out of Purchas, saying that if grown men among those people had no beards they were accounted fools and men of no credit, *and some of them refuse to buy and sell with such and say they have no wit, and that they will not beleeve them.* Doughty, in his *Arabia Deserta,* noted that among the Arabs a well bearded man was still looked upon as one who *had never hungered.* However, we will leave the later history of Islam and return for a moment to the Crusades, for these afford some notable contrasts in the matter of beards, and may help to explain some of the changes that we shall presently observe in Western fashions.

In the first Crusade of 1096, so William of Malmesbury tells us, the most savage countries collaborated, and he enumerates them. The Welshman (says he) left his hunting, the Scot his communion with vermin, the Dane his cups and the Norseman his raw fish. To the Venetians the Holy War was openly recommended by their Doge *on grounds of religion—and of commercial utility* (I steal the words of Brown's *Venetian Republic*, as quoted by F. J. Hudleston). To the cultured Arab the whole array must have appeared very much like the barbarian invasions had appeared to the people of the Roman Empire.

Great Beards flourish in the time of Great Queens

And among the strange things about these savages from the West was the fact that so many of them shaved. T. A. Archer, in *The Crusade of Richard I*, has an interesting note on this subject. The third Crusade (1189-92) took place when fashions were already changing in the West ; and it may well be that the two previous Crusades had helped to bring about the changes, for we shall presently have to consider the curious and rapid transformation of (e.g.) the Normans, of the Conquest—close cropped and close shaven—into the Normans of the next generation, with long locks and often long beards as well. But at no time in the Middle Ages did the beard have that universal vogue in England which it came to have (significantly ?) under two noted Queens. It is to the Elizabethan and the Victorian that we must look for our best beards. Throughout the Middle Ages there is a long battle between the Beards and the Anti-Beards, which ends, in the last century of feudalism, with a shaven age, the razor having triumphed.

So, although beards were worn by some of the crusaders in Cœur de Lion's time, there were enough shaven faces to cause comment from the Saracens and their historians. Pogonotrophy had, in fact, become as characteristically Moslem and Oriental as shaving (no matter how many examples of beards may be cited to the contrary) was peculiarly Occidental and Christian. The Crusades may have influenced the temporary revival of the beard in the time of the later Normans and the earlier Plantagenets, but the greater was the scandal—for it was the Saracen beard that was imitated by the returning Crusaders, or so many Christians regarded the matter. Bishop Serlo, as we shall see, in his violent onslaught on the bearded nobles of his time, compared them to Saracens. How far the practice of shavery among the Latin clergy influenced this identification of shaving with Christianity, it would be hard to say. But quite certainly some Christian authorities considered that the ban on whiskers included the laity—whether by extension from clerical practice, or out of jealousy, or for some other reason I will not attempt at present to conjecture.

To return, then, to the Crusades : the Arab historian Yusuf Ibn Rafi *alias* Ibn Shaddad *alias* Baha Al-Din or Bohadin, as he is called in the West, in speaking of one of the warriors from the West (Henfrid de Toron) says that *he had his beard shaven in accordance with the fashion of his nation*. And did not Abu Bekr, the little son of the Sultan Salah ed-Din, shed tears of terror when he saw the shaven faces of the Crusaders—the Franks, as they called them ?

A Special Passport for a Beard

When we consider, in our next chapter, the changing fashions of the West, this impact of the two civilisations must be borne in mind. It was the knight Templar who, through all these changes, continued to wear his *barba prolixa*, surely on account of the long connection of his Order with the East. And when beards were most rare in the West, among the few exceptions recognised was that of the pilgrim to the Holy Land. According to Strutt, one Peter Auger, valet to Edward II, obtained letters of safe conduct from his monarch and employer when he was about to visit the Holy Places as a pilgrim and had made a vow not to shave his beard. He evidently felt that the beard required a special passport, and the certificate that he was a *bona fide* pilgrim was clearly sufficient—though his principal apprehension appears to have been that he should be mistaken for a Templar. (Having become increasingly unpopular—regarded with suspicion by the Church and hostility by certain temporal powers—the Templars were finally suppressed in 1314, the year of Bannockburn.) In later years a similar convention survived in the concession granted to Catholic priests, who are to this day permitted to grow beards if they are living in the Levant or in any place where a shaven face is liable to be regarded with contempt.

Hence it is not surprising that the first three Frankish kings of Jerusalem should have been bearded. The third of these,

Baldwin II, before his accession to the throne, figured in an episode which we shall consider later—the pawning of a beard ; and even a Christian beard was still considered, on occasion, sacred enough to give weight to a seal. Du Cange (under the words *Barba* and *Pilus*) gives two separate instances, from the twelfth century, of documents sealed with three hairs of a man's beard, whereby it was evidently conceived that some additional sanctity accrued. Thus a French royal charter of 1121 is found to be sealed *cum tribus pilis barbæ meæ*. But the consideration of royal beards, and especially those of Emperors, almost deserves a book to itself.

The pagan Beard of the Emperor Julian

We have already observed that the first Roman emperors were not bearded. Hadrian took to a beard to conceal scars,[1] two of his successors because they were philosophers, Julian as a mark of his apostasy (which greatly occupied his time and monopolised his memory in later ages). Julian's famous *Misopogon* was a reply to his turbulent subjects at Antioch. In Bury's Gibbon (1900, vol. ii, 485) the matter is referred to with numerous learned references :

> The streets of the city (writes the historian) resounded with insolent songs, which derided the laws, the religion, the personal conduct, and even the *beard* (the italics are Gibbon's own) of the Emperor.

The author of the *Decline and Fall* considered this beard worth some discussion. It was his view that Julian wore it as a philosopher and a disciple of Socrates, in short that it was an illustration for one of Horace's satires, where he uses the words *sapientem pascere barbam*, to nourish a wise beard, or in other words to study Stoic philosophy. Gibbon considered the *Misopogon* a singular monument of the resentment, the wit, the humanity and the indiscretion of Julian. It was exposed before the gates of the palace, he tells us—that is to say, the Imperial Palace at Antioch.

---

[1] Aelius Spartianus says in his *Vita Hadriani* that the beard was worn *ut vulnera quæ in facie naturalia erant, tegeret*. See also Dion Cassius LXVIII, 15.

The Beard of Charlemagne

We read the treatise eagerly and were disappointed. There was a good deal about the effeminacy of the men of Antioch (instancing their shaven chins) but really very little in the essay that directly concerned the beard. But it may be noted that Julian, in contrasting his own face with the shaven ones of his critics, remarked : *I like neither to give nor to receive kisses.* However, we will pass on. The beard appeared and disappeared, and then appeared again ; and so in rhyme we reach the time of Mighty Charlemagne. For it is necessary, after all this dodging to and fro, to begin with Charlemagne in the next chapter if we are to understand the records of Bayeux and to form a true picture of what really happened in 1066. To Julian the beard spelt pagan dignity when even the Asiatic subjects of the Empire were shaven ; and most Christians appear to have followed the fashion. To the sons of Islam the beard was also a mark of distinction from Christian priests, who shaved, and Christian laymen who frequently followed their example. But what shall we say of the fabulous beard of Charles the Great ? Or of those sacred hairs in the seals of the twelfth century ?

CHAPTER IV

1066 : BEARDS VERSUS BAYEUX

Carolus Magnus habuitne barbam, an puro fuit mento ?
J. F. W. Pagenstecher

*In former times penitents, captives and pilgrims usually went
unshaved and wore long beards, as an outward mark of their
penance or captivity or pilgrimage. Now almost all men wear
curled hair and beards, bearing upon their faces the tokens of their
filthy lust, like stinking goats.*   Orderic Vitalis

OF the ancient Britons Cæsar wrote laboriously (*De Bello Gallico*,
V, 14) concerning their habits : *omni parte corporis rasa, præter caput
et labrum superius.* In which passage he also mentions woad.

Advantages of the Moustache

We have already observed this fact : they shaved everything
except the hair of the head and the moustache. So also, as we
have seen, the Welsh long retained a similar appearance, as
Giraldus Cambrensis describes them in the twelfth century :
Barbam viri, præter gernobada solum, radere solent ; the men are
accustomed to shave the beard, save only the moustaches. Thus,
in his *Descriptio Cambriæ,* he shows us a people much like the
modern Breton peasant, with his large and bushy moustachios.
Such were the original peoples of France and Britain. The
peculiar advantages of leaving the moustache unshaven were
described by Diodorus Siculus, who said that the hairs of the Gauls
became involved with their food and served as a sieve for their
drink.

The Teutonic conquerors of Gaul and Britain, of Spain and
Northern Italy, no doubt experienced the same advantages. But
we have seen that many of them originally wore not only moustaches, but chin beards. The very word *barbarian* has by some
been derived from *barba* and *rus,* a reminder that the Nordic
invaders were unshaven and rural—as distinct from the shaven,
town-bred Roman Christians and those provincials who had
accepted Roman civilisation with its State Religion. (In that case

it might be compared with the word pagan, from *paganus*, a peasant).[1]

Bitter fate of Rotharis

Such were those Lombards at whose laws we have already glanced. They were converted to Christianity, but secretly worshipped a golden serpent ; and as late as A.D. 663 we read that this snake was melted down by St. Barbatus—significant name. As to their own name, according to Higden's *Polychronicon* it was derived *a longis barbis quas fovebant* (or, as one of Higden's early translators has it, *of the longe berdes whom thei noryschede*).[2] Rotharis, who promulgated the first code of the *Lex Langobardorum* by his edict of 643—the result of a diet held at Pavia, when the wise laws against beard-pulling were evolved—was himself the victim of a bitter fate. The Abbé Fangé gives Paulus Warnefridus, author of the *Historia Langobardorum,* as the authority for the story that he was captured and forcibly subjected to a shave and a hair cut.

The Squalid Beards of Ravenna

But sadder was the fate of the whole race in the time of Charlemagne. In 773 Charles invaded Italy, captured Pavia and overthrew the Lombard Kingdom, the title of which he added to his own collection. Some of the Lombard dukes were allowed to remain as vassals of the Frankish King, and of these the most important was the Duke of Benevento. A certain Grimoald held this title, which Charlemagne refused to confirm unless Grimoald compelled the men of the Duchy to shave. And of Ravenna we read (in the *Liber Pontificalis Ecclesiæ Ravennatis* of Andreas Agnellus) that the people there had already been forced to cut short their *squallid beards.*

[1] The author is well aware, or ought to be, that this derivation of *Barbarian* is quite preposterous. The word was in use among the Greeks before it ever became Latinised, and was of onomatopoeic origin, signifying the apparently meaningless hibber-gibber of an unknown, and therefore uncivilised, language.

[2] *Dicitur a longis ea Longobardia barbis* (Pagenstecher)—but the derivation has been disputed. There is a story that the Lombard women, when this nation was at war, would accompany the men, arranging their hair in such fashion as to resemble beards. A similar story is told of the Athenian women by Suidas.

Now, if this be so, what are we to make of that solicitude for the beards of his ambassadors which the great Charles is alleged to have shown in a story to which we have already referred ? And (even more perplexing) what are we to make of the great beards with which Charlemagne and his Peers were credited by the ancient chroniclers, or by the writer of the *Chanson de Roland*, who said of them : *Fair of form and proud of mien they are, white and waving both their hair and beard.* (I quote from Professor Brandin's translation.) The date of the Song of Roland is a matter of dispute ; but for my part I do not believe those words could have been written until the Normans had begun to wear beards, about the beginning of the twelfth century, as we shall see. Surely no such lines were ever sung by Taillefer to the shaven warriors at Hastings.

The pardonable hyperbole of Eginhard

In any event the *Chanson* may be dismissed (if you will) as the work of a romancer who lived too late to know what he was talking about. But Eginhard, who was in a position to know, says much the same—though some doubt has been thrown upon his testimony by the Abbé Fangé, who points out that many of the long-bearded *rois fainéants* of Charlemagne's secretary must have been fabulous, since most of them died too young for such a thing to have been possible. [1] Nevertheless I say and affirm that Eginhard must at least have known whether his master and his contemporaries wore beards or no, however much he may have been tempted into hyperbole regarding their alleged prolixity. And the story of Charlemagne's beard is a very persistent one, coupled with the useful information that the beards of the Peers of France were worn outside their armour and not—as one might suppose—neatly tucked in.

We have therefore to reconcile the existence of this famous beard, which is indeed almost a matter of faith so far as I am concerned, with the Frankish Misopogon who forced the Lombards to remove those *longe berdes*. And not only so, but we must reconcile it with at least one representation of Charlemagne

[1] Clothaire III, Clovis III, Dagobert and Childeric III died in their 'teens, Clovis II and Childeric II in their early twenties.

showing him unbearded but with an enormous guardsman's
moustache. This moustached Charlemagne will be found among
the illustrations to *The First Europe,* by the late Delisle Burns, in a
plate made from an old copy (1738) of a mosaic at the Lateran ;
and as the mosaic dates from A.D. 800 the evidence is tolerably
good.

Solution of 𝕯𝖆𝖘 𝕭𝖆𝖗𝖙𝖕𝖗𝖔𝖇𝖑𝖊𝖒𝖊 𝕶𝖆𝖗𝖑𝖘 𝖉𝖊𝖘 𝕲𝖗𝖔𝖘𝖘𝖊𝖓

But it was in November, 800, that Charles went to Rome prior
to his coronation as Emperor in December of that year. And
here is surely the clue to the whole matter. For it was after he
became Emperor that Charlemagne must have grown his beard,
the beard royal and imperial, the beard of the Father of the World,
a beard worthy of the pomp and circumstance with which Leo III
had endowed the king of the Franks.[1]

One of the Byzantine Emperors, Constantine *Pogonatus,* had
already impressed his beard upon human history. Henceforward
the Emperors of the West were frequently to emphasise their
personalities in the same manner. Some have expressed the view
that the *soubriquet* of *Pogonatus* marks Constantine IV as an inno-
vator. Certainly the Great Justinian, who lived over a century
earlier, was *at one time* clean-shaven—or so he is represented in a
mosaic of about A.D. 547 in the Church of St. Vitale, Ravenna (a
contemporary work of art executed by the command of Justinian
himself). The era of Constantine Pogonatus may have marked
the final return of the Eastern Empire to the wearing of the beard,
so conspicuously unusual even in the East at the time of Julian the
Apostate, though we shall see that in the matter of beards
Justinian himself led the way. In much the same way the beard
which Charlemagne grew after his elevation to the throne of the
Cæsars set a fashion which many of his successors were to follow.
Otto I (crowned in 936) was bearded ; and (though his immediate
successor shaved) there is, on the whole, an imposing collection
of Holy Roman beards including, of course, that of Barbarossa.
But while the Byzantine Emperors restored a universal fashion

[1] It must be admitted that later seals show Charlemagne with little or no
beard. But I have done my best for him and decline to discuss the matter any
further.

and began a long unbroken tradition, those of the West seem to have been continually in conflict with a hidden hand : something in Western civilisation has always disliked and opposed the beard, and all the bearded emperors of history have not succeeded in finally defeating that prejudice. On the contrary, the last word appears at the moment to lie with the razor.

What, in fact, was it that made Charlemagne himself, before his coronation as Emperor, so hostile to the beards of Benevento ? This is far more significant than his changed opinions of later years. One cannot escape the conjecture that, however debatable is Professor Rolleston's identification of pogonotrophy with hippophagy, the connection he traces between pogonotrophy and paganism held good in Western Europe in spite of all efforts to break it down. The quotation from Orderic Vitalis at the head of our chapter is typical of many which emphatically express this point of view, though we shall see that many Occidental writers were equally strongly of the opposite opinion.

The Mark of the Beast

As to early mediæval customs Delisle Burns (*op. cit.*) furnishes several examples. A mosaic in the church of St. Maria Maggiore, Rome (*circa* A.D. 435) shows the Magi as clean-shaven. A psalter (Utrecht, *circa* 800) shows clean-shaven warriors about the time of Charlemagne's coronation. Such examples can be multiplied from many sources to show that the clean shave was a common practice in the West, which appears to have been adopted by the Christians in the time of the Roman Empire and regarded perhaps as a distinguishing mark when the heathen hordes with their barbaric beards or no less terrifying *grennones spiculati*, their twirled moustachios, overran the western Mediterranean. Then, as Christianity slowly spread northward once more, it appears to have brought with it the habits of the Latin peoples and—in an insidious, indefinable way—shaving became characteristically Christian and the beard or moustache something very like the Mark of the Beast. They were found on the Moslem and the Jew, on the pagans of Scandinavia and Germany, and the Barbarians with a thin veneer of Christianity who inhabited the British Isles. They were consequently regarded with suspicion.

An odd comment is afforded by the word *Barbazatus*, which will be found in Du Cange's *Glossarium*. The Sieur Du Cange considered that the word was a mistaken rendering of *Baptizatus*, as it clearly referred to Jews and Moslems converted to Christianity. *Judæi multi* (he quotes from an old document) *eo anno præ timore Barbazati sunt*. Why, says Du Cange, should they have shaved their beards when confessing the Christian faith? Surely for the same reason that a *Cathar* who recanted was compelled to renounce the heresy of vegetarianism by the ceremonial eating of flesh. The beard was sacred to the Jew and the Moslem, and to shave it off a proof that a religion which sanctified the beard had been renounced.

Shaving and Circumcision

From such an assumption, entirely in keeping with the explicit opinions of Bishop Serlo, it would not be too great a step to consider shaving as having a positive virtue *per se*, like circumcision among the Jews. It was quite as decisive an action for a Jew or a Moslem to shave as for a Gentile to be circumcised—though less drastic. Alexander cannot have inflicted such pain upon his army as the gentleman mentioned by Tristram Shandy's father, who circumcised his whole army in one morning. Indeed, it comes to my mind that the perils of mass circumcision were experienced by the unfortunate subjects of Hamor the Hivite, whose story will be found in Genesis XXXIV. The men of this tribe were treacherously persuaded to follow the custom of the Israelites, beguiled for a purpose by the sons of Jacob—true chips off the old block—*And it came to pass on the third day, when they were sore, that two of the sons of Jacob, Simeon and Levi . . . came upon the city boldly and slew all the males.*

Where the Hebrew chronicler found boldness in this massacre of defenceless victims I cannot imagine. Jacob took it badly, not because it was treacherously done (that would have been a criticism of parental example in a man who owed everything to having deceived his brother, his father and his father-in-law) but because the Israelites were outnumbered. (*Ye have troubled me to make me to stink among the inhabitants of the land,* he said, *and I being few in number, they shall gather themselves together against me, and slay me.*) In short, we may conclude that Ilus took a risk with his army—I refer the reader to *Tristram Shandy*, Book V, Chapter XXVIII, and to the doubtful testimony of the Phœnician History attributed to Sanchoniathon. (Compare Joshua V. 3—the Jewish General took the same risk.)

Forcible Shaving of Jews

Alexander of Macedonia acted upon the opposite principle of taking no risks at all ; and I doubt if the *Barbazati* really had much of which to complain as regards being shaved. Yet I am assured that the forcible shaving of Polish Jews by the Germans in the years 1914-1918 was counted among the worst possible crimes. The German object on this occasion appears to have been purely hygienic ; yet some Polish Jews considered that this forcible shaving was worse than all they had suffered at the hands of the Cossacks. Others saw in it later the beginnings of the persecution which developed afterwards in the days of the *Dritte Reich*.

This was in eastern Europe, where Gentile custom had traditionally respected the beard, and Jews had not found it difficult— except for one or two episodes which we shall review later—to maintain the Levitical regulations. [1] In Western countries many Jews from the earliest times appear to have clipped their beards short, making a fine distinction between the use of scissors and that of the forbidden razor. Indeed, Leviticus XIX, 27, is itself capable of more than one interpretation. Such chicanery in the matter of the sacred beard was itself evidence of the pressure of opinion against wearing one ; and it is manifest that those Jews who removed their beards in the Middle Ages must have done so for reasons very similar to those which today prompt a Negro to de-kink his hair—for (during any of the periodic cycles of shaving which have occurred in Western Europe) one was liable to insult and injury if one wore this offending ornament. But while a Negro may seek immunity by attempting to pass for a White, the mediæval Jew not merely found it safer to resemble a Gentile in appearance, as far as he could—he was in positive danger of being

[1] Under Cabalist influence. The *Cabala* of Isaac Luria, who never combed or so much as *touched* his beard (for fear of losing a hair from it) had great influence in Poland.

forced to abandon both his beard and his faith if he did not dissimulate the latter by scrapping the former. The effective use of scissors would have given nearly as clean a trimming as could be obtained with the razor (before soap came into general use about the fourteenth century) and such trimming made a man less conspicuous in a shaven world.

There are some other curious words in the *Glossarium Mediæ et Infimæ Latinitatis*. *Barbanus* is a paternal uncle (in legal and common usage among the Lombards, characteristically enough, according to Du Cange). *Barbascere* is to-begin-to-grow-a-beard and *Barbula* an adolescent—both pleasant words to play with. *Barbuquet* is a blow on the chin—though Littré says it is not derived from *barbe*. But there is one word upon which we must pause a moment, for it may give a further clue to the way in which Ye Olde Berde was regarded by Mediæval Man. That word is *Barbatus*.

Barbatus=Epilepticus=*a lunatic*

We shall soon meet this word *Barbatus* applied to lay brothers in a monastic order and to the bearded Franciscan friars, the Capuchins of later years. But a secondary, and perhaps earlier, meaning is given by Du Cange. It is *Epilepticus*. And the meaning is made even clearer with the quotation : *Hos etiam Lunaticos vulgus vocat . . . iidem et Barbati dicuntur*. This is of great interest, surely, for it lumps epileptics, lunatics and bearded men together in one category. To be a *Barbatus* is to be an epileptic, and those whom the common herd call lunatics are also termed *Bearded Ones*. Such a usage could only have been acquired in an age when a man was considered out of his senses if he let his beard grow, just as he was surely possessed by the Devil if he had the falling sickness. At no time until the eighteenth century did shaving really become practically universal in the West, but the prejudice against beards which then showed itself at its strongest is of very ancient origin.

Mystical Significance of Beards and of Shaving

The beard of Charlemagne represents the pull in the opposite direction, for at no time in Western history is the case for the beard without advocates and exponents. Even, as we shall observe, the smooth-faced gentry of the eighteenth century had barbigerous heretics in their midst. In Charlemagne the beard is clearly an attribute of majesty : *Du coté de la barbe est la toute-puissance* as Arnolphe said. The mystical significance of beards and beardlessness alike is emphasised in the coronation of one of Charlemagne's successors (Henry II, called the Saint) in 1014. According to the *Chronicon* of Dithmar von Walbeck, Bishop of Merseburg :

Henricus dei gratia Rex inclytus a senatoribus duodecim vallatus quorum sex rasi barba alii prolixa Mystace incedebant.

It was evidently a matter of the highest significance that six of the Senators were shaved and six bearded ; and we must note that they proceeded *mystace*, that is to say *graviter* (Du Cange) or surely one might almost say *with a mysterious carriage*. Sterne says somewhere that gravity is a mysterious carriage of the body to cover the defects of the mind ; and what could better contribute to such mystery than a beard ? I note that *mystaceberbes* is a name coined by Ulmus (*De Fine Barbæ Humanæ*), and certainly nothing will better conceal a defect of the face than a mysterious growth on the chin. Indeed, I am tempted to remind the reader that *mystace* has also some dim connection with the word *moustache*, which the mediæval writers correctly assumed to be of Greek origin. (The lexicographers have found it hard enough to graft it on to another stem.) Both words are from the same Greek root, as every ventriloquist knows from experience.

So to Saint Henry both beards and shaven faces were mystic symbols. Baldwin IV of Flanders was called *Honesta Barba* by King Robert of France, who proudly wore his own beard outside his cuirass, like the knights in the *Chanson de Roland*. Two barons mentioned by Du Cange were known as *Gernobadati* (dog Latin) *propter barbæ prolixitatem*, on account of the prolixity of the beard. The first Dukes of Normandy were bearded—Rollo and William of the Long Sword, and Richard his son ; but these were Norsemen, only recently brought within the pale of the Church. Alfred Canel, among his studies of Norman history, wrote an *Histoire de la Barbe et des Cheveux en Normandie*, from which I glean some fragments out of the second edition of 1874.

In Normandy, as in most Western countries, most churchmen were at one time opposed to beards, and eventually the converted pirates meekly submitted to be shorn. By the middle of the eleventh century beards had become so rare that any exception to the rule served as a distinguishing mark,[1] and we read of Hugues-à-le-Barbe, of Roger-à-la-Barbe, evidently marked men as unrepentant pogonotrophists. Geoffrey III of Anjou (who succeeded to the Countship in 1060) was also distinguished as *the Bearded*. The army which conquered England is described by Robert Wace in the *Roman de Rou* as being shaven so that not so much as a moustache was left—a slight exaggeration, as there were some exceptions on record. Rodolphus Glaber (Rudolf the Bald) has described for us the introduction of hair cropping and shaving in the north of France under Ecclesiastical influence, and Gaufridus, Prior of Vigeois, also discusses the matter. But there remains a mystery regarding the habits of the Anglo-Saxons, in spite of the bland assurance of the *Encyclopædia Britannica* that the shaving of the chin was introduced before the Conquest—this in the otherwise reliable article on Beards (14th Edition).

Mystery of the Anglo-Saxons

We have already observed that the Anglo-Saxons were originally a bearded people, and have recorded the prejudice, on Alcuin's authority, that in his time shaving marked a man as a catamite.[2] Evidence for the early eleventh century is not prolific. Alleged portraits are too easily accepted as evidence, merely because we have become accustomed to them ; but further examination will often throw more than doubt upon their value.

If, for example, the reader looks through the plates of Henry Holland's *Baziliωlogia* (1618) he will find William Rufus correctly represented as clean-shaven. Henry I is also depicted with some accuracy at least in respect to the long hair and beard to which Bishop Serlo objected. Stephen and (more doubtfully) Henry II

[1] Shaving was common at this time in other parts of Western Europe. A late eleventh century MS. at the British Museum, for example (MS. Additional 11695) shows Spanish warriors as clean-shaven.

[2] *Sunt effeminati*, he wrote, *qui vel barbas non habent sive* . . . (The rest is unfit for these chaste pages, but is quoted in full by Du Cange under *Effeminati*.)

are bearded in these illustrations, and so are John and Henry III ; but Cœur de Lion has only a slight suggestion of a moustache. The first Edward appears to have shaved with a blunt razor, but Edward II and III are bearded, also the Black Prince. There is some attempt at correctness in the case of Richard II, whose portrait, with the small tuft on the chin, must have been familiar to Holland's artist, Renold Elstracke. Bolingbroke is missing in the B.M. copy, but Henry V and Henry VI are shown clean shaven, as they should be—also Edward IV, Richard Crookback and the first of the Tudors. These, and the faces that follow, would have been familiar to early seventeenth century artists from the available contemporary representations. The earlier heads are clearly mainly inventions by Elstacke, who did not even know the dress or armour in use at each period, and contrived to give to most of his kings a distinctly Tudor appearance—representing (no doubt) the earliest age he could remember, and for which he could find suitable models. But how far astray Elstracke could wander is best shown in the engraving purporting to represent William the Conqueror, who appears with a long beard and side whiskers. [1]

Let us turn, then, to the available pictorial evidence for the English before the Conquest. The Bayeux Beard of Edward the Confessor resembles, in one episode, so many rows of carrots or radishes (to borrow the description of J. A. Repton, in a work to which I shall refer later) but he is also shown, in another episode, with the common forked beard of his race, accompanied by a drooping moustache. When we compare these representations with others, the discrepancies are even greater. An illustrated article in the *Gentleman's Magazine* (second volume for 1825, pages 301-306) shows us the Confessor as he once appeared in a painting in Westminster Abbey. (This painting was already a victim of vandalism, the sport of idle boys, as the writer explains ; but the plate which illustrates the article was made from a drawing by Schnebbelie before the panel was ruined.) This portrait is considered to agree with the stone figure of the king in Henry VII's chapel and with the woodcut in Wynken de Worde's edition of

[1] In later years he did grow a moustache and *barbiches* (small tufts). Canel even considers him as the originator of the new Norman fashions in the time of his sons, for motives such as I have suggested in the case of Henry I.

the *Golden Legend* (both of which may have been copied from it). But it does not accord with either of the Bayeux figures, unless we assume that the king's beard was overdue for a perm when he posed for the artist. Bayeux should be the more reliable ; but if the embroidery itself cannot speak decisively we are at once in difficulties.

The unreliability of artists

The truth is that many of the portraits upon which even Repton, Fairholt and others relied were executed generations or centuries after the death of their subjects. This is clearly indicated in the case of the Confessor, who was shown in the painting at Westminster Abbey dressed in a style altogether out of period. Even the pointed arch of the panel betrays the late date of the work. And even contemporary artists must often have worked from memory. Moreover, within a single generation men often changed their bearded or beardless fashions as women change their hair styles. When modes have been changing, as they were in the time of Henry VIII, we may expect to see the king in a series of styles for which doubtless he himself did much to set the pace. So also in Victorian times the same man may appear in a sequence of portraits, showing all the seven ages—of which five may well demonstrate different fashions in beards or beardlessness. (Browning wore almost every style in turn.)

To make matters harder, we have the inability of artists in the past to realise (any more than writers) the *modus vivendi* of an earlier age—a lack of any historical sense that made Shakespeare's Greeks and Romans, his mediæval barons, his Macbeths and Hamlets Elizabethan gentlemen to a man. By the same token the biblical characters carved, painted, or portrayed in stained glass were always the mirrors of their own age ; and those who looked no further back than a century found it beyond their imagination to picture a fashion they had not seen used or to conceive of people who thought in other terms than their own. (I have often wondered when and how this historical sense began, and how far it has carried us. The Victorians certainly thought they had it, and were doubtless attentive to sartorial detail in a stage play ; yet their mediæval romances are merely fairy stories about themselves, rigged up in fancy dress and waving property Excaliburs. Will our own work look any more convincing to the irreverent gallery of Posterity ?)

So, then, we must be wary of portraits. Even if contemporary, they may err. And if accurate, they show no more than a phase in a man's life and beard.

The case against Bayeux

The celebrated sampler of Bayeux is commonly accepted as authentic in all matters of fashion and costume ; but the difficulty about this, when we consider face fashions, is that the Bayeux evidence contradicts almost every written record we have with regard to the Saxons. That the Normans of the Conquest were shaven we have already observed. A few wore short moustaches, but beards were very rare—thus far the old embroidery coincides with written testimony, for almost all the Norman chins are shown as beardless.

But—apart from the beard of Edward the Confessor—the Saxons look much the same. In outlines that resemble the art of Edward Lear, and show the true source of his inspiration, the Saxons on the old sampler (for surely it is time we stopped calling it tapestry) resemble closely their Norman enemies. Sometimes on the upper lip of a Saxon or a Norman there appears the suggestion of a moustache. More often there is no such suggestion. Very seldom does one come across a stray beard. Perhaps a close study of the original would yield one or two more, but the point is immaterial. In general the figures in this embroidery (and we shall do well to remember that it is a Norman job, perhaps executed by Norman needle-women who had never set foot in England or seen a Saxon) conform to whatever independent knowledge we have of Norman fashions. With regard to the Saxons the story is very different.

Early tradition, as recorded by William of Malmesbury (who nevertheless confused the Saxons with Cæsar's Britons), insists that the spies sent out by Harold reported *pene omnes in exercitu illo Presbyteros videri*—they almost all seemed to be priests (not Presbyterians—a fantasy far more terrifying) *quod totam faciem cum utroque labio rasam haberent*. But why should such a thought have occurred to Harold's *speculatores* if there was as little difference in face foliage between the two armies as the Norman needle-work shows us? The Saxons, too, could be taken for an army of priests if the testimony of Bayeux is to be believed, for they are almost as often depicted with both lips shaved.[1]

The Norman French verses of Wace to which we have already alluded apply the story exclusively to the shaven upper lips of the Normans.

> Un des Engleis qui ont veu
> Les Normans tout reis tondu
> Cuida que tuit prevoires fussent
> Et que Messes chanter peussent
> Que tuit erent tondus et reis
> Ne leur estoit Guernon remeis . . .

Of the shaving of priests in the Latin Church we shall have more to say anon. Here we need only note that we have a second source for the tradition that the English were surprised at the absence of even so much as a moustache on most of the Norman faces.

The Origin of Algy

Moustaches were certainly rare enough among the Normans at that time, as Wace's word *guernon* serves to remind us. *Als Gernons*, with moustaches, was the *soubriquet* of William de Percy, one of the Conqueror's fellow-gangsters; and it is evident that this distinguishing mark was then sufficiently rare to serve as a description. (The same title, *Als Gernons* or *aux Gernons* distinguished another of William the Bastard's freebooters, Eustace II, Count of Boulogne, from his father, Eustace I.) The Christian name of Algernon,[2] or Algy, as known to the Percy family centuries later and to the peerage of modern pantomime, derives from the robber baron William, *cognomento Asgernuns*, as one record

[1] The monastic chroniclers speak of Norman influence on Saxon habits, especially in the South, before the Conquest. But there is no mention of this influence having extended to the beard—a point which would surely have been noticed. See, however, Appendix G for my own doubts in this matter.

[2] For further information on Algernon see *Notes and Queries*, 9th Series, vol. ii, pp. 248, 289, 293, 454 and 517.

tells us. But what evidence does the Bayeux embroidery afford for the supposition that even the rarity of moustaches among the Normans would have astonished the Saxons in any way? Once more the text and the texture are at variance.

Credulity of an historian

The monk Aelnoth should have known something of the habits of his countrymen, having lived himself at the very time which we are considering. He was among the English exiles who took refuge in Denmark after the Conquest, and (in his *Historia Ortus, Vitæ et Passionis S. Canuti*) he speaks of the English, about twenty years *after* the battle of Hastings, as shaving their beards. This he records among the devices used by them for much the same reasons that led many Jews to take similar steps in the Middle Ages. The implication is clear enough, that the beard had been normal among the English; but such has been the prestige of Bayeux that Freeman quoted this passage from Aelnoth in a footnote to his *Norman Conquest* (1876, IV, 685-686) with two corroborative statements from Matthew Paris and had no more to say on the whole matter than a query as to how such evidence could be reconciled with the sacrosanct *Tapestry,* as he called it.

He might as well have asked how we can reconcile the laws of perspective with Bayeux. The testimony of Matthew Paris would be of little value without the earlier records; but the great chronicler of St. Albans himself lived in a time when the distinctive characteristics of the Anglo-Saxons were more than a dim memory of the past. What does Matthew say of this matter? In the *Gesta Abbatum* the English nobles, *tam milites quam prælati,* go into exile when the ruthless Normans take their lands; and these exiles are described as holy men, well-born and bountiful, *qui more orientalium, et maxime Trojanorum, barbas et comas nutriebant.* They cultivated their beards and their hair in the manner of the Orient, and of the Trojans in particular. The exploits of Abbot Frithric, in whose life this passage will be found, were no doubt as fabulous as Freeman indicates. But the remarks about the hair and beards of the English nobles must surely have been based upon a strong tradition at least, if not on an earlier account which Matthew Paris merely edited or re-wrote.

The tradition is, in fact, far too persistent to be easily dismissed. Elsewhere in the *Gesta* (I.42 in the Rolls Series) Matthew tells us of English nobles who were compelled *barbas radere cincinnos tondere* in the Norman manner. (*Cincinnus*, a lock or curl, is an interesting reminder that Cincinnatus, the ploughman-dictator-hero of ancient Rome, and represented as a tough and simple type, took his cognomen from a word almost synonymous with effeminacy.) So the English are again represented as shaving their beards as though this were something unusual—*more Normannorum*. And again, William of the Long Beard, who raised a revolt of the Londoners, in the days of Cœur de Lion, is worth some attention.

William of the Long Beard

This man—William Fitzosbert—was executed in 1196 ; and Matthew Paris must have known many who could speak of him from personal recollection. Regarding Fitzosbert's family Matthew says that *ob indignationem Normannorum radere barbam contempsit*, on account of their hatred for the Normans they scorned to shave their beards. It is a little strange, observes Freeman, that (in such case) this man should have borne the name of William. Stranger, I may add, that he should have been called Fitzosbert. But not many years were to pass before a foreigner, one Simon de Montfort, was to become the leader of an English movement, just as Disraeli was one day to qualify as *Nature's Englishman*. So a family of Norman, or partly Norman, origin could possibly have identified itself with England and the English people, in a sense which was not yet true of the Plantagenets and their gallimaufry of locusts—Normans, Angevins, Bretons and other odds and ends.

His Beard a Symbol

Why, if not, does Matthew write with such enthusiasm both of William's beard (by which he was known in his time) and of his deeds ? William of the Long Beard resisted the unjust incidence of taxation and died a shameful death for upholding (says Matthew) the cause of truth and of the poor. So whatever his name or lineage, his beard (which is said to have reached to his waist) and his politics agreed both with one another and with the racial and social struggle as Matthew Paris still saw it, writing in the succeeding generation. Needless to say, the beard in itself no longer had any great significance in an age when the Normans themselves had taken to wearing it—the importance of the story lies in the assertion that it was a family trait, a deliberate identification with a Saxon past of which a strong tradition lingered.

Indeed, the last infiltration of foreign blood before 1066 had come from Denmark ; and here (as in the case of the Saxons) all that we know of the people confirms the view that they were bearded. We read of Sweyne Fork-Beard, and that seems to have described the usual style, Fosbroke noting that the fork had sometimes as many as six prongs. Saxon tradition was similar, and deeply rooted, there being *no record of any notable change* among the Saxons or the Anglo-Danes before 1066. So that all the *prima facie* evidence is against Bayeux.

Parallel cases of misleading works of art

As to the possibility of error in contemporary art, consider any of the numerous European efforts to depict Saracens in the time of the Crusades. The *Encyclopædia Britannica* (14th Edition VI, 771) reproduces an illustration of combats between Christians and Saracens in stained-glass windows (now destroyed) formerly in the Abbey of St. Denis, at Paris. For form's sake there is some slight difference in the armour given to the opposing forces, but *all the combatants are clean-shaven* ; and though the Christian army was no doubt a true enough representation, the Saracens do not, in fact, remotely resemble Saracens, who would certainly have been bearded.

Indeed, on page 782 of the same volume of the *Encyclopædia* the reader may find a reproduction from an illumination to an Arab manuscript, and see how Arabs pictured themselves. Here, once more, we are shown an army (thirteenth century) so the comparison is a fair one. The whole appearance is entirely different in dress and every other particular, conforming (as we should expect) to fashions which have changed very little in hundreds of years. Only two of the figures are without beards, and these may well be intended for women or for eunuchs.

The main point, however, is that a comparison illustrates vividly the inaccuracies which can creep into art which is nevertheless relied upon because it is contemporary with the men, the mode or the event. Space was at least as important as time in a world that was mercifully preserved from our slick communications. Why, therefore, should one assume that those industrious women in Normandy knew any more about the actual appearance of a Saxon than the designers of those windows knew about Saracens?

Saxon Influence and the Beard Revival

Finally it may be pointed out that the Normans, with remarkable rapidity, abandoned their fashions after the Conquest. Is it too much to suppose that in this return to the wearing of long hair and beards in the time of Henry I, the conquerors were influenced by the customs of the conquered? It would not have been the first or the last time such a thing had occurred, from the days when the Romans learnt Greek philosophy to the time when the nabobs of John Company revolutionised the habits of the English upper classes by the Brahminical institution of the morning bath. Or there was Alexander the Great, who conquered the Persians and was conquered by their garb, as Tertullian said (*De Pallio*). It is even, perhaps, significant that the beard became fashionable at court in the reign of Henry I, who made a point of flattering his Saxon subjects in many ways. But this change in the Normans must next occupy our close attention, as the return of the beard was itself the signal for one of the most violent and successful campaigns on the part of the Anti-Beard Party.

Curious errors of Mr. Williamson and of the Encyclopædia Britannica

Mr. Hugh Ross Williamson, in *The Arrow and the Sword*, has recently stated that the ecclesiastical chroniclers, in the time of the Conqueror's sons, deplored the habit of shaving, which he supposes to have been practised by the courtiers *so that their beards should not chafe their friends when they kissed*. The passage is clearly based upon a complete misreading of Orderic Vitalis, who complained *not against shaving* but *against beards*, recording also the words of Bishop Serlo's famous sermon on the subject. The actual words of the Bishop, as reported by Orderic (*Hist. Eccles.* lib XI, cap. XI) were :

> *Barbas suas radere devitant, ne pili suas in osculis amicas præcisi pungant, et setosi Saracenos magis se quam Christianos simulant.*

That is to say, they *avoid* shaving their beards lest the bristles (*pili præcisi*) prick their friends in kissing them ; and *so hairy are they* that *they resemble Saracens* rather than Christians. This passage has even been misread by the writer of the article on William Rufus in the *Encyclopædia Britannica* (Editions of 1929 and 1945). At the very end of this article the writer, who gives Vitalis among his references, says that the king's *long locks and clean shaven face marked his predilection for the newfangled fashions which contemporary ecclesiastics were never weary of denouncing.*

There was nothing new-fangled in the fact that William Rufus shaved, nor was this practice denounced by the Church. On the contrary, as we have seen, the razor had been imposed upon Northern France by the Church itself and was already well established. The novelty lay in the long locks ; and further novelty was soon to appear in the form of the beard. Before explaining the circumstances of Serlo's onslaught it may be well to consider the source of misunderstanding regarding his words, as quoted above.

Of bristles and paramours

Freeman comments (*William Rufus II*, Appendix Note G) that seemingly the shaving of the ancient heroes of Normandy was but rare, perhaps weekly. That will hardly suffice to explain the allusion to bristles ; for if the nobles were such fops as Serlo maintained, and disliked presenting a bristly mouth to their girl-friends (*amicas*—the feminine is used, which disposes of another of Mr. Williamson's assumptions) the remedy was obvious. They had only to shave more often, if we accept Freeman's explanation ; and that is precisely what we should expect any reasonable person to do, let alone the gallants described by Serlo. Since the Bishop was clearly concerned with inducing his congregation to shave, one might almost have expected him to urge that by doing so frequently enough the disadvantages of the bristles could be overcome . . .

Shaving in the Middle Ages was certainly not the daily business that it is today. Few could shave themselves—for self-shaving did not become common until soap was cheap, plentiful and of good quality. The later advent of the safety razor is an event of even greater importance. As late as the year 1522 we find a regulation that *No man shalbe made fre unlesse he . . . shave hys upper lipe wicklye.* Once over weekly was evidently considered standard practice. But it is abundantly clear that even a fresh shave was far from a close one, leaving a shaven face in the Middle Ages as smooth as a toothbrush. Consider, for example, the case of the Knight in Chaucer's *Marchantes Tale.* (This merchant himself wore a *forkèd berd*, like his Saxon ancestors.)

The knight in the story is a Lombard, whose race, when the tale begins, has long abandoned the *insignia* of its name and fame. Himself elderly, he has all his life

> . . . *folwed ay his bodily delyt*
> *On wommen ther as was his appetyt*

But at the age of sixty he decides to marry a young and beautiful girl. That he is evidently not the man he was, and aware of the fact, is made patent in the account of his precautions, which I emphasise only to make it clear that so painstaking a groom would at least have added as good a shave as the best barber could give him, if he shaved at all—which he evidently did.

The said precautions are detailed :

> *He drynketh ypocras, claree and vernáge*
> *Of spyces hote, t'encreessen his coráge ;*
> *And many a letuarie hath he ful fyn*
> *Swiche as the cursed monk, dan Constantyn*
> *Hath writen in his book* De Coitu . . .

But when we come to his person, the best the knight could do for cheek and chin was surely enough to scare the bride from his bed :

He lulleth hire, he kisseth hire ful ofte
With thikke bristles of his berd unsofte,
Like to the skyn of houndfyssh sharpe as brere,
For he was shave al newe in his manere.

If these bristles when he had *shave al newe* were all that a bride-groom could manage (*in his manere*) in the fourteenth century, when soap was beginning to come into use, we may safely assume that shaving two hundred years earlier was even less effective. This explains quite simply why the courtiers of Henry I let their beards grow out of consideration for their concubines.

Even in Shakespeare's time the clean shave as we know it can hardly have been usual. In Henry IV, Part I, I, 3, where Hotspur describes the courtier who so offended him after the fight at Holmedon, this effeminate cub had clearly done his best with clothes and perfume. Yet of his efforts (or the barber's) at shaving his face Hotspur says that

his chin new reapt
Show'd like a stubble-land at harvest-home.

Manifestly it was to this appearance, and even more to certain other inconveniences attending what we should consider a three days' growth, that the courtiers in the time of Henry I objected. And their remedy was to give up shaving—a fashion in which the king himself led the way.

William Rufus toyed with Judaism

William Rufus, who was not so revolutionary, merely grew long hair ; but had his flirtation with the Jews gone further (he hinted at one time that he might take up Judaism, but I think it was said merely to alarm the Bishops) we might have seen the Levitical code implanted in England and the beard with it. It was left to William's brother to restore the beard ; and, though there was no suggestion that this restoration was part of an anti-Christian movement, some churchmen certainly regarded it as such.

The Church Militant

Among these was Orderic Vitalis, who was born in England some ten years after the Norman Conquest and included the events of his own time in his Ecclesiastical History. He objected strongly to men wearing long hair (like harlots, he said) and he lamented the departure in this matter from the apostolic precept (*apostoli præceptum*)—referred to also by William of Malmesbury, who noticed the change in fashion with disapproval in the first book of his *Historia Novella*, cap. 4, quoting the Apostle Paul (*Vir si comam nutrierit, ignominia est illi*). William of Malmesbury tells the story of a knight who dreamed he was being strangled with his own locks and woke to cut them off in a fright. This story he thought suitable for the fops of his time *qui obliti quid nati sunt, libenter in muliebris habitum transformant*—such as, forgetful of their natural sex, transform their appearance to that of women. The chronicler even claimed that the fame of that awful dream had spread throughout England, causing long-haired warriors all over the country to follow the knight's example and crop their hair. But the panic had not lasted long, and the ringlets had soon returned—even false ones for those who could not produce enough of the home-grown product. The English Bishop Wulfstan of Worcester waged war on this custom, keeping a knife handy for direct action ; and Archbishop Anselm even used the weapon of excommunication against men who persisted in wearing long hair.

War and Disease the punishment for long hair and beards

Indeed, as early as the year 1102, a Council held at London, under the presidency of the Archbishop, had found it necessary to decree *ut criniti sic tondeantur ut pars aurium appareat et oculi non tegantur*—that the hair should be cut in such a way that part of the ears should be visible and the eyes should not be covered. But the beard is often the target of even fiercer attacks, in language that only monks, priests and prophets can use with an appearance of decency. Orderic Vitalis (who himself regarded war and disease in his time as God's punishment for human wickedness in wearing long hair and beards) has favoured us with an account of the most dramatic move attempted at this time against the new fashions.

Serlo, Bishop of Séez, may have felt more than the usual load of responsibility for preaching the gospel of the razor, for

(according to Alfred Canel) one of his predecessors wore a beard
—a delinquency far more reprehensible in a bishop than it was
in a layman. This claim is made by Canel in his *Histoire de la
Barbe et des Cheveux en Normandie* with regard to Yves de Bellesmes
(Bishop of Séez from 1052-1070) on the grounds that a beard was
found on the Bishop when he was exhumed in 1601. I am not
entirely convinced by this argument, and in the absence of the
defendant I wish to plead on behalf of my client that astonishing
stories are told of the posthumous growth of the hair and beard
such as might account for the most meticulously shorn cleric
being discovered *in flagrante barbascendo* some time after his burial.
Wolferus, the chronicler of Hildesheim, tells of a woman
buried at Nuremberg, whose grave was opened forty-three years
later, when hair was found growing through all clefts in her coffin ;
and I submit to the jury that there are many such examples,
some of which will be found in Winter's *Trichologia* (London
1869).[1]

Robert of Normandy—his crimes

Be that as it may, Bishop Serlo certainly considered that he had a
mission to fulfil, and the weight of ecclesiastical authority was on
his side. When our Henry I arrived in Normandy, engaged in
the family pastime of invading the dominions of Robert Curthose,
it was Serlo who acted as principal Army Chaplain and preached
at Carentan a militant sermon against Henry's brother. The
crimes of Robert, as enumerated by Serlo, were indeed formidable.
It was revealed that the Duke of Normandy often lay in bed till
three p.m. for lack of bread—nay more (as his agnomen implied) he spent the greater part of his time among the bed-clothes
for want of the means to drape his person, the wretched Duke being
without trousers, stockings or shoes. For this reason Robert
was prevented from going to Church, which doubtless made the
most important count in Serlo's indictment.[2]

[1] See also the *Medical Record* (New York, 1877, xii, 515) for article on *Hair
grown after death*.

[2] The age of Army Chaplains appears to have begun with Henry I. Another
of his protegés was Roger, later Bishop of Salisbury and Justiciar. He owed his
fortune to the speed with which he could get through a Mass—a great advantage
in an army.

Having thus established the fact that he was on the right side in the fraternal fracas, the Bishop took advantage of the prestige gained by his fiery denunciation of the Duke of Normandy's poverty to censure the king of England and his courtiers for their beards and long hair. He reminded them that it was not for ornament or pleasure that penitents had been ordered to let their hair and beards grow, but as a symbol of the ugliness of their sins in the sight of God. The unkempt hair of such penitents *denotes the deformity of the soul by outward ignominy*, he said.

The Shears of Bishop Serlo

No sign of sorrow for sin are the beards the Bishop sees before him. Like his chronicler he says that by such courtly beards the wearers take after goats, *whose filthy lasciviousness is shamefully imitated by fornicators and sodomites*. Good men properly regard them with abhorrence, on account of the odious foulness of their lusts. There follows a reminder that Popes and Bishops have condemned such innovations, but these hardened sinners . . . and then follows the passage in which Serlo attributes beards to the fact that women dislike bristly kisses. Such people have been foretold in the Revelation of St. John, the prelate concluded.

The King and Robert de Beaumont, Count of Meulan (the latter being the fashionable pattern of the age) wilted and succumbed. From beneath his robes the bishop produced a pair of shears ; and in the sight of God, *coram publico*, he removed the offending hair and beards before the king and his nobles had leisure to repent of their repentance.[1] Surely no rabbi could have performed his office with more eagerness.

[1] There is a seal of Henry I in which he is represented as shaven—perhaps dating from this episode, of which Mabillon gives an interesting account. (Equally high-handed action was taken by Godfrey, Bishop of Amiens, who on Christmas Day, 1105, refused the communion to all who wore beards. Even barbarossa is said to have submitted at one time to this clerical campaign.)

CHAPTER V

RADAT AND FILIOQUE

Goddes Angell shove away his berde.
John Lydgate

My text is from Lydgate's *Falls of Princes*, rhymes royal on themes derived from Boccaccio, filtered through a French translation. No matter; it serves its purpose. We must see for ourselves next what Goddes angells have to do with the matter, for our talk is now of theology.

Of weighty matters

Twice before the Reformation was the Christian Church split, once for a letter which left few traces and once for a word which stayed. When the battle was all between Arians and Athanasians a single letter flared, shook, trembled, spluttered and was snuffed out. Henceforward it was established that the nature of the Trinity was *homoousion* and not *homoiousion*.

The Council of Nicæa determined the matter; but a few centuries later some Western Christians, not satisfied with the Holy Ghost of the Nicene Creed, which proceeded from the Father, added the word *filioque—and from the Son*. The innovation spread from Spain over Western Europe, but Constantinople barred the gates of the East. They would not have *filioque*. A Pope hesitated and temporised, but the eastern Patriarchs were adamant. Out of that *filioque* came the Great Schism, severing the Western Church from the Eastern.

The double procession of the Paraclete was therefore the source of a greater controversy and a greater cleavage than the Protestant Reformation. It was a distant echo of the old controversy of *homo* and *homoi*, for the Spanish innovators were doing their best to contravert the lurking Arianism of the Western Goths. The Eastern Church was as soundly Athanasian as Latin Christendom, but too conservative of tradition to allow such tinkering with a creed laid down by the Holy Fathers. Therefore for the sake of one word was the seamless robe rent in two ; and all other differences between East and West are subsidiary to the problem of *filioque*.

The Beard Schismatic

But the moment the split occurred, each side, as is the nature of persons engaged in controversy, began to look for further delinquencies in its opponents. They had not to look much further than the ends of their noses, for one difference was immediately apparent : that the Eastern clergy wore beards, and the priests of the West did not. This might be considered a matter of personal taste or national custom, but neither side was prepared to regard it in this way, once the fight was on. The Greeks, in particular, were inclined to make a big issue of the matter, and regarded shaving as one of the major sins of their Latin brethren. As an old English poem tells us (*The Pilgrimage and the Ways of Jerusalem*—about A.D. 1500)

> *That is the geyse of that contre,*
> *The lenger the berde, the bettyr is he.*

Two centuries before the Great Schism a similar controversy had been settled on English soil. The major issue between the Roman missionaries and those of the Irish Church, who had pleaded their respective cases before king Oswy at the Synod of Whitby (A.D. 664), was the right time for keeping Easter. But here again a matter of apparently minor importance had been allowed to take a prominent part in the subsequent discussions, the secondary controversy on this occasion having concerned the correct tonsure of a clerical or monastic head.

A digression on the Tonsure

Irish practice, introduced into Scotland and Northumbria, had always been to shave the front of the head, in a crescent, from ear to ear. (This tonsure resembled that of the ancient Hebrews when mourning, and perhaps it also resembled the cut used by certain Oriental idolators ; which may help to account for the fact that the Roman missionaries called it the Tonsure of Simon Magus.) The Romans themselves shaved a circle on the crown of the head[1]—the now familiar tonsure of the mediæval monk and priest—which they called the tonsure of St. Peter, saying that the ring of hair round their bald pates stood for the crown of thorns. So another aspect of shaving had already helped to divide Christians, and no one can read Bede's *Historia Ecclesiastica* without realising the importance that once attached to controversy on the tonsure. Sixty years after the Synod of Whitby we still find Abbot Ceolfrid writing to the king of the Picts, those evanescent barbarians known to most of us only as occasional nuisances against whose depredations Roman walls were built or Saxon aid invoked by the helpless Britons. The Picts, however, in the reign of King Naitan, were Christians, converted at first by Irish missionaries and now re-converted under Roman influence to keep the canonical prescription for the observance of Easter.

But the Abbot was anxious that the Picts should also observe the canonical tonsure (though he explained that the difference was not so vital as that respecting Easter) and he pointed out how important it was to avoid any resemblance to the charlatan who sought to buy for filthy lucre the gift of the Holy Ghost. The tonsure, he says, must be upon the top of the head, which is the highest part of the body—an argument which has a semblance of logic, without any clear premises. And, for the matter of that, I cannot find why Simon Magus was credited with the crescent tonsure or any tonsure at all (unless those critics are right who assume that the Simon Magus story is largely a caricature of St. Paul, in which case we have definite evidence that the Apostle once polled his head), nor do any of the Roman apologists attempt to explain the reason for attributing this tonsure to the Magician. The argument becomes harder to follow the further we proceed, but I am glad to record that the good abbot concludes by conceding that he does not mean to imply that those who use this tonsure are to be damned; and for this I will give Abbot Ceolfrid good marks.

Was Photius a eunuch ?

Not so the bearded Greeks, as they glared at the shaven

[1] It is curious that in Mexico under the Aztecs such a tonsure was regarded as destructive of the power of sorcery and enchantment—see Frazer's *Folklore in the Old Testament*, in his admirable chapter on Samson.

protagonists of *filioque*. Photius, the learned and quarrelsome Byzantine, who was more responsible than any other person for the Great Schism, was particularly violent on the subject of shaving among the Western Clergy, although (according to Cardinal Baronius) he was himself a smooth-faced eunuch (*cum alioquin ipse esset eunuchus glaber*). I have failed to discover where Baronius picked up this trifle, for which he supplies no reference, and I cannot myself confirm it from any other source ; though I notice that it was repeated, on the Cardinal's sole authority, by the Most Rev. Charles Seghers in the *American Catholic Quarterly Review* in 1882 (Vol. VII, page 282). I hesitate to believe that, in a Church where so much was made of beards in general, and the beard clerical and patriarchal in particular, any *eunuchus glaber* could have held priestly office, still less attained the distinction among his bearded fellows which Photius achieved. [1]

Curious moderation of Ratramnus

Also, how would a eunuch have dared to choose such dangerous ground for combat ? When his contemporary, Ratramnus of Corbie, replied to Photius (*Contra Græcorum opposita Romanam ecclesiam infamantium, A.D. 868*) he did not ask his opponent what had become of his own whiskers, if they were so essential to priesthood. On the contrary he argued (with commendable moderation) that too much was made of the matter, altogether, salvation being independent of the question, to shave or not to shave (*barbæ detonsio aut conservatio*). This was that same Ratram-

[1] That pedantic critic of the errors of other people, G. F. R. Molé, was so misled by this story of Photius that he revised centuries of ecclesiastical history to fit in with it. In his account of beards in his *Histoire des Modes Françaises* he actually represented the Eastern clergy as shaven priests who abused their Latin brethren, at the time of the schism, for wearing beards (*op. cit.* 155-156). This book was published in 1773, and it is astonishing to relate that when the chapter on beards was re-published with further notes in 1826 this classical howler stood uncorrected. The Photius legend may be compared with that which Erastus circulated about Paracelsus, giving as evidence the statement that Paracelsus had no beard and detested women. Portraits of Paracelsus differ radically, but that of Tintoretto definitely gives the lie to Erastus, for he represented the great physician with a small beard.

nus, or Bertram, who coined the word *stercoranist* to describe Paschasius Radbertus, when the latter wrote that the consecrated elements were *nec alia quam quæ nata est de Maria, passa in cruce, resurrexit de sepulchro;* of which matter I have had somewhat to say in another place, but I mention it to show that he could hit hard below the belt when he had a mind for all-in controversy. Yet here he roars as gently as any sucking dove.

In a Church founded upon tradition there can be little doubt that the Greeks could cite older authorities, which may partly account for the more moderate tone of the Latin champions, and their insistance that the matter was not of prime importance. As in the case of *filioque*, the innovators were clearly the Western clergy, the conservatives being those of the Orient—and it may be no accident that ever since that time one Church has emphasised before everything its Catholicity, the other its Orthodoxy. On the side of the Orthodox there was Leviticus, with the testimony of Clement of Alexandria and many facts commonly accepted by a majority on both sides, such as the probability or certainty that Christ and the Apostles were bearded, after the Jewish fashion. (Some artists and others, as we shall observe, took an independent line on this question; but most theologians do not appear to have considered it a matter for dispute.)

A Venerable Forgery

There were also the *Apostolical Constitutions*, a very venerable forgery which the Greeks considered as highly authoritative, because it purported to set out the scheme of Christian discipline laid down by the Apostles themselves. I quote from the edition of 1563, published at Venice, *cum privilegio summi Pontificis* (which was very nice of him) and I add a warning that there are other versions with variable wordings, though the sense of them all is much the same :

Neque vero licet barbæ pilos corrumpere : neque hominis figuram præter naturam mutare . . . Hoc enim mulieribus decens Creator Deus statuit, viris indecorum esse indicavit. (Lib. I, Cap. IV.)

Nor is it permissible (reads the text) to destroy the hair of the beard, and unnaturally to change the form of a man . . . for God the Creator has decreed this to be decent for women, but determined that it is unsuitable for man. The authority given for this is—of course—Leviticus xix, 27. Authorship has been claimed, upon flimsy evidence, for St. Clement, called Romanus, who is said to have been the fourth Pope and (according to one version) was ordained as a priest by St. Peter himself. The style and sentiments resemble those of his namesake of Alexandria, whose writings may have influenced this work if its date is as late as many suppose. The *Constitutiones* declare that the smallest hair of the beard must on no account be clipped. God, who created us after his own likeness, would load with his hatred those who violated his law by shaving their chins.

Testimony of St. Epiphanius against shaving

But this section of the *Constitutiones Apostolicæ* is explicitly concerned with the laity ; and those who take great account of this authority may consider whether observations specifically addressed to laymen were intended to apply equally to priests, which is certainly not equally clear. The passages quoted above were, however, used by St. Epiphanius in a fierce denunciation of shaven faces—and his words achieved immortality among the classical clichés of the Pro-Beard Party of later years. This Epiphanius, who lived in the fourth century, was much troubled by the sartorial and tonsorial habits of the Massalian heretics, which he regarded as the outward and visible sign of their inner corruption (though from all I can discover about the sect, they appear to have been sober and decent people, much like the early Quakers in many respects). In his great opus *contra octoginta hæreses* Epiphanius says specifically of some Mesopotamian monks who had fallen into this heresy, that they removed their beards and let their hair grow long, and he then quotes the *Apostolical Constitutions* against this practice : *Atque quod ad barbam attinet, in Apostolorum Constitutionibus divino sermone ac dogmate præscribitur ne ea corrumpatur ; hoc est, ne barba ponatur neve meretricius cultus et ornatus usurpetur.* Was there anything, asked the Saint, more contrary to good morals than the custom of those who defied these ordinances ?

Testimony of Tertullian

Tertullian's authority would, of course, have been accepted by neither side, since he had died in a strong odour of heresy (a very priggish and uncharitable heresy, at that ; so that I hope God had more mercy on him than he would have had on his fellow men). But Tertullian does at least give us some idea of the way Christians regarded the beard about 200 years after the birth of Christ ; and if anyone should urge that Tertullian, when writing *De Pallio*, spoke as a puritan heretic and no Catholic Christian, I will reply, firstly that he wrote his defence of his philosopher's mantle at least two years before he left the Church (or, more probably, was kicked out of it) and secondly that *De Pallio* is remarkably free from Tertullian's habitual failings. It is astonishingly light-hearted, gay and witty—a literary *tour de force* without any theological axe-grinding. Here, then, he speaks with some evident contempt of his Numidian neighbours, whose faces were close-shaven, while their locks hung as long as nature would allow—or even longer, with the aid of horse-hair. With these habits he couples the use of resin and of pincers, for depilation.

St. Jerome and St. Cyprian

But I cannot speak of Tertullian without calling to mind his tract *de Cultu Feminarum*, where (in the seventh chapter of Book II) he acknowledged among masculine failings the over-neat trimming of the beard, the plucking of hairs from the face and the shaving of (it would appear) the moustache : the word he uses is *circumradere*. St. Jerome also objected to shaving, and even to the tonsure (urging in both matters an avoidance of extremes by the wearing of short beards and of a short hair cut). And St. Cyprian, among the vices of his time—the third century— wrote in his *Liber de Lapsis* of men who cut off their beards and women who painted their faces. He quotes Leviticus, mentions depilation and concludes : *Thus, to please the world, they are not afraid to displease God.* He does not indicate that priests are exempt from this displeasure, but leaves a loop-hole to which we will refer later.

Indeed, as late as the fifth century we have evidence that even in the West, a beard was held by some to be the proper ornament of a priest. Sidonius Apollinaris, who lived in those days, was no model of virtue, for he was (before he became Bishop of Clermont) a politician who turned his coat as often as expediency dictated a change in allegiance. But his evidence must surely reflect contemporary opinion when he speaks of his friend Maximus Palatinus, newly ordained a priest. His clothes (wrote Sidonius[1]) his gait, his modesty, his countenance and conversation, were religious ; as to his hair, it was short and his beard long (*tum coma brevis, barba prolixa*). This model priest was also a vegetarian.

Problem of the Roman Church

Against such evidence as this the Western Church was hard put to it to discover any suitable precedent for its custom of shaving. It could be urged that Leviticus belonged to the Old Dispensation and that some other references cited did not necessarily apply to the clergy ; or it could be argued that too much was being made of too small a point. But as the practice of shaving was practically universal in the Latin Church of the ninth century, and for six hundred years after the Great Schism, positive authority had to be found for the *fait accompli*. It was found in the most extraordinary manner.

Among the many ancient records of the Church there exist certain canons attributed to the Fourth Council of Carthage, said to have been held about A.D. 398. How vague is our knowledge of this Council may be realised by comparing two articles in the same edition of the *Catholic Encyclopedia* (1907). The article on *Canons* speaks of this Council of Carthage as an historical event, and says that it confirmed the *Breviarium* of the Canons of Hippo in A.D. 393. On the other hand, the article on *Beards* refers to this Council as the *so-called Fourth Council of Carthage* and says that it *in reality represents the synodical decrees of some council in Southern Gaul in the time of St. Cæsarius of Arles (c. 503)*.[2]

[1] Lib. IV, Ep. 24. His works were edited by Jean Savaron, who commented on this passage, which he considered important evidence.

[2] See Hefele's *History of the Councils of the Church* (1876, vol. ii, 409-410) where serious reasons are put forward that this Council never took place.

The famous forty-fourth canon

From this authority of doubtful origin we have what the *Catholic Encyclopedia* describes as *the earliest positive legislation on the subject for clerics*—that is to say, on beards. And the forty-fourth canon is then quoted as follows in the article on this subject :

Clericus nec comam nutriat nec barbam

That is to say, *a priest shall not nourish his hair nor his beard.* But I deeply regret to record that the *Catholic Encyclopedia* says little more on this subject except that the prohibition was probably directed only against beards of excessive length, and that it was widely quoted and included in the *Corpus juris.*

Now I am surprised that Father Herbert Thurston, who wrote this article on Beards, did not consider it necessary to inform his readers that the wording of the forty-fourth canon is and has been hotly disputed. For it is alleged by some writers that, about the time when *filioque* was slipped into the creed, the word *radat* was as neatly amputated from the alleged canon of the alleged council. *Aliquis misopogon,* wrote Cornelius à Lapide, *radat erasit.* That is to say, it has been claimed that the words should, in fact, read :

Clericus nec comam nutriat nec barbam radat

which, being translated, has a directly opposite sense, so far as beards are concerned, for it signifies that *a priest shall not nourish his hair nor shave his beard.*

The matter has been learnedly thrashed *pro* and *con*, the case for *radat* being summarised from the works of many authorities by the Rev. Joseph Bingham in his *Origines Ecclesiasticæ* (Vol. I, Book VI, Cap. IV, Section 15). I confess I have neither the scholarship, nor yet the inclination, to follow the controversy[1] far afield, still less do I desire to drag the reluctant reader with

[1] The *nec radat* party does appear to have a stronger case, which their opponents have never really answered. But Barbier de Montault in *Le Costume et les usages ecclésiastiques* (1898, vol. 1, 186) quotes evidence from the *Peristephanon* of Prudentius Clemens that a fourth century priest in Carthage shaved. The evidence, however, is not conclusive, and does not dispose of the MSS. quoted by the other party.

me, though I must admit to some preference for the amended reading as the more likely Latin construction. It appears also more probable that—if any ruling was ever laid down about the year 500 or earlier—it would have been in order to insist upon clerical beards rather than to prohibit their growth. But I warn all but the stoutest hearted against exploring this particular mare's nest. *Radat* must once have rivalled *filioque* as a theological shuttlecock, and the wells of obscure references to the controversy are as yet almost unplumbed.

Beards in Babel

To make matters worse, some authors quote the sentence in the plural, *Clerici nec comam nutriant nec barbam (radant)*, everyone manifestly re-writing it to suit his taste, singular or plural, with the *radat* or without, while Laurentius Surius is quoted by Rudolf Hospinian (*De Monachis*) with *Clericus nec comam nutriat, nec barbam tondeat*, which differs once more in the actual verb supposed to have been omitted. The Abbé Fangé, in his *Mémoires pour servir à l'Histoire de la Barbe de l'Homme*, makes the best of both worlds. On page 253 he quotes the usual version, without the *radat* : *Clericus nec comam nutriat, nec Barbam*. This, with good reason, he attributes to the *third* Council of Carthage—for on page 258 he quotes the same tag, adding *radat* and says that it is now the *fourth* Council that he is quoting. The coincidence that in each case he claims the forty-fourth canon as his reference does not appear to have worried him any more than the contradiction which he implies between the two Councils, until (in a later section of the same work) he suddenly turns to discussing the controversy, as though unaware of the fact that he has already pontificated on both sides—an unusual feat of controversial gymnastics.

Precarious predicament of the Latin case

Here, then, we have a Council which may never have taken place, the rulings of which (as Father James Broderick S.J. reminds me in a letter) would have had only local significance, being no more than a provincial synod. The wording of the vital canon in this unimportant and somewhat hypothetical Council is disputed ; and even if the wording as Father Thurston gives it be accepted, he himself states that the meaning is not very clear, as the prohibition (in that reading) is merely to the effect that a priest shall not *nourish* (*nutrire*) a beard. A cleric might presumably—as some later priests and even Popes in fact did—grow some kind of beard and still claim that he did not *nourish* it. And yet—*mirabile dictu*—the principal weapon of the Latin armoury in the great beard question, was originally and historically this supposed forty-fourth canon of the Fourth Council of Carthage. The case for the shaven clergy was allowed to hang for six centuries on an arbitrary reading of an ambiguous version of a disputed text of a mere provincial synod which may never have taken place. And this—I quote Father Thurston once more, from the *Catholic Encyclopedia*—*was widely quoted* and *had great influence in creating a precedent.*[1]

Modern Catholic apologists have long ceased to base their case for a shaven clergy upon such flimsy foundations. It is, they insist, a matter merely of Catholic practice, and not of canonical law. In search of information on this subject I was shocked to discover that the British Museum Library contained no copy of the latest digest of the canon law by Wernz and Vidal (*Jus Canonicum*, Rome 1928) though I understand that one is now being obtained. In the meantime, by the kindness of Father James Brodrick, I have consulted the copy in the Jesuit Church at Farm Street.

According to this authority there is no doubt that Christ and the Apostles wore the full beard usual among the Jews and other Oriental peoples at that time. The early fathers also were bearded, and this practice continued in the East. But in the West, from the fourth and fifth centuries onwards, there was a practice of not nourishing the beard, but rather of cutting it off, and (in point of fact) of shaving it—*barbam . . . potius tondendi atque adeo radendi*. Then follows a reference to the invectives of Photius against the Latin clergy *quod barbas radere non abnuerunt*,

[1] I must admit that the other party was often equally unscrupulous in its method of reasoning—witness J. A. Dulaure, who quotes the opinion of Tertullian on the Fourth Council of Carthage, which took place (if it ever did) nearly 200 years after Tertullian's death.

and a reference to Cardinal Humbertus, Legate of Leo IX at Constantinople in the ninth century, who said that the Greeks would not have communion with those *qui comas tondent et secundum institutionem Romæ Ecclesiæ barbam radunt*—those who cut the hair and shave the beard after the manner of the Roman Church.

The Greeks refuse to have communion with the shaven

That was true enough. The Greeks were prepared to carry their prejudices to the point of excommunicating all who did not conform to them. In a series of attacks the Greek clergy began to abuse their Latin brethren for the habit of shaving, and Michael Cœrularius made a big point of this reprehensible practice in his work against the Papal supremacy. The Romans replied with quotations from Holy Writ, to show that the Nazarites shaved when they had fulfilled their vows (though I cannot myself discover that their shaving, which applied primarily to the head, was extended to the beard). And had not Ezekiel, in the famous passage (Chap. V. 1-2) shaved off his beard *in misterio,* and disposed of it *partim ad combustionem, partim ad concisionem, partim ad dispensionem,* to signify what should become of Israel ?

True origin of the shaven clergy

We have observed that the fashion of shaving among the western clergy was copied from the common habits of the urban population in the time of the Empire—a fashion which had remained quite common even when Hadrian and other emperors had worn beards though the evidence of sculpture shows that it was by no means universal. Father Seghers, in the article already mentioned (*American Catholic Quarterly Review,* 1882) was quite clear on this point, giving for comparison the Roman toga, which became the Roman cassock of later years. In much the same way judges, policemen, liveried servants and other functionaries reflect in their costumes the culture of the place and period in which those costumes were stabilised. (Incidentally no judge or butler wears a beard today for the same reason.) Father Seghers was nevertheless stretching a point when he followed Baronius in attempting to prove the shaven habits of the Romans, in the time of the Empire, by citing a passage from the *Noctes Attica* of Aulus Gellius. This passage (lib. iii, cap. iv) clearly refers only to the custom of Roman nobles in the time of Scipio Africanus—and that only of young and middle-aged men (*in medio ætatis*,[1] which presumes that the elderly at that time wore beards).

The Riddle of Justinian's chin

The Most Rev. Father was also so anxious to prove his case that he claimed Constantine Pogonatus as the first bearded Emperor of Byzantium, saying that Justinian shaved. But this simplification is contradicted by a mosaic above the king's door in the narthex of Santa Sophia, Constantinople, which shows Justinian quite unmistakably bearded. Father Seghers has on his side the mosaics at Ravenna (in addition to that at St. Vitale there is one at St. Apollinare in Urbe) ; and it is possible that the Italian versions and that of Constantinople may all have been correct in their time. The Hagia Sophia was begun in 532 and consecrated in 537 ; there was plenty of time between the completion of that job and the date of the mosaic at St. Vitale (about 547) for Justinian to remove his beard. But the fact remains that he wore one previously, and that he did so after his coronation as Emperor.[2] So that the theory of *Pogonatus* as the first bearded emperor of the East will not hold any shaving water. On the other hand, with those Ravenna mosaics in mind, I am equally inclined to doubt Fosbroke's statement in his *Encyclopædia of Antiquities* that the bearded fashion of the Eastern Emperors began with Justinian and continued without interruption till the fall of Constantinople. Justinian is reported to have had at least one shaven successor in the Emperor Heraclius, said to have removed an enormous beard and cut short his hair (*qui est Imperatorum habitus*) when he seized the throne in 610 A.D. The tradition still seems to have had some weight at that time.

[1] Since writing this I have realised that Aulus Gellius may have meant that Romans then shaved *after* middle age, younger men being bearded. Pliny appears to confirm this.

[2] There is also said to be an illustration in the *Imperium Orientale* of Anselmo Banduri, which shows Justinian without a beard but sporting a moustache. I cannot find this plate from the reference offered by Fosbroke.

An Emperor without a nose

(This paragraph, beginning in parenthesis, must come to an end before a thought carries me too far—the brackets putting a term to some dangerous serendipity. But I cannot let *Pogonatus* pass again without remarking that his son, Justinian II, was known as *Rhinotmetus*, because his enemies cut his nose off. I did not think, when reflecting in Chapter I on the comparative incidence of beards and noses in the human species that I would find a family history so suited to my text. But mark that no person is remembered in history for the mere possession of a nose or solely for the lack of a beard.)[1]

The main contention of Father Seghers was probably right, however, and he correctly compared the imitation of current fashion with the common practice of Roman priests ever since in identifying themselves, as far as possible, with the people among whom they live and work. Indeed, it may not be entirely without significance that the line of bearded emperors who followed Hadrian ended—until the Empire had ceased to be Roman in anything but name—with Constantine the Great. He it was who established shaving at the same time that he established Christianity as the State Religion ; and it must have been this fact which Julian had in mind when he identified his whiskers with his apostasy, as though the razor had been comprehended in the alleged *donatio*—the fatal gift attributed to his uncle. Even Julian himself shaved when first invested with the rank of Cæsar, in the life-time of his cousin Constantius—ceremonially

[1] Since writing this I have noticed that C. L'Estrange Ewen, in his *Origin of British Surnames* (London, 1938, p. 101) mentions an Israelite known as *Moses cum Naso*, but I doubt if the insistence that he had a nose was intended to imply anything unusual in the mere possession of one. On the other hand the same authority mentions *Aelfsige mid tham berde* in the eleventh century—clearly one of the bolder Saxons who became conspicuous by sticking to his beard under the tyranny of the shaven Normans. *Rob. cum barba* (1247), *Rob. ove la Barbe* (1286), *W. with the Berde* (1315) are other examples cited, the last reappearing in the same year as a single word in the Assize Rolls—*W. Wyththeberd*. L'Estrange Ewen also refers to an elegant person, *Hugh Belebarb* (1205) and to a certain lady—*Alice Barbe Dor*—whose golden beard flourished in 1247. (*Flourished* is the ideal word, from *floreo*, which had a secondary meaning of sprouting whiskers in adolescence.)

removing his philosopher's beard, as Gibbon recalls, because it was already considered incompatible with the character of a Roman prince. It was not until Constantius was safely dead, and Julian was crowned as Augustus, that he liberated his beard and paraded his apostasy. So already the Christians had conformed to (and helped to establish) the normality of shaving. After a single generation of shaven Christianity it is clear that it was the bearded Julian who was the crank, the outsider.

Where Romans may wear beards

True to this principle of observing local custom where possible, the Catholic Church has never been rigid in its allegiance to the razor, but allowed practice to vary according to place and circumstance ; though in this it has not been entirely consistent. Catholic priests who work in the Near East are, in fact, permitted by tacit or express privilege to grow beards like the neighbouring Schismatics (so the *Catholic Encyclopedia* informs us) because there *a smooth face carries with it the suggestion of effeminacy*. The same authority also states that Catholic missionaries are allowed the same privilege in the East *and in other barbarous countries* where the *conveniences of civilisation cannot be found*. In the *Jus Canonicum* (Wernz and Vidal, 1928) Tom. II *De Personis*, there is also a learned scholion upon this subject, showing the exception made for priests of the Latin rite *in regionibus orientalibus* and in certain other cases on a special dispensation from the Apostolic See. What is not explained is the inconsistency with regard to variations in western custom ; for we shall see that in the bearded sixteenth century beards became very common among the higher Roman clergy ; but in the equally bearded mid-Victorian period no attempt was made by Rome to conform with contemporary western practice among laymen.

To return to the origin of this custom, even the precise date of the Fourth Council of Carthage, if it ever took place, has been a matter of dispute. It was said to have been called by Aurelius, Bishop of Carthage, some say while St. Siricius was Pope (in A.D. 397), though others make it later, in the time of Pope Anastasius I (399-401). But Dulaure, in his *Pogonologie*, quotes from the canons of a later Council held at Barcelona in

540, a ruling that no priest should nourish his hair or shave his beard (*Ut nullus Clericorum comam nutriat, aut barbam radat*[1]— apart from the decline in the Latin, the sense is that of the amended reading of the Carthaginian Canon, and appears to be modelled on it ; so that there is further reason here to suspect the deletion of *radat* in the Carthaginian ruling). And it is equally difficult to trace the official development of policy at headquarters.

Carelessness of Cardinal Baronius

Cardinal Baronius claimed that Pope Clement I shaved in the first century A.D., and (as we shall see) an even earlier claim was made by the Council of Limoges in 1031. So little is known of Clement Romanus that the Cardinal offered no evidence, and in fact he could not have offered any worth examination ; indeed, as Father Seghers points out, the Cardinal was himself so careless as to allow the engraver who illustrated his *Annales* to depict Clement as bearded. Why Baronius was so anxious to establish the antiquity of shaving among the clergy I am at a loss to explain ; many have drawn attention to his errors, but none has noted the curious paradox of a bearded priest defending the propriety of shaving. For Cæsar Baronius lived in that strange period, of which we shall speak later, when Popes, Cardinals and Bishops commonly wore beards ; and he was no exception, as is shown by the likeness reproduced in the *Catholic Encyclopedia* (article on Baronius). As to Clement Romanus, his reputed authorship of the *Apostolical Constitutions* might have been considered as presumptive evidence that he wore the beard which he was supposed to have advocated for others. But enough has been said of that doubtful document. Much the same may be said of the claim that Clement's alleged predecessor, Anacletus, instituted shaving—even his precise name is uncertain.

Some Bearded Popes

Leo III, who was the first Pope to pronounce in favour of *filioque*, is also credited by some (appropriately enough) with being the first pontiff to shave ; but his dates (he was a contemporary of Charlemagne) seem incredibly late. Many subsequent

[1] Even Seghers admits the authenticity of this canon.

Popes of the early Middle Ages wore beards[1]—John XII (Pope from 955 to 964) was one of these; and engravings in the *Acta Sanctorum* (the famous *Propylæum* for the month of May, which was banned by the Spanish Inquisition) show a number of bearded Popes up to the middle of the twelfth century : Damasus II, Leo IX and Victor II all wearing beards, for what this evidence is worth, when even laymen had abandoned them (under clerical pressure) in the north of France. Even stranger, Honorius IV, Innocent II and Eugenius III, who together covered all but two years of the period 1124-1153 in their years of office, are all represented as bearded. This is hard to explain, if it can be believed, in view of the campaign against beards which had been launched by Gregory VII (Pope from 1073—1085, of whom we shall speak later), a campaign which was energetically conducted throughout the Church.

Hadrian IV : *let Erin remember*

Both Fangé and Dulaure profess to rely on Daniel van Papenbroeck's *Propylæum* for another odd, and perhaps inaccurate, piece of information—that Anastasius IV (Pope from 1153-1154) was the first shaven pontiff in the twelfth century. But two of his predecessors (Celestine II and Lucius II) are represented as shaven in Papenbroeck's *Propylæum*—both twelfth century Popes. Pascal II,

[1] There was a certain Vigilius, who was made Pope by Justinian's Generalissimo, Belisarius, in A.D. 537. (He was, in effect, Anti-Pope until the death of his legitimate predecessor, Silverius, whom he sent into exile—but that did not prevent him from being recognised as the Vicar of Christ by the Church, both in his time and since.) This Vigilius, being ordered to Constantinople by his Boss, Justinian, spent there eight miserable years ; and among the persuasive tactics used by the Byzantine Emperor to induce papal agreement in matters theological, Vigilius was dragged about by the beard—a game which seems to have amused the brutal and licentious soldiery. Father Seghers thinks he grew a beard because he was a prisoner, deprived of a razor. I am more inclined to the view that he followed the principle, when you are in Byzantium, do as Byzantines do. According to an engraving in the *Effigies Pontificum Romanorum cum eorum vitis in compendium redactis*, in the British Museum, Innocent VI appears with side-whiskers and a moustache in the middle of the fourteenth century ; and John Trithenius (1462-1516) is represented in Thevet's *Livre de Vrais Portraits* (1584) with a long, straggling forked beard—curious in a Benedictine abbot of that period.

who occupied the Holy See from the end of the eleventh century until 1118, denounceed long hair.   And, although his omission of any mention of beards might be considered significant, the engraving in the *Propylæum* shows him as shaven. Also Hadrian IV, whose *bull* (let Erin remember !) *Laudabiliter* authorised and encouraged King Henry II to conquer Ireland, is bearded in the engravings of the *Propylæum*.   The authenticity of this *bull* about Ireland has been disputed, but the evidence is overwhelming. [1] According to John of Salisbury, Hadrian based the gift on Constantine's *Donation*, and subsequent Popes made it explicitly clear that they supported English brigandage up to the time of the Reformation—even after, in Mary Tudor's reign.   The *bull*, in fact, found a nineteenth century apologist in Cardinal Newman ;   so it little matters what Hadrian IV intended originally. Other engravings show Lucius III, Honorius III, Alexander IV, Hadrian V, John XXI, Nicholas III and Martin IV (who died in 1285) wearing beards of various sizes and shapes.

Though it is impossible to weigh accurately much of the available evidence, it is certain that the anti-beard party on the whole made steady progress during the middle-ages—and that in spite of the clearest evidence that it was going against the tradition of the Early Fathers.   Much that Clement of Alexandria wrote can be so interpreted as to apply only to laymen, but not his plain statement that shaven men were indistinguishable from women unless one could see them naked (*et certe, nisi quis eos nudos videret mulieres esse putaverit*).   Nevertheless, the controversy as to what a man meant can never be brought to an end so long as there is any ambiguity in language and so long as persons with different interests are anxious to justify them.   The great Christian scholar, Cornelius à Lapide, considered that Clement of Alexandria's words held good for the clergy.   The Most Rev. Charles Seghers, in the article we have quoted (*The Practice of Shaving in the Latin Church*) was equally clear that the words of Clement, no less than those of the *Apostolical Constitutions*, were intended only for the laity (*American Catholic Quarterly Review*, Vol. VII, pp. 282-283).   But while the Greeks and other protagonists of

[1] For Irish readers it may be enough to know that this Pope was an Englishman—Nicholas Breakspear, the only Sassenach who ever made the grade.

pogonotrophy have been able to show old authorities that could, at least, be reasonably interpreted as admonishing all to wear beards, clergy and laity alike, the champions of Roman tradition have been incapable of producing any genuine authorities of real antiquity that appear to have ordained shaving with the same clarity and emphasis. This may account for the confusion of Latin practice and its numerous inconsistencies.

Bearded Baronius defends shaving

Severely handicapped by that beard of his, Baronius in his *Annales Ecclesiastici* (Jesu Christi Annus 58, CXXXVIII) very neatly evades both Epiphanius and the *Apostolical Constitutions*—that is to say, he quotes the one, mentions the other, answers neither and considers the matter sufficiently discussed. But under Cap. CXXXIX for the same year (*Barbam Radendi Mysteria*) the Cardinal goes somewhat further. Shaving he finds not only to be permitted by Holy Writ and ancient usage among the clergy, but it has a mystical significance, and was practised for this reason among Western priests in the time of Sidonius Apollinaris. In view of the evidence of Sidonius himself, this is a somewhat tall statement, and one which Henri de Sponde took occasion to correct in his digest of the *Annales* (Cologne 1690).[1]

The Barbarous English

In the seventh century Western practice appears to have become more uniform—on the shaven model. Walter Farquhar Hook, in his *Lives of the Archbishops of Canterbury* (Vol. I, 142-144) tells of the Pope's emissary Hadrian, an African who was sent to England in 668 to find a suitable candidate for the Archbishopric of Canterbury. A Roman of that age, said Dean Hook, *was not likely to suppose that there was much difference between an African and an Englishman ; both were barbarians.* But a difference existed, for many Africans clearly followed Eastern fashions in some respects. Hadrian, we are told, had to wait for his hair to grow in order to wear the correct Latin tonsure when going to England, *also to*

[1] In a letter (to Petreius) Sidonius does, it is true, refer to a shaven priest. Practice was evidently not uniform at the time ; but Seghers' attempt to explain away the bearded bishop is a poor effort.

curtail the licentious prolixity of his beard. The reference to the tonsure makes it clear that the crescent tonsure was still in use in parts of Africa—a fashion that would have horrified the Latinised clergy of England, hot from their victory at Whitby, though it would have rejoiced the defeated Celtic party. (The Celtic bishops, wrote Hook, traced their Christianity to the preaching of Oriental missionaries, and professed to agree with the Eastern Churches respecting the celebration of Easter.)

There is one point that is skilfully exploited by some defenders of what eventually came to be the almost universal practice of the Latin clergy. They have maintained that a distinction between shaving and *plucking* might well have been made by the early Fathers, and Baronius found himself *easily persuaded* that Christians had objected to this effeminate habit.

Of shaving and depilation

As to what Tertullian and Cyprian meant, there is at least one passage by the former (*De Spectaculis,* XXIII) which is beyond ambiguity, for though he was writing of the Roman games he in no way restricted his censure to laymen or to depilation. *Will God,* he says, *be pleased with him who applies the razor to himself* (he says nothing of plucking) *and completely changes his features ?* Note that this could not refer to the shaving of the body. Such shaven visages seemed to a Christian in about 200 A.D. (and it is immaterial that the writer died a heretic) an imitation of Saturn, Isis and Bacchus, for such was Tertullian's comparison. Cyprian, it is true, gives more scope for the supposition that he opposed depilation rather than shaving. In *De Lapsis* (cap. XXX) the word *vellere* is used—and the man who *barbam vellit,* plucks out his beard, is specifically associated with those immoral places, the public baths. He is, in fact, the man who frequents bathing places with women ; and no early Christian approved of mixed bathing. Hence Cyprian's *corrupta barba in viris* could well mean defaced beards in this sense—plucked out by the roots. Elsewhere Cyprian used the same word *vellere,* showing that it may indeed have been his main obsession. But the evidence of Epiphanius, Sidonius and others could not have been, and still cannot be, so easily dismissed.

However, Baronius claims, for what his evidence is worth (and on this question of beards it seems strangely unreliable), that no one reproached the Latin Church on account of shaving until Photius, the Schismatic Bishop of Constantinople, wrote to Pope Nicholas to abuse the beardless Romans. As Nicholas himself expressed it, in a letter to Hincmar, Bishop of Rheims, and the other Bishops of France (A.D. 867): *Moreover they* (the Greeks) *endeavour to throw blame on us because the clergy who are under our authority do not refuse to be shaved*. Hincmar refers to this letter and mentions celibacy among the other crimes charged against the Romans.

Theory of the Abbé Fangé

In attempting to sort out the chronology of beards and beardlessness, and at the same time to account for the variations observed, I am inclined to the view of Père Fangé, who suggested that beards disappeared from the Vatican with the severance of the Holy See from the Byzantine Empire—a reasonable supposition—and that they re-appeared spasmodically with the rise of the Holy Roman Empire in the West, as a subtle from of *homenaje* to the Teutonic predilection for bushy chins. The bearded Otto the Great (who restored the Empire known as Holy and Roman) was crowned by John XII—said to have been the first Pope to wear a beard after Leo III began the shaven fashion (if he did) with the *filioque*—and this account would fit Fangé's theory, though Otto and John XII subsequently quarrelled, and not all Holy Roman Emperors wore beards.

The same principle applied, no doubt, in reverse, during these tedious brawls between the Papacy and the Empire which later became a normal feature of medieval power politics. Then the clergy must surely have increasingly emphasised their shaven tradition in contrast to the bearded Hohenstaufens, or whatever dynasty was supreme beyond the Alps. Hence, perhaps, the German saying *um des kaisers Barb streiten*. At one time, we know, the bearded imperialists would insult—or even attack—a beardless man at sight, regarding him as belonging to the other party by *prima facie* evidence. Once more we have an inevitable political association: the beard marks the Ghibelline, the shaven chin is likely to betray the Guelph or Hwelp or Whelp. (I am grateful to the *Encyclopædia Britannica* for the etymological data, which is very apposite, in spite of bearded Guelphs at Buckingham Palace or elsewhere at one time or another.)

Did St. Peter shave ?

A series of Church Councils dictated so emphatically on the subject of beards that those rows of bearded Popes in the *Acta Sanctorum* engravings must be considered highly suspect. The Council of Limoges (1031) discussed the Great Schism and the Beard,[1] coming—I know not by what devious reasoning— to the conclusion that St. Peter himself had shaved, having apparently beaten both Anacletus and St. Clement Romanus in this papal competition. I was amazed to discover that Father Seghers actually (as late as 1882) took this tradition of the shaven Peter quite gravely, on the authority of old legends which tell of Peter's martyrdom, when he was supposed to have been shaved of his hair and beard before being put to death. This (according to *the anonymous author of a very old chronology*—the vagueness is that of Father Seghers—*quoted by Christianus Lupus*), became ecclesiastical practice *in mysterio*. The Most Rev. Father hinted that he could *adduce such weight of testimony as would force the scales down*, in favour of this story. Instead of attempting to do this, he wisely contented himself with a few fairy stories. Firstly, he called on the testimony of St. Gregory of Tours, which must be allowed great weight, for St. Gregory lived only 500 years after Peter's time, so was almost an eye-witness. Unfortunately this impeccable testimony still failed to cover the beard question, for Gregory only indicated that Peter used the tonsure, and this (it seems) of his own free will, out of humility, which hardly helps to establish the first version of the story.

Next (believe me, I have not quite forgotten Limoges) Father Seghers produces a heavenly vision out of the writings of the venerable Bede, in which a boy *saw* St. Peter with a shaven face. This vision should have been conclusive, but another vision

[1] In the same year the Council of Bourges also forbade beards, and similar orders were issued by the Council of Coyac (Spain, 1050) also by the Council of Toulouse in 1119.

(on the authority of St. Peter Damian) had to be produced to clinch the matter. All that needs to be added is that yet another legend, not quoted by Father Seghers, will be found in Mgr. Paul Guérin's *Vies des Saints*, published in 1882, while the American Father was making out his case for shaving.[1] In Vol. IV, page 452, is a story that Peter was sent to Jerusalem to announce the coming of the Messiah. The Jews seized him, *et par dérision lui coupèrent les cheveux en rond sur le haut de la tête.* This story is told on the authority of Germanus of Constantinople (born in the seventh century) who, however, gave no indication of its source.

Origin and decline of the tonsure

So it seems that Peter was tonsured by the Jews, tonsured and shaved by the Romans, and (when not being persecuted) shaved or tonsured himself as a mark of humility. It is curious that the tonsure, so intimately connected with the shaving of the beard, should have passed completely out of use among the secular clergy of Rome, while the shaving of the beard has remained.

In addition to the various origins given above, all on such good authorities, many other reasons have been advanced in defence of the tonsure, though their combined force was not sufficient to preserve its use. The reader may recall the arguments put forward on behalf of the Roman tonsure in a previous

[1] The controversial technique of Father Seghers is much to be admired. First (p. 289) he says that he will *not decide* whether the story of St. Peter being shaved is historical, but that he *could adduce such weight of testimony* and so forth. Next he produces the stories summarised above. On page 308 he returns to the subject, with the statement that *we have already proved it* (i.e., the shaving of St. Peter by the Pagans) *by the testimony of Peter, Patriarch of Antioch, St. Peter Damian, Ratramnus, the Venerable Bede, St. Gregory of Tours, and a very ancient chronology.* The proof consists of the matter which I have summarised, plus the testimonies of Ratramnus (ninth century) and Peter of Antioch (eleventh century) which are quoted later—obviously mere echoes of a legend, with regard to which they could speak with no more knowledge than Father Seghers or myself. On his own admission Seghers cites no authority older than Gregory of Tours (late sixth century), but the weakness of the case is not so remarkable as the method used to put it across—the reader is first disarmed by a declaration that the Most Rev. Father does not intend to contest the issue ; and having listened indulgently, not too critically, to these old wives' tales he is suddenly informed that Fr. Seghers has proved the point he undertook to leave undecided.

chapter—it was so superior to that of the Celts because it symbolised the crown of thorns. Guérin's *Vies des Saints* (Vol. 336) supplies yet another reason—the bald pate is a reminder that God can see what is going on inside the head, symbolically uncovered to his view. It is sad to reflect that an institution so sacred and symbolic should have disappeared because it exposed those who maintained it to a more hostile scrutiny (not of God, but of man) and to persecution, in Protestant countries—for such was the reason for the rule regarding the tonsure falling into disuse among the secular clergy. In those days of persecution many Catholic priests wore beards, which must have furthered the same end of remaining inconspicuous in a bearded age—i.e. the Elizabethan period. But the priestly beards disappeared in time ; the shaven chin returned. Not so the tonsure, among the secular clergy of England and Ireland.

A curious inconsistency

But, of course—the Council of Limoges. It also affirmed that shaving provided a *necessary distinction* from the laity—a curious reason to give in view of the origin of the custom (in imitation of Roman laymen). Indeed, if it were true, one would have expected the Latin priests, for the same reason, to have grown beards themselves when they had persuaded laymen to shave—as they did about that time and later—and certainly *not* to have adopted beards when working among bearded peoples, as explained in the *Jus Canonicum*. The Council of Limoges was nevertheless remarkable for the soft answer with which it sought to turn away the wrath of the Greeks. These schismatics, they said,

> *have chosen the custom of not shaving ; they ground their choice upon the example of the Apostles Paul and James, the brother of the Lord, saying with reason (for nothing should be concealed) that the clergy, like the laity, ought to preserve on their faces this ornament of virility, as a dignity of the human condition, a dignity created by God himself, and with which he has been pleased to honour man alone . . . The Greeks add likewise that Our Lord of Nazareth always wore his beard . . .*

Therefore, with commendable tolerance, and admonition to

toleration on the other side, the Council concluded that, in such circumstances, neither side ought to censure the other— *Et hac in re neque illi nos, neque nos possumus reprehendere illos.*

Enforcement of the comprehensive tonsure

The Council of Limoges nevertheless ordered all clergy within its jurisdiction to shave. So did the Council of Bourges, held the same year, which (in its seventh canon) ordained *ut Archidiaconi Abbates Præpositi . . . et omnes qui ministerium intra sanctam Ecclesiam tractant, tonsuram ecclesiasticam habeant, hoc est, Barbam rasam, et coronam in capite.* The ecclesiastical *tonsure* is thus assumed to *include* the removal of the beard.

When Hildebrand was crowned as Pope Gregory VII he found among the *mansionarii* of St. Peter's sixty Roman citizens who were either married or had concubines, and these gentry passed themselves off as Cardinal priests because they shaved and wore mitres. The impostors were ejected by the good Pope, but their existence was in itself an interesting comment on the complaint of Saint Peter Damian,[1] a contemporary of Gregory, that the *Barbirasium* alone distinguished the clergy from the laity. This same Pope had much trouble with one of his own prelates, who insisted on wearing a beard.[2] In 1075, two years after he was crowned, Gregory found it necessary to write to Orzoc, the *Podestà* or Judge of Cagliari, in Sardinia, about this bishop. I call him a bishop, although Gregory unquestionably referred to him as primate (*frater noster, vester Archiepiscopus*); but the *Catholic Encyclopedia* assures me that the bishopric of Cagliari was not raised to a primacy until later in the century, when Victor III was Pope (see article on Cagliari, 1908, Vol. III). So Gregory VII must have used the title as one says *Herr Ober* to the *Kellner* in the *biergarten*; or maybe he was just muddled by so much ecclesiastical taradiddle.

[1] Letter to Pope Alexander II. Text given by Seghers.

[2] An odd comment on Gregory's opposition to the beard is afforded by a statue of him at Salerno, in which he is represented as wearing one himself. The statue is of uncertain date and the Bollandists would not commit themselves as to its authenticity. See the *Acta S. Gregorii VII* in Migne (Latin Series cxlviii, 22).

N'importe . . . The Pope wrote to the Podestà and said that the *Archiepiscopus* in those parts ought to shave in the same way that every priest of the Western Church *ab ipsis fidei Christianæ primordiis* (a tall statement that) had held to the fashion of shaving the beard. Indeed, one letter was not enough ; and in 1082 Gregory had to repeat his demand that the secular power in Sardinia should bring the bearded prelate to heel. All the Sardinian Clergy, said the Sovereign Pontiff, were to shave in the same way (the bad habits of the bishop had evidently been imitated by his subordinates) and this order was to be enforced on pain of confiscation of the property of these priests. Evidently this was their personal property, of which (in the best tradition) they must have had plenty, for the punitive measure was to be *to the profit of the Church of Cagliari.* The Pope who could bring an Emperor to his knees (that celebrated capitulation at Canossa) was not to be beaten, surely, by a mere bishop.

Excommunicated beards and forcible shaving

Gregory was a great enemy of marriage among the clergy and of the beard. He rigorously enforced celibacy and (perhaps by association ?) maintained that any priest who wore a beard was guilty of a serious crime. In 1073 he called a Council where a canon against priestly beards was among the decisions made (*Synodus Gerundensis*, can. VII). In 1119 a Council at Toulouse went so far as to threaten with excommunication clerics who let their hair and beards grow. Pope Alexander III is quoted by the *Catholic Encyclopedia* (1907, II, 363) as saying that such priests were to be shorn forcibly, if necessary, by the Archdeacon[1]—a ruling later incorporated in the Canon Law among the Decretals of Gregory IX.[2] (I am willing to believe almost anything of this same Pope Alexander, for he further and very fully sanctioned the conquest of Ireland by Henry II, confirming that *bull* of Hadrian IV . . . Perhaps the Irish clergy wore beards.)

[1] *Clerici qui comam nutriant et barbam* (wrote the Pope to the Archbishop of Canterbury) *etiam inviti a suis archdiaconis tondeantur.* But *et barbam* may be a later insertion.

[2] He also included in the Decretals the orthodox version of the 44th Canon of the 4th Council of Carthage.

Before leaving Alexander and the *Catholic Encyclopedia*, I am tempted to quote from this same source (X, 125-6) some observations apropos of the Council of Tours, called by Alexander III, where it was decided that the shedding of blood was incompatible with the Holy Office of the clergy. How this squared with the rich record of fighting bishops (and Popes) I do not know : but at the time it was interpreted as meaning that they might no longer practise phlebotomy. So, after this Council, in 1163, blood letting and surgery (the latter specifically forbidden to priests once more by the Fourth Synod of the Lateran, in 1213) became functions of the barber. Hence the Barber-Chirurgeons of fame, as met later in the pages of *Don Quixote* (and, of course, Sweeney Todd). The *Catholic Encyclopedia*, in pointing out that these prohibitions on the part of the Church did not imply any hostility to medicine, mentions a curious practice which was banned by Boniface VIII in 1299-1300—that of boiling the corpses of notable persons who had died abroad, in order that their bones might be more conveniently transported to the ancestral tomb. This prohibitory rule, says the *Encyclopedia*, had reference only to cases of death in Christian countries, while in the Orient (e.g. during the Crusades) the usage seems to have been tacitly allowed to continue.

Fatal results of facial fertility

As we have already hinted, these same Crusaders (such as brought back their bones unboiled) were responsible for the long-haired and long-bearded fashions which marked the twelfth century. The growing rigidity of the clerical rule in the West at this time stands in marked contrast to this infiltration among laymen of Oriental customs, regarded by the Church as vaguely heathen, schismatic or heretical. In 1098, when most Western Christians still shaved, the contrast between them and their Saracen enemies had been sufficient to warrant that the beard could be relied upon as a distinguishing mark in a conflict. Hence this was assumed in the night attack made upon Antioch in that year, by the Crusaders—though the darkness proved so impenetrable that many Crusaders were killed by their own allies, the more readily because there had been little recent opportunity to shave, so that those whose chins were most fertile were easily mistaken for infidels. But the Cardinal-historian of the Crusades, Jacques de Vitry, writing over a century later, found the Latin Christians who had followed the Cross to the Holy Land quite riddled with Oriental vices. In his *Historia Orientalis*, that curious work which describes the magnetic compass (known to the Arabs but as yet no more than a fable among Christians) the Cardinal expresses his disapproval of the fashions— including those of hair and face—adopted by the Frankish Christians in the East. (This Jacques de Vitry was a great persecutor of the wretched Albigenses and believed that Crusades should begin at home ; but I do not think the Albigenses included beards among their heresies.)

It was from the East that the Western Christians learnt not only to wear beards again, but to treat them with a peculiar respect. The Charlemagne of the *Chanson* who is made to swear

By this my beard and this moustache of mine

is a creation of the new fashion against which the Church waged war. Clearly it was not a Christian oath but a Saracenic invocation. The significance of Bishop Serlo's sermon becomes clearer when the hair and beard controversy is viewed in the light of the Great Schism and of the struggle with Islam, though there was a third reason, in the case of the clergy, which I shall discuss in the next chapter.

Long beards banned in Venice

A decree of the Venetian Senate, in 1102, ordered the cutting of all long beards. In England local prejudice among laymen clung to the beard perhaps more than in most countries—as I have already suggested, its revival at court may have been out of flattery towards Anglo-Saxon sentiment. The clerical rule was nevertheless accepted, perhaps earlier and more universally than it was on the Continent. The dooms of King Alfred, already quoted, show that a priest was then assumed to be shaven. Indeed, he was called a *bescoren man* in the Kentish laws of Wihtred (A.D. 696), only a hundred years after a bearded Pope—Gregory the Great—had sent the first Roman missionaries to England. A Canon of King Edgar's time warns every clerk in holy orders not to *let himself be mis-shaven nor keep his beard for any time*, and there seems to be little doubt that English priests and monks kept the shaving rule more consistently than the Popes. The difficulty of the anti-beard party in England was always with the laymen, as we have seen. They were much addicted also to long hair, centuries before Anselm came over from Bec with Bell, Book and Candle for the love-locks of the later Normans. (The wearers of long hair, by a canon of 1096, were *excluded from religious worship while living and denied the benefit of prayers after death.*)[1]

On the Continent many priests appear to have resisted the enforcement of shaving, just as there was a great outcry against the enforcement of celibacy. That there must have been considerable laxity is shown by the frequent repetition of prohibitory regulations. The Church of Béziers, as Jacques Dulaure shows in his *Pogonologie*, was obliged to repeat its orders in 1323, 1332 and 1351. A synodical statute of the Church of Orléans, in 1323, ruled against priests wearing *long* beards (evidently a concession) on pain of excommunication. Similar regulations were issued at Avignon (1337) and at London (1342), while a provincial synod at Paris in 1333 forbade the clergy to grow *barbas prolixas* under penalties ranging from suspension to refusal of communion. As late as 1361 we find similar instructions issued at Rouen ; and in 1370 the Bishop of St. Malo (Pierre Benoit) was still trying to bring his stubborn Breton priests to heel, forbidding them to grow long beards and those drooping moustaches so dear to the people of Brittany. It may be that only the (almost universal) habit of shaving which prevailed in the following century finally cured the Breton clergy of this impropriety.

Common association of hair with sin

The learned Durand, whose views on hair and sin we noticed in our first chapter, was by no means alone in his association

[1] An interesting list could be made of the offences for which ex-communication has been merited. According to J. J. Blunt (*Vestiges of Ancient Manners*, etc., 1823) it was threatened—following an ancient pagan custom—against those who made use of churches (or their walls) to relieve themselves, at Florence and Bologna. Similar threats are said to have been necessary at Genoa in the Middle Ages.

of these two phenomena. We have already observed that the Egyptians shaved the whole body, from motives of cleanliness, which in all the great religions (save one) has had, from the beginning, some association with holiness. Monier Williams, in his *Religious Thought and Life in India*, mentions the ritual of shaving the body as part of the formal process of expiation by pilgrimage to a sacred stream, the shave and the bath together rejuvenating the guilty soul. All that is odd in the teaching of Durand, and others of like mind, concerning the beard is that these hairs of the face are treated separately and with such distinction, unknown to the simpler taboos of savages. And among the hairs of the face it is abundantly clear that what worried the clerical mind, during this long campaign against sin and whiskers, was not primarily the beard proper—as we now understand it—but the *moustache*.

Peculiar wickedness of the moustache

A learned friend of mine, Mr. Ben Vincent, remarks in a letter that :

> In the New Forest, and (so far as I know) throughout England, in the middle of the last century, a moustache was said to be the Mark of the Beast. On the other hand shaving was, in country districts, a painful and laborious process, and a waste of good water. So the countryman (especially the non-conformist) shaved off the Mark of the Beast, *but* allowed his beard to grow. This is the origin, unless I am misinformed, of the Varmer Joiles type of whiskers which comically frame the face, giving it an apelike appearance.

Mr. Vincent's authority for this statement was his father-in-law, a Methodist minister who lived near Lyndhurst, in Hampshire. The origin of this remarkable *taboo* is of great antiquity ; but its exploration must be left till our next chapter, when we will attempt among other things, to elucidate the history of *Bigotes*, those moustaches which the Bishop of St. Malo must have found even more obnoxious than hairy chins, when displayed by the recalcitrant clergy in his diocese.

CHAPTER VI

BEARDS AND BIGOTS

The vision of Christ that thou dost see
Is my vision's greatest enemy.
Thine has a great hook nose like thine ;
Mine has a snub nose like to mine . . .

William Blake

Bigot, n. One who holds irrespective of reason, and attaches
disproportionate weight to, some creed or view . . .
(F. etym. dub ; *Visigoth* and Sp. *bigote,* moustache,
have been suggested).

The Concise Oxford Dictionary

IN order to consider my next problem, which concerns the
representation of biblical characters in art, I must take leave for
a moment to return to Adam.

Suggested origin of Adam's Beard

According to the Abbé de Grécourt, in some verses quoted
by Père Fangé, the origin of the beard was in this wise. Adam,
finding Eve quite unbearable, as well he might without other
company (except Satan in his various disguises)

Car il n'avoit que la femme et le diable,

complained to his Creator with great bitterness, asking him to
return his rib and take this woman back. Efforts having been
made in vain to console the unhappy man, whose miseries aroused
nothing but mockery in the unfeeling choir of Heaven (for what,
indeed, did they know of our forefather's troubles ?) God alone
had pity and proposed a remedy :

Prends, lui dit-il, cette huile souveraine,
Vas t'en frotter le visage en secret ;
Tel en sera le salutaire effet
Qu'il te rendra la face redoutable
Et te fera l'air male et respectable.

125

Adam took both the oil and the advice, and, applying the former to his face, was gratified by instantaneous results such as may hardly be believed except by those who have proved by experiment the efficacy of a hair-restorative and ·the accuracy of the claims made in advertising it.   He upon whom

> le moindre coton
> N'avoit encore ombragé son menton

felt now the sudden and miraculous growth of that which proclaims the adolescence of his descendants, *nous annoncer la saison des plaisirs*.   Not unnaturally, in this Just-so Story, his fingers being still oily, we are informed that *il essuya ses mains en maints endroits*, with similar results, and, as you may well imagine,

> *Alors, tout fier de sa toison nouvelle,*
> *Il sut trouver l'intraitable femelle.*

Its effect upon Eve

His appearance occasioned such surprise to Eve that it is not difficult to credit the assurance that she became *douce, tendre et docile* in face of her husband's novel and *redoutable aspect*.   How Eve herself later discovered the magic oil, what use she made of it and by what accident she failed to provide herself with a beard, the reader may discover for himself, for such matters are beyond the scope of my present discourse.   I merely produce the Abbé's evidence as a further contribution to the controversy as to whether Adam was born bearded.   The Abbé maintains that he was not ; but (unlike Van Helmont) he makes this growth antecedent to the Fall.

Regarding the value attached to the beard by so many who wear it ;   and even attached to the capacity for growing it by many who shave it off (such as will tell you that they are under the necessity of shaving twice daily, as though there were some cause for pride in the fact) this peculiar value set upon hairs is not universal.   John Bulwar may have underestimated in stating that *the Chinoyse also have very thin Beards, consisting not of above twenty or thirty haires, a thing wonderfull to behold*.   But from all I have heard he was right enough when he added that when the

Chinese *would describe a deformed man, they paint him with a thick Beard.*

Shock caused by bearded missionaries

So also among the Bantu the beardlessness of these people is by them regarded as one of the distinguishing marks between a man and a monkey. The appearance of the first missionaries among them (bearded, I am told) created something of a shock—or so I am informed by Mr. Ben Vincent, this time on the authority of his father, long resident in Kenya. Mr. Vincent remarks that the Teutonic languages must sound very guttural to the Bantu, whose speech is even more euphonious than Italian ; so that the bearded missionaries, with their straight hair and unchipped teeth must have appeared to the simple savages as horribly overdressed baboons uttering guttural wisdom. And how were the Bantu to know any better since they could not be sure whether the newcomers were a bright blue beneath their pants ?

I cannot follow the learned Mr. Vincent any further, as he proceeds to argue that the desire to solve this problem may have been the origin of de-bagging. Mine is a serious work. I merely mention the matter of the Bantu to show that the respect paid by many to the beard, or at least to the capacity to grow one, is not universal. Those races which produce good beards regard them as a sign of superiority, while those which cannot grow them look upon the beard as the mark of a lower animal or an inferior civilisation.

Beard and moustache of the Creator

The controversy between the Greek and Latin Churches was not, of course, concerned with the propriety of man being naturally barbigerous or otherwise. But in the Latin Church there was (not infrequently) a tendency to depict in art the prejudice which the Romans nourished against the wearing of a beard. At Chartres Cathedral—according to a portfolio of reproductions which I have before me—the artists of the twelfth century depicted the shepherds in the story of the Nativity as shaven, though a thirteenth century St. Peter wears a curly beard and a moustache with all the vestments of a bishop, *pace* those who have argued to the contrary. There are, in fact, some very presentable beards in evidence among these reproductions, but I am concerned here chiefly with irregularities and exceptions. The Creator wears a short, well-trimmed beard, but appears generally to have shaved his upper lip—an important point of which we shall shortly consider the significance. When creating the Heaven and the Earth he seems, however, to have shaved off only one half of his moustache, doubtless from mere inadvertence in the confusion of the primeval Chaos ; and he later appears with distinct moustaches (both sides) when creating the moon and the sun.

But when we see God making Adam there is direct support for Van Helmont and the Abbé de Grécourt in the beardless man who evolves from the clay—a thirteenth century Adam, as smooth as a child. Here is man before the Fall—without sin and without whiskers, or so the art of medieval Chartres believed him to be.

Hans Memling, in the fifteenth century (when beards were rare indeed in the West), painted the Magi as beardless, and even depicted shaven Jewish priests, taking shocking liberties with history. We have already noticed the clean-shaven Magi in S. Maria Maggiore. The late Delisle Burns, in *The First Europe*, has a reproduction of a shaven Christ, and four other beardless Christs will be found in Wilhelm Worringer's *Formprobleme der Gotick*. The first of these, from the Abbey of Werden (eighth to ninth century) wears a moustache only, the other three being clean shaven. One is a fine carving in ivory, of the eleventh century, the others being dated about 1400 (Göttingen) and about 1440 (Erfurt).

Some clean-shaven Apostles

Worringer also shows a symbol of St. Matthew, very clean shaven and clerical (eighth century) and a similar representation of St. Timothy, from the Cluny Museum at Paris, looking every inch a curate. St. John appears well shaved in St. Stephen's, Mainz ; and of two evangelists in a twelfth century gospel book (Munich State Library) one is clean shaven while the other wears a moustache only. The head of an Apostle, by Hans Tilman Riemenschneider (1460-1531) is also clean shaven.

It is perhaps significant that—in contrast to the shaven eighth century Matthew—Worringer reproduced two bearded Matthews, one of about the same date (770) of Saxon design. My countrymen were perhaps not so easily persuaded that the apostles shaved. The representation of Christ and the apostles in art has been discussed with Teutonic thoroughness by Weiss-Liebersdorff in *Christus und Apostelbilder* (Freiburg, 1902) and I am only concerned here to show the extent to which Western fashions were reflected in a retroactive *radat* which even cleaned up the founders of the Church. Such works of art inevitably caused great scandal in the eyes of the Greeks, who viewed with horror the shaven saints in the Latin churches.

Objections to the moustache

In the examples mentioned above the reader will have noted that in some cases the artist who denied a beard to his subject allowed him a moustache—a thing (as we have already hinted) far more reprehensible than the beard proper. Those who have experimented with a large moustache must have learnt from that experience the difficulties which it can create, as described already in the case of the Gauls and Britons. It was possible that this fact was partly responsible for the nineteenth century *Varmer Joiles* style of beard, as described at the end of the last chapter. It has been said that Abraham Lincoln adopted a similar fashion merely in order to avoid unnecessary complications with the soup, and one has only to recall Covetousness, as described in *Piers Plowman*—*His beard, like a bumpkin's, bedraggled with bacon*, as Coghill renders it. With such considerations in mind we come next to consider the objection which Fosbroke mentions in his *British Monachism*. The moustache was to be removed, he said, *lest the Eucharist should be violated by it*.

Even that famous pogonophil, Clement of Alexandria, compromised on the subject of the moustache. The hairs of the upper lip, he said (*Pædagogus* iii,ii) *tondendi sunt, non novacula (est enim illiberale) sed tonsorum forcibus*—they were to be removed, not with the razor (that was not genteel) but with tweezers—a curious concession to depilation, which the Fathers generally considered so much more criminal than shaving. (Clement advocated this course only in so far as the moustache interfered with eating.) And even in the sixteenth century, when clerical beards became common in the Roman Church, the *Catholic Encyclopedia* mentions the continued insistence on the necessity for the clergy not *allowing the hair on their upper lip to impede the drinking of the chalice*. On this point the same authority (article on Beards) adds that it *has always been accounted a solid reason in favour of the practice of shaving*.[1]

Explanation by a Bishop

Ernulphus, Bishop of Rochester—that same prelate whose form of excommunication Tristram Shandy's father considered to be a digest of the art of swearing, compiled with as much learning and diligence as the Justinian Code—this Ernulphus is quoted by Fangé on the subject of moustaches and their disadvantages. *Evenit enim frequenter,* he said, it happens indeed frequently, *ut barbati et prolixos habentes granos,* that Bearded Ones having long moustaches, *dum poculum inter epulas sumunt, prius liquore pilos inficiant quam ore liquorem infundant*—they dip their whiskers into their drink before they swallow it. It is surprising that Ernulphus, in that very comprehensive *omnibus* anathema —wherein he damned the excommunicated in the hair of their heads and in every part of the body down to the toe-nails, in eating and drinking, walking and sleeping and every conceivable activity of the human body, mentionable and otherwise, by the authority of the Trinity, the Virgin, the Apostles, the angels and archangels—omitted to curse them in their moustaches. It is also a little odd, in view of such strong objections to the moustache, that Father Seghers should have mentioned (among the exceptions to the Latin rule) that Catholic priests in Albania,

[1] Manuel Calecas, a Greek who went over to the Roman rite, wrote several books against his countrymen. In one of these, *De Tonsura Crinium,* he gives this same reason for shaving the beard, i.e., that it might interfere with the taking of the sacraments, *atque ita non parvus error sit.* According to Genesis XLIII, 32, the Egyptians considered it an abomination to eat with the Hebrews ; and it may be that even in those days fastidious people like the Egyptians were revolted at the sight of these bearded visitors, mingling their whiskers with their food and their food with their whiskers. The prejudice must surely be older than the sacraments.

at the time when he was writing, were permitted to wear moustaches. (Indeed, they still wear them in those parts). But I can no longer delay consideration of my own original theory—that the moustache was also *homoiousian*, i.e. that it was suspect of Arian tendencies.

We have already observed that the beard came at one time to be regarded as a mark of barbarity. St. Ennodius, Bishop of Pavia, writing about five centuries after the birth of Christ, lampooned one of his countrymen for wearing a Gothic beard (*barbam Gothicam*) and a Roman cloak. But I am not sure that the Gothic beard was necessarily a true beard, as we should now understand it—the ancients were not so particular in fine distinctions between the beard and the moustache ; and the moustache rather than the beard as we now use the term, was more characteristically Gothic at that time. Indeed, as late as the eighteenth century the word *beard* is used by Defoe to describe the moustache. Randle Holme (the third of that dynasty of genealogists, in his *Academy of Armory*) wrote in 1688 of the moustached Britons in the days of the Roman Conquest : *The British Beard hath long Mochedoes on the higher lip, hanging down either side the chin, all the rest of the face being bare.* In considering the attitude of Ennodius and others towards Gothic whiskers it is of some importance to remember that these same Goths—the Visigoths—were also Arian heretics, and that Latin opinion at quite an early date may have begun to associate *homoiousian* theology with the aforesaid Gothic moustaches.

The origin of bigotry

This theory is not necessarily too delicately spun to stand a strain. A clue may perhaps be found in the word *bigot*, for the origin of which I take leave to quote Murray's *New English Dictionary*. According to this authority the word *bigot* is first found in the twelfth century as a proper name of some people, apparently in the south of Gaul (a district colonised by the Goths and at one time ruled by their kings). It was therefore suggested in the seventeenth century that the word *bigot* might be an Old French rendering of *Wisigothus*, a Visigoth, with the implication that this corruption of the name had come to acquire an evil sense among the Catholic Franks. On this theory the lexicographer throws some doubt, but admits that the medieval Latin form *Bigothi*, found in Du Cange's *Glossarium*, gives some slender support to the supposition.

Gothic, *a term of abuse*

The Goths were a curious people, who conquered in turn almost every country in Europe, yet left their name nowhere except on forms of architecture that developed some 350 years after the last Gothic kingdom had fallen. The one living association of the word *Gothic* is, in short, based upon a fable and a calumny; for the men of the New Learning, unable to understand or appreciate the civilisation of their medieval ancestors, attributed it to the barbarism of the Goths, whom they debited with the destruction of the classical culture. Indeed, it was the merest chance that the buildings we now describe as Gothic did not come to be known as specimens of Vandal Architecture upon the same hypothesis. The diarist Evelyn expressed no more than seventeenth century *zeitgeist* when he spoke of what is called Gothic architecture as a *fantastical and licentious manner of building* : *congestions of heavy, dark, melancholy, monkish piles, without any just proportion, use or beauty.*

Few nations, indeed, seem to have been the subjects of more unreasonable prejudice than these same Goths, especially the Visigoths, whom Gregory of Tours accused of conducting bloody persecutions of the Catholic Church, whereas history records that the Arian Gothic kings were remarkable for their toleration of those (the great majority of their non-Gothic subjects in Spain and Gaul) who accepted the Nicene Creed. This view is now sustained by Catholic historians, and was even maintained in the fifth century by Salvian of Marseilles (*De Gubernatione Dei*) who contrasted the piety, chastity and tolerance of these heretical barbarians with the vices of his Roman and Catholic countrymen.

It would not, therefore, have been a remarkable thing if a people who were first falsely accused by Catholics of persecuting the Catholic Church, and then charged by Protestants with criminal responsibility for the existence of our finest Catholic Cathedrals, should have acquired such an ill name as to become a by-word for intolerance. To be a Goth implied to the Roman, barbarism ; to the Catholic Arianism ; and to the Protestant of later years it recalled those heavy, dark, melancholy, monkish piles. What more natural than that such a name should become synonymous with some vice ? And what vice more handy to attribute (it is a universal law of slander) than one's own personal failing ?

A Vindication of the Vandals

(I cannot proceed to the point at issue without taking liberty to refer the reader, for comparison, to Beck and Hodgkin's brief but admirable article on the *Vandals* in the *Encyclopædia Britannica*, where he will find a similar vindication. These writers could find no justification for the common use of the word *Vandalism* in the capture of Rome by the Vandal King Gaiseric, who merely plied his trade industriously as a pirate and empire builder, setting out to attack *the dwellings of the men with whom God is angry*. Although the article to which we refer makes it clear that the direction of the Divine wrath was—very properly—determined by the prevalent winds, the writers describe the capture of Rome as an unspectacular performance : *He took the city without difficulty, and for fourteen days, in a calm and business-like manner, emptied it of all its movable wealth.* Gaiseric merely collected reparations, but was falsely accused of wanton destruction on account of his persecution of the Catholics—a charge from which I cannot absolve him, though the measures which he took were very mild in comparison with those which the Catholics had already taken against the Priscillianists, and mere play by comparison with the persecutions on which Catholics embarked at a later date.)

Were the Visigoths the original Bigots ?

So, then, these Visigoths may well have been the true and original *Bigothi* or *Bigots*, the *V* having changed to a *B*, just as the *Barba, Barbe, Bart, Barf, Beard, Baard* or *Bars*[1] of the Romans,

---

[1] In Russian it is *Boroda*, and the chin is *Podborodok* (*that which goes under the beard*). Similarly in Polish we have *Broda* and *Podbrodek*—an interesting comment on the universality of beards in these countries at one time. In Celtic *Bar* is a variant of *fear* (= *vir*, i.e., a man), and *barb* in Breton means virile.

French, Germans, Celts, English, Flemings or Tartars became
(by an opposite process) the *Varve* of the Gascons. But there are
other claimants, whom we must consider, and be sure that they
will lead us back again to beards, for the next is the Spanish
bigote, a moustache, which is mentioned by Murray as a possible
source for the word *Bigot*. Before discussing this I will, however,
list the other claimants.

Peculiar English of Duke Rollo

Firstly we have the authority of an old chronicle for an English
origin, or what the chronicler took for English. The story (of
which a version will be found in Duchesne's *Historiæ Normannorum*, and also in Du Cange) is that when Rolf or Rollo, the first
Duke of the Normans, was asked to do homage to Charles the
Simple, King of France, by kissing the king's foot, *Hic non est
dignatus pedem Caroli osculari ;* and personally I cannot blame him.
Indeed, I will remind you that the first Norman dukes were
bearded, which would have added to the indignity. (When one
of Rollo's successors defeated Hugo, Count of Châlons, in
battle, the latter threw himself at the Norman duke's feet, with
a saddle on his back, in token of submission. With his long
beard the Count was said to have looked more like a goat than a
horse, according to evidence cited by Père Fangé.) So Rollo
refused the honour, and the twelfth century historian of this
drama says that he

> *lingua Anglica respondit, Ne se Bigot, quod interpretatur,
> Ne per Deum*

A strange statement, indeed—the Duke replied in English, *Ne se
Bigot*, which is, translated, *No by God*.

The Duke's English was certainly a little queer, but why he
should have spoken English at all is not explained. However,
Du Cange offers this as one attempted explanation of the word
Bigot, for the chronicler claims that the Normans were thence-
forward known as *By Gods* or *Bigots*, just as the English came to be
known in France, at a later date, as *Goddams* or *Goddems*. (Referring to Murray I find the following from the *Athenæum* of
November 25, 1893 : *The English . . . confiscated . . . even the small*

possessions of farmers and burgesses in order to people their new colonies with fresh-imported God-dams, *red-bearded . . . foreign-tongued . . .* The lines refer to the Hundred Years War, and fascinate me chiefly because of the ubiquity of the beard in literature. Note that these English ones were described as *red*, of which we shall have more to say later—also of the Hundred Years War itself, which began with an injudicious shave . . .)

The Bigot and the Bastard

Where were we? *Ne se Bigot*: neither Murray nor Littré allows this improbable derivation, which savours of a story invented to explain a name, as Littré suggests, though the conclusion of the old chronicle (*apud* Duchesne iii, 360)—*unde Normanni adhuc Bigothi vocantur*—appears to have some support from Wace, who claimed that the French in his time applied the word *bigos* or *bigoz* in opprobrium to the Normans, as may be seen in the *Roman de Rou*. Here the French call the Normans *bigos et draschiers*, the latter word meaning (*dit-on*) beer drinkers, though beer was never naturalised in Normandy or England until centuries later, when it began to oust ale. As a family name we must also admit that this epithet *bigot* was worn gracefully by Robert le Bigot (or Bigod), a Norman contemporary of William the Bastard, whose family played a big part in English history, after the Conquest, when they acquired the earldom of Norfolk. It seems not unsuitable that the Bastard and the Bigot should have been so prominent in the share-out of the Saxon swag.

The next claimant is *Beguta* or *Bigutta*, which Du Cange gives as a variant of Béguine. The word offers a perfect example of a philological wild-goose chase. Littré traces the name of the Béguines, a lay sisterhood which originated in the Low Countries, to the word *Béguard*, a member of a brotherhood similar in character, thus deriving the feminine form from the masculine. This in turn he derives from a Flemish verb *beggen*, and English *beg*, since begging was the profession of the Béguards. At this Murray shows the utmost surprise, denies the existence of any such Flemish verb as *beggen*, but conversely derives our English *beg* and *beggar* from the Béguards and Béguines. He also reverses the natural order by deriving the masculine form from the feminine, and produces as the origin of the whole tangle a certain Lambert le Bègue (that is to say, the Stammerer) who started these women on their path of holiness. In short, Monsieur Littré is caught begging the question.

Claim of the Béguines rejected

But I cannot accept Murray's own suggestion, on the strength of Speght's notes on Chaucer (where he identifies *bigin* with *bigot*, and both with superstition and hypocritical women) that these Béguards and Béguines throw any light upon the word *bigot*, a word in use (as we have seen in the case of the Norman conquerors) long before the Béguards became a proscribed sect, suppressed by the Catholic Church and abused by the Protestants. It was in the fourteenth century that the Church disowned the Béguards and the Inquisition began to persecute them ; and obviously it was much later that the name Béguine became a term of abuse among Protestants. (Bilious Bale in his *Apologye . . . agaynste a ranke Papyst* coupled the name of these good women with wanton wenches, and a later writer linked them with *nuns and naughty packs*.) But Robert le Bigot wore his title before the Béguines ever came into existence, let alone disrepute.

I offer next the name *Bigerra*—a wild guess, but fascinating, because it takes us back to Spain, and doubtless to the Goths. Note that of four bids, the first leads direct to the Goths (*Visigothi*), the second to the moustache (*bigote*) which is the same thing. Ruling out the story of *Ne se, Bigot* as preposterous, and the Béguines as chronologically impossible, every solution so far points to the Goths, to moustaches, or to Spain ; for Bigerra was a town in the Pyrenees, at that time part of Hispania Tarraconensis. Now it should be noticed that there may be some connection between this name Bigerra and *bigote*, a moustache, for the *bigerrica* worn by the Bigeriones, was *a shaggy or hairy garment*. Sulpicius Severus, a native of Aquitaine (*circa* 363-*circa* 425) twice refers to these garments and comments upon their hairiness. The scent seems for a moment to lead us towards Bigerra, for the name is modernised as *Bigorre* : why should not Bigorre be the original home of bigotry ?

The inevitability of hairiness

But here a fresh cross-current carries us back once more to an inevitable connection with moustaches, for Du Cange cites an old authority who derives *bigerrica* from the German *beharich* (modern German *behaart*), that is to say—*hairy*. The links grow stronger. Why should not the town have taken its name from the characteristic garment of the wandering tribe that settled there, and both the garment and the moustache have borrowed a name from the same root? There seems no reason to connect these shaggy-coated people with bigotry, but they have at least given us a thought as to the origin of *bigote*.

I will pass over *Bigo*. Du Cange quotes : *le mary d'icelle femme curoit et nettoyoit l'estable de ses vaches à ung engin appelé Bigot*—the husband of this woman scraped and cleaned the stable of his cows with an engine, called *Bigot*. I thought for a wild moment that the man was using his moustache as a broom for the cow-shed ; but it seems the word *bigo* or *bigot* here means a mattock. No luck there. The classical Latin word *Bigus* is given by Lewis and Short as a contraction of *Bijugus* (two yoked together) which might describe a pair of moustaches ; but I think not. And it takes us no nearer to Bigotry, anyway.

Does Bizarre *signify Bearded ?*

I had reached this point in my researches, and was feeling the strain in the form of Dictionary Dizziness or Verbal Vertigo, when the word *Bizarre* not unnaturally came to my mind, merely as descriptive of my own tangled speculations. But being by then too confused even to spell this word, I had recourse once more to a hair of the dog—that is to say, I returned to a dictionary. The result was more than surprising, for it appears that *bizarre* is from the Spanish *bizarro*, which the *New Velasquez Dictionary* translates as *gallant, brave, high-spirited* or (alternatively) *generous, liberal, high-minded*. But Littré traces the word through the Spanish to a Basque word, *bizarra*, meaning a BEARD, though he offers a less likely alternative from the Arabic :

Deux étymologies s'offrent : le basque *bizarra*, barbe, décomposé par Larramendi en *biz arra* (qu'il soit un homme) ;

et l'arabe *bāshāret*, beauté, élégance, d'où vaillant, chevaleresque, puis le sens de colère, emporté, extravagant.

Who in his senses would choose the Arabic derivation ? How could beauty and elegance turn to anger ? For note that this word *bizarre* is also connected with *bigearrer*, to argue, and the Italian *bizárro*, high mettled or even quarrelsome. Now a beard can signify many things—to one it is beautiful (e.g. to the owner) to another it is not ; to one it is a badge of courage, to another a warning of wanton aggressiveness. And above all, to some it is merely odd or fantastic—*bizarre*, in fact. Even the cautious Murray quotes the Basque derivation from Littré and ignores the Arabic theory. He will not commit himself, but compares this supposed adaptation of *bizarra*, a beard (to mean anything from *handsome* to *choleric* and *quarrelsome*) with the Spanish *hombre de bigote*—literally a moustached man, but signifying a *man of spirit*. So we are back again with these inevitable *bigotes*.

All roads lead to Spain, the Goths, whiskers and Arianism

Now here indeed is a parallel too close to be ignored. On the one hand it is suggested that a word meaning *beard* has come to be associated with everything from a compliment to a reproach. And on the other hand a word meaning *moustache* is associated with pride in one's good qualities, whilst it is also suggested that it is linked with a term of abuse—*bigot*. And both *bizarre* and *bigot* point to a Spanish origin. In fact, whether we trace bigotry through *bigotes*, Visigoths or even Bigerra, we get back to Spain, the Goths, moustaches and Arianism. The whole complex seems inescapable and is closely comparable to the bizarre story of the Basque beard. But always there is this dual meaning— what (indeed) more natural, when that which was the pride of the Arian barbarians in the Iberian Peninsula was for the same reason a thing of horror to their enemies ? Both the beard and the moustache may have filled such a double rôle ; but especially the moustache.

Ripley in *The Races of Europe* spoke of the Basques shaving their chins and growing side-whiskers, in order (he said) to emphasise their facial characteristics, i.e. their long chins. I find no reason to suppose that this was always their practice, and mistrust evidence of this sort, based upon the habits of a people at a particular period in history. (Ripley's work was published in 1900.) A pointed beard would emphasise a long chin even more aggressively than a clean-shave ; and I'll warrant a Basque braggart in the halcyon days of the conquistadors would have wagged as boisterous a *bizarra* (was it not derived from *biz arra*, according to Littré, signifying the very mark of manhood ?) as any Castillian caballero. And *bigotes*, to boot : look only at the riches of the *New Velasquez* to see all that a pair of whiskers has meant to an Iberian. *Tener bigotes* (to have a moustache) signifies *to be firm and undaunted* (in one's own eyes, that is—note that to an opponent it would appear as *bigotry*, the same thing viewed differently). Even a woman's face may be praised by the gratifying hyperbole that she has *buenas bigoteras*.

Leather cases for the moustache

Velasquez gives *bigotera* for a leather case, designed specially to preserve the *perm* (so to speak) in one's moustache, at night. Littré quotes from the *Dictionnaire de l'Académie* (1696) :

> *Bigotelle* ou *bigotère*, pièce d'étoffe ou de cuir dont on se sert pour tenir la moustache relevée.

So a special case, then, was used to preserve these precious ornaments ; and the name shows that the device originated beyond the Pyrenees, though it clearly spread to France. It is perhaps hardly necessary to add that the moustache was as jealously protected by law (among peoples who valued it) as was the beard. The *Lex Frisionum*, for example, ordained a fine of two gold coins for anyone who cut off another person's moustache.[1]

The Moustache political and national

The pride which the Spaniards took in their *bigotes* must therefore be considered a heritage from the Visigoths ; and when Pope, in his *Moral Essays*, called Philip V of Spain a bigot, he was actually bestowing a compliment, though one that Philip did

[1] Sidonius says that the Franks in his time *combed* their moustaches—giving some indication of their length.

not deserve, for it was he who started the clean-shaven fashion among the Spaniards at the beginning of the eighteenth century. A Spaniard with no *bigotes* and no beard was no longer *bizarro*—not bearded, brave and handsome. Hence the saying which Dulaure quotes : *Des que los Españoles no llevan bigotes, no . . .* but the rest is hardly repeatable : we will leave it that since the Spaniards lost their whiskers they were not the men they used to be.[1] Their rebel subjects in the Low Countries must have appreciated the importance of a moustache when fighting the Spaniards in the sixteenth century. *The Historie of the Low-Countrey Warres* (translated by Sir Robert Stapylton from the work of the celebrated Jesuit, Famianus Strada) describes the confederacy of the *Gheuses* or *Gueux* against the Spaniards with much emphasis upon the fact that, though these confederates called themselves *beggars* (we are perilously near those *béguards* again) and affected to dress as such, they *began to cut their beards leaving onely great mustachios turned up like Turks.*

It was a political emblem, often to be imitated in later centuries. The moustache was the badge of freedom and of national pride, presented in a form not new to the Spanish enemy. *I suppose* (the narrative continues) *their meaning was to take away the contempt of their beggars clothes by the terrour of their upper lips, and to shew themselves at once humble and formidable.* Sitting very close behind a guardsman's moustache (to steal a phrase I heard but yesterday) these sturdy beggars could mock themselves of the Spaniards.

Opinion of J. A. Dulaure

This Gothic pride in the moustache is deeply rooted, finding its expression in our own time in the opinion of Mr. Osbert Lancaster, who thinks nothing of moustaches which are not

[1] Charles Mackay, in *Memoirs of Extraordinary Popular Delusions*, quotes a more presentable version of the saying, applied, however, to the beard : *Desde que no hay barba, no hay mas alma*—since we have lost our beards we no longer have souls. *The Spectator* (No. 331) quoted the *Sueños* of Quevedo to illustrate the proverbial pride of Spaniards in their *bigotes*. One such, having been sentenced in the last Judgment, was led off by two imps of hell : but they chanced to disorder his moustachios, and could not prevail upon their prisoner to proceed further until they had repaired the damage with the aid of curling irons.

visible from the rear.[1]   And *The Handlebar Club*, as it is called, exists today entirely to stimulate the prolixity of moustaches by an annual competition for the longest span.   Dulaure, writing in a beardless age, lamented the passing of the beard, but even more he pined for the moustache.   As a beardless face, he said, is a sign of puerility and weakness, so is a bearded chin of virility and prudence ;   in like manner whiskers, which hold the middle course between these two extremes, announce youth and desires.   The moustache, to this writer, gave to the face *a stately vigorous, fiery look, which characterises the young man, and is not displeasing to the ladies*.   The tending of his moustache he considered productive of manly, courageous ideas.   Indeed,

It was highly flattering to a lady to have it in her power to praise the beauty of her lover's whiskers, which, far from being disgusting, gave his person an air of vivacity.   Several even thought it an incitement to love.

The qualities of prophets

And yet it was a woman (Queen Victoria) who, when beards returned once more to fashion, banned moustaches in the British Navy.   The Queen would doubtless have been offended had it been suggested that she was on the side of the Catholic Church, but Catholics, in their insistence, above all, on priests shaving the upper lip, could have claimed support from even stranger company.   The Prophet of Mecca was no friend of the razor, but according to Hughes' *Dictionary of Islam* (under *Fitrah*), Mohamet is related to have said :

There are ten qualities of the prophets—*clipping the mustachios, so that they do not enter the mouth* ;   not cutting or shaving the beard ;   cleansing the teeth ;   cleansing the nostrils with water at the usual ablutions ;   cutting the nails ;   cleaning the finger joints ;   pulling out the hairs under the arm-pits ;   shaving the hairs of the privates ;   washing with water after passing urine ;   and cleansing the mouth with water at the time of ablution.

[1] Mr. Lancaster's object may be contrasted with that of the White Knight :
> But I was thinking of a plan
>   To dye one's whiskers green,
> And always use so large a fan
>   *That they could not be seen*.   (Our italics)

Since we are here concerned only with the first two attributes of a prophet (appertaining to his moustache and his beard) we must resist the temptation to comment upon the others, except to add the explanation given by Mr. Hughes regarding the cleansing of the nostrils. The nose, he says, is to be washed in this manner because it is supposed that the devil resides there during the night ; which puts me in mind of an ancient objection of the people of Wallachia to execution by hanging—because (so they say) it prevented the soul from escaping by the more honourable openings. But to return to the upper lip (and above all to avoid the controversial subject of noses) Plutarch, in his *Morals*, makes this statement regarding the Spartans, which I quote as it was Englished by Philemon Holland :

At Lacedæmon (says he) the high controllers called *Ephori*, so soone as they be installed in their magistracie, cause proclamation to be published by sound of trumpet, that no man should weare mustaches or nourish the haire on their [*sic*] upper lips. [1]

The ancient monuments of Greece (like those of Cyprus and Tuscany) show that this practice was common among those peoples. On the other hand John Bulwer (who makes some comment on this edict of the Ephori in his *Anthropometamorphosis*) being himself of the opinion that the moustache was the most venerable and sacred part of the facial hair, wrote that *All other Nations who shave the other Barball parts of the face refraine from this, because reason it selfe seems to perswade this verity, that this renowned part is not to be violated.*

Bulwer on the Barball parts

The reason which Bulwer gives for this especial value attached to the moustache is that (so he claims) :

[1] A very odd reason is given in Frazer's *Folklore in the Old Testament* (1918, vol. iii, 236) for the men in the Nicobar Islands removing these hairs with tweezers. This is done after a death, to disguise one's self, in order to avoid being troubled by the spirit of the deceased. No doubt this is as good as any other reason.

They are most according to Nature, which if not alwaies, yet at least do often happen ; and . . . if men have any Beard they have some on the upper lip . . . although the other barball parts be bare . . . such men being looked upon as monsters who are destitute by Nature of the Beard in the upper Lip and Chin, and have some under their Chin, and upon their Cheeks. These are rare in mankind, and with the tyranny of no Rasor can you ever extort or fright out of the mind of men that ingrafted admiration whereby they prosecute such men who are utterly void of haire upon the Region of their upper Lip.

Similar views were expressed by Saunders, the astrologer,[1] who found such men of an ill nature. To this argument from the *natura rerum* Bulwer adds another, from the testimony of Montaigne, who found in his mustachios a perfumed nose-bag that would retain any scent he gave to them and hold it neatly below the nostrils. And to this is added the argument which we have already considered in relation to beards generally, that they can conceal the deformity of our features. For Bulwer speaks of a gentleman of good worth, whom he knew, a man who, having lost all his teeth, *wore his Mustachoes thick and standing up, to conceale that lapse of his Visage.*

Some errors in the Anthropometamorphosis

Among Mohammedans who did not follow the practice of the Prophet in the matter of moustaches, Bulwer notices the Persians. For he says (quoting a reference from *Purchas His Pilgrimes*) that the Tartars shave their upper Lips and warre with the Persians for not doing so. And again he says of them : The Persians allow no part of the body haire, the upper lip excepted, which grows very long and thick. And much the same Bulwer said of the Turks in his time, also of the Arabians, of whom he wrote that they shaved their beards, though he allowed that some of them suffered their beards to grow and never cut

[1] *Phisiognomie, Chiromancie*, etc., by R. Saunders (1653). I am puzzled by a remark in Archbishop Sancroft's MS. Notebooks (quoted in *Notes and Queries*, 11th S., XI, 262) to the effect that Englishmen were once—period unstated—in the habit of cutting the hair of the upper lip, *which everywhere else was thought unmanly.*

them. But as Bulwer's authority for the habits of the Arabians was Pliny, who lived nearly six centuries before the Hegira, it is no wonder that he should have been so wide of the mark. Indeed, he was almost as much at fault in the case of the Turks, whom he later admitted to shave their slaves as a mark of their servitude, and to scoff at Christians for cutting off their beards. (It is true that the Sultan Selim I, in the early sixteenth century, broke all precedents by shaving off his own beard, so that his Grand Vizier should have nothing to lead him by—so he said ; but he was notable in his time only as a scandalous exception to the rule.) Turkish moustaches were certainly of proverbial length, nature having endowed the Turk with prolific propensities in this respect ;   but nature (and custom until recent years) would appear to have favoured Turkish beards also.[1] Busbequius, incidentally, claimed that he saw a Janissary at Constantinople, with hair so thick that a musket shot could not wound him.

Bulwer's assertion regarding Persian shaving will stand closer investigation, at least as regards their chins. His authority was Thomas Herbert's *Description of the Persian Monarchy*, first published in 1634—better evidence than Pliny could offer—but I find his explanation of the war between the Persians and the Tartars in conflict with another version of this quarrel, and have been unable to unravel the whole truth. The account given by T. S. Gowing (I know not from what source) in his *Philosophy of Beards* was that

One of the points of Persian heresy is preferring a black beard (that is, to a red one, as favoured by the Prophet himself) *and a particular cut . . . they once waged a cruel war with the Uzbec Tartars, in which they were accustomed to lay their enemies' beards as trophies at the feet of the Shah.*

A comparison with David's marriage offering
This sounds like a less revolting version of King David's battle trophies, brought as a gift to his royal father-in-law on the

[1] Aaron Hill's *Account of the Ottoman Empire* (1709) makes it clear that the Turks, in distinction from the Persians, grew long beards at that time. The case of Selim I is mentioned by Bacon as an evident exception (*Works*, 1872, vii, 157).

occasion of his marriage (I Samuel xviii, 27 and II Samuel iii, 14, make it clear that David regarded his nasty offering as the purchase price of his wife ; and I am told that Mr. D. H. Lawrence wrote a play about David in which he insisted on introducing the incident, to the dismay of a London producer, who did not feel able to contemplate such realism in a West End performance). The story is credible—beard collecting is also not unlike scalp-hunting. Fangé's version appears to throw the blame for the war on the Tartars. The *Bukkariens*, he says, *espèce de Tartares*, quarrel perpetually with their neighbours, because the latter will not shave the upper lip as the Tartars do. They call such moustached Moslems *caffres*, that is to say, *infidels*, as they do the Christians. (Modern Christians appropriately use the same word *kaffir* for some of their pagan idols, I mean their mining shares in South Africa.)

The moustache question the cause of the trouble

Well, whichever way one looks at it, this question of *fungus facialis communis* seems to have been taken somewhat seriously by the Tartars and the Persians, and the weight of opinion appears to lie with the theory that it was the moustache question that caused the trouble. Many Persian paintings belonging to the centuries which followed the Arab conquest show clean-shaven Persians, though the moustache without the beard certainly appears the most common usage. The Venetian traveller Giovanni Maria Angiollo so described the Persian Sophy, Ismail, who finally defeated the Uzbecs in 1510 ; and it is curious that the reason for the Persians shaving off the beard below the lips, according to Père Fangé, was the same as that usually advanced for removing the moustache (which they preserved)—*par principe de propreté*, says the abbé. Sir John Chardin (1643-1713), whose *Travels in Persia and the East Indies* is reckoned one of the most reliable accounts of Persia in the seventeenth century, was ordered by the Shah to conform to the national custom during his sojourn at Ispahan—compliance with this involving the loss of a fine long beard.[1] But as to the Uzbecs, it is my private

[1] Chardin's own statement regarding the Persians in the seventeenth century was prefaced by some excellent observations on the difficulty of generalising as

opinion that the Persians made war against them because they
were Uzbecs and because they were a nuisance.

Bulwer also mentions the Hungarians as a people who shaved
off their beards, leaving their *Mustachoes, the which are sometimes
very long.* Those Hungarian moustaches were among the few
survivors in Europe of the eighteenth century holocaust and
(becoming eventually a fashion among cavalry regiments) helped
to bring back whiskers in the great nineteenth century revival.

The original Moslem prejudice against the hairs of the upper
lip, though abandoned by the Turks and the Persians, was found
as far afield as the Maldive Islands by François Pyrard de Laval,
who left some records of their habits in his *Observations*, having
been ship-wrecked in those parts in 1602 and lived five years
among the islanders. His account, translated into English and
abbreviated, will be found in *Purchas His Pilgrimes* (vol. IX, page
507 *et seq* in the edition of 1905—and having found it I will put
in a *caveat* warning all against ever trying to pick out a reference
in this edition ; and I wish I had gone straight to an older one
before the Glasgow University editors had played hop-scotch
with the text).

Fastidious habits of the Maldives

These Maldive Islanders are here described as being (the men
among them) hairy over all the bodie, yea so thicke as more cannot
be imagined. Hereof (says the writer) they boast, as if it were
the strength of nature . . . *and if a man bee not so hairy, they say,*

to national characteristics. Having made that clear, he described the Shah, the
great officers and the soldiers as wearing *only long whiskers on the upper lip, which,
joined to a tuft of hair on the upper part of their cheeks, grow to a very enormous size,
insomuch that some, it is said, are near half a foot long.* Their *maulas* and what he
terms religious people wore long beards, and the common people wore beards
clipped short. Chardin confirms the statement that they removed all hair from
the body. (See Pinkerton, 1811, Vol. IX, 201). The seventeenth century
drawing of an old man with a long beard (by Riza-i-'Abbasi) which Dimand
reproduces on p. 54 of his *Handbook of Muhammadan Art* (1947) may be a *religious
person* within the meaning of the act. It is worth noting that Sir Robert
Sherley, who was the Shah's ambassador to Pope Paul V, is represented in
Richardson's illustrations to Granger wearing Persian clothes and clean shaven.
The date is 1609.

that hee rather resembles a woman then a man, and despise him for it.
(Here, indeed, is man's pride in his hairiness, and a proper
contempt for women.) But as to the hairs around the mouth,
the Maldives shaved them away, leaving only side-whiskers and
the lower beard,[1]

> because they would not for any thing being eating or drinking
> touch a haire, being the greatest nastinesse and filthinesse in
> the world : wherefore they have no haire about their mouth ;
> and I have often seene that for finding onely one haire in a
> platter of meat, they would not touch it, and remained rather
> without eating.

And yet these same people, who so abhorred their own hairs
if they should mingle with their food, were most careful to
preserve their clippings and shavings, as John Bulwer explains.
As to their method of shaving their moustaches, Monsieur de
Laval (or rather the indefatigable Samuel Purchas, in doing him
into English) curiously comments upon it.

> They are verie hardie and insensible in all this (says he)
> and use no hot water in shaving them ; their razors cut verie
> naughtily, and they doe nothing but poure a little cold water
> upon it ; and whatsoever hurt they do, they complaine not,
> and say it paines them not : All this comes of custome to
> them, for else they would be as sensible as we.

Which, as Euclid or somebody used to say, would be absurd.
It seems a sober and satisfactory thought upon which to end a
chapter.

[1] The same principle was evidently accepted by the Boers in the Orange
Free State, who preserved the *clean mouth*—in distinction from the full beards
of the Transvaalers. Of the beardless eighteenth century Max von Boehn notes
that only actors could wear moustaches, and then *only when impersonating
murderers or highwaymen.*

CHAPTER VII

OF PRAYERS FOR SHAVING AND OF OTHER MATTERS, INCLUDING FALSE BEARDS

Dominus vobiscum.

Oremus, Dilectissimi, Deum Patrem omnipotentem, ut huic Famulo suo N., quem ad juvenilem perducere est ætatem, benedictionis suæ dona concedat ; ut, sicut exemplo Beati Petri, Principis Apostolorum, ei exteriora, pro Christi amore, sunt attondenda juventutis auspicia, ita præcordiorum divellantur interiorum superflua, ac felicitatis æternæ percipiat incrementa. Per eum qui unus in Trinitate perfecta vivit & gloriatur Deus per immortalia sæcula sæculorum. Amen.

Benedictio ad Barbam Tondendam.

A collect used in the Abbey of Bec

Monks not to sleep with naked legs

Monastic shaving was not considered a matter of individual discretion. Indeed, it was assumed in a monastery that everything was to be regulated which was capable of regulation. Bishop Hugo Gratianopolitanus even gave strict orders that monks should remove their boots when going to bed (*ut de caligis pedules abscinderentur*). They were, however, to sleep in their clothes and to wear socks, *nam dolebat nonnullos in religioso habitu ad sanctitatis injuriam tibiis dormire nudatis*—for it grieved not a few who were in orders to sleep with naked legs, to the detriment of sanctity. A canon of the Second Council of Carthage even decreed that any priest or monk who made a joke should be anathematised.

The proper days and periods for shaving were determined with the same precision. A convocation held at Aix-La-Chapelle in A.D. 817 decided that French monks should shave once a fortnight, but forbade the use of the razor at certain times and seasons (*ut in quadragesima, nisi in sabbatho sancto, non radantur, in alio autem tempore semel per quindecim dies, & in octavis Paschæ*). Fosbroke, in his *British Monachism* says that under the Sempringham rule the canons were shaved seventeen times in the year, but he adds that one of the *Inquirenda* of King Henry VIII's visitors was *whether ye bee wyckely shaven.*

Unshaven monks to be whipped

Rules relating to the beard existed in all the monastic orders. The Carthusians, who only shaved six times a year, cannot have been clean-shaven by any modern standards during the greater part of the year—perhaps at no time, for the shaving was evidently somewhat crude. The rule of St. Columbanus states that the deacon whose beard is not shaved (*diaconus cui barba tonsa non fuerit*) shall be punished with six lashes (*sex percussionibus*) for his fault. The period (about A.D. 590) lends some importance to this ferocious regulation, and its existence throws much doubt on the usual representations of St. Columbanus as wearing a beard himself.

As to the manner of this shaving, we read that the monks of St. Augustine's, Canterbury, were wont to shave one another until 1266, when it was decided to hire professional barbers owing to the numerous casualties. According to Fosbroke the same history was repeated in other houses. A form of barber's soap appears to have been in use, though by no means universally, and those who enjoyed its benefit knew the lather under the name of *lascivium*. Some monasteries we are assured (in a document quoted by Du Cange) also employed aromatic herbs, which they cultivated for this purpose. Normally shaving took place in the cloisters, the razors being handed out to those who were to use them (where professionals were not employed) and kept, at other times, under lock and key.

Order of Psalms for Shaving

Not only the face needed to be periodically shaved, but the crown of the head, where the tonsure required weeding, save only on those pates where Nature had abandoned the unequal contest. (Why is it only the hair of the head that withers with the years? For the rest, *Naturam expellas furca, tamen usque recurret,* you may drive off Nature with a razor, but she will always come back.) While chin and crown underwent the periodic ritual, those not actually engaged in shaving or being shaved chanted psalms, following the

Ordo Psalmorum ad Rasuram (for not even this could be left to chance). One can very well imagine them chanting the hundred and thirty-third :

> *Sicut unguentum in capite, quod descendit*
> *in Barbam, Barbam Aaron . . .*

—a strange simile indeed in the liturgy of these shaven Levites. Suddenly the great bell would sound and (mindful, says Monsieur Fangé, of the motto *nihil operi Dei præponatur*, that nothing should take precedence before the work of God) all would hasten to the chapel, the shaven, the unshaven, and the half-shaven—these last to stand in a place apart, and not to mingle with the brethren in the choir.

But the first shaving of a brother at his initiation was an occasion of especial pomp. For this were such prayers written as that which heads my chapter, for use when the shorn hair and beard were consecrated at the altar; of which prayers the industry of Fangé has collected many examples, with the sources from which he gathered them, all of which the curious reader may find for himself in the last chapter of the *Mémoires*. And here indeed is Barba Aaron again—*Pour forth, O Lord, thy benediction upon him and let it flow over his head and beard like the ointment which descended . . .*

For the lay brothers, hewers and drawers to the shaven clerics, there was no such ceremony. *Barbam non decurtent, nec rasoriis grenones radant,* runs the Carthusian Rule relating to the *conversi*, the lay brothers : they were positively forbidden to cut off their beards or shave their moustaches : though another account (both are quoted by Du Cange under *Grenones*) appears to contradict this. Here the ancient Carthusian custom is said to have been *ut toties radantur conversi et eorum Grenoneæ auferantur.* Their *grenoneæ* or *grenones* or *grani* were to be removed—the word is identical with *guernon* in the Norman French, as the text proceeds to explain : *sic appellamus barbam superiorem*, the upper beard, or moustache. Generally, however, it is clear that the lay-brothers did not originally shave.

Lay-brothers called Illiterati *or* Barbati

Hence the *conversi*, otherwise known as *Illiterati* or even *Idioti* and other unflattering names, were above all things the *Barbati*, the Bearded Ones. The word is also used, it is true, for epileptics and lunatics (as we have seen) and for the bearded Franciscans (later formed into a separate order as the Capuchins) and a few other orders which did not shave—one is mentioned by Du Cange—but generally it signifies the lay brothers of a shaven order. [1]

Such were the *fratres barbati* of Gramont, who revolted against their shaven brothers and established a temporary pogonocracy [2]— *luctuosum in Ecclesia Dei spectaculum*, wrote Stephen, Bishop of Tournay, who described with horror the ascendancy of the monastic proletariat, brandishing their beards like horns. To bring these *Barbati* to order our King John was induced to intervene on behalf of Papal authority, as Crop-eared Prynne recalled in his *Antiquæ Constitutiones Regni Angliæ*, throwing in the correspondence to show how insidious had been the encroachment of Rome upon English liberty—though none but he knew the relevance of the matter. In at least one order the indefatigable Fangé notes that these lay-beards (abandoned in most of the orders of his time) had already fallen into disuse at the beginning of the tenth century, when Bernard of Cluny laid down his rule for the reformed Benedictine houses. *Pro signo Laici*, wrote Bernard, *mentum tene cum dextra, propter Barbam quam antiquitus non raserat id genus hominum*—the word *antiquitus* showing that the custom was already extinct among the Benedictines when Bernard drew up the new Rule.

The early Franciscans

As to the Franciscans, whilst the founder himself was commonly represented with a long beard, his immediate followers do not appear to have worn one ; a fact which is made clear by a Bull of Honorius III, in the time of St. Francis, permitting the brothers to wear their beards when preaching the Gospel to the Saracens. [3]

[1] For other bearded orders see Du Cange (v, *Barbatus*) and Fangé, pp. 310-311.

[2] Father Seghers mentions this revolt and gives some interesting facts about the *Barbati* in the article I have so often quoted.

[3] But, according to Matthew Paris, Innocent III refused to confirm the Rule of this order because of the long beards worn by the brothers. The whole story is very confused.

This special privilege (as we have observed) has at all times been allowed by the Roman Church for those whose duties took them to the East—a delicate concession to Oriental prejudice. Thus, when beards were most rare, Fosbroke notes in his *British Monachism* that the peasants only, and those who had travelled to the Holy Land, did not shave, after the custom of the Orientals ; to which he adds this quotation from Joseph Strutt (*Dresses and Habits of the English People* II, 318 seq.) *that it was dangerous at the commencement of the thirteenth century for a stranger to appear with a beard.* Of this we have already commented ; but we shall note here the fact that the Capuchin Beard was clearly an innovation which had no place in the rules of the Saint, though it probably found hospitality on his own chin, and that it was even counted among the austerities practised by Father Elias, during his retirement, after his deposition (but clearly, by deduction, not during his reign) that he grew whiskers. Like the Church itself, the Franciscan order split on various issues, and one of them was the beard question.

Conflicting views with regard to laymen

The Capuchin beard[1] was therefore in some sense apocryphal and peculiar eventually to this branch of the Order, though (long before the days of the Franciscan friars) the monks of the eighth century wore beards commonly enough. The Templars were a bearded order, but as they came to a Bad End their custom can have done no service to the Cause. In conflict with the tendency which we have noted, on the part of some clerics, to induce laymen to follow their own practice (perhaps an instance of sour grapes) there is a quite contrary tendency that will be found in certain medieval Church historians. These regarded shaving among the laity as effeminate—indeed they found it even worse than effeminate. They felt it to be in some sense impious or sacrilegious for the laymen to adopt a fashion which was the prerogative of monks and clergy. The Benedictine Rule (Cap. I, 27) describes the tonsure on the head of a layman as a lie to God, and the shaving of the face in anyone not in orders as soft and effeminate.

[1] See Appendix C.

Hence one tale, of the eleventh century, informs us of a layman who shaved and had the misfortune to be tried by ordeal on a charge of theft. He was innocent, but the verdict of cold water went against him. What was the cause? On consulting a priest he was told that the judgment of Heaven had condemned him for removing his beard, a privilege confined to his spiritual superiors. The story will be found in Migne's *Patrologiæ*, Tom. CXLVI, in the *Liber de Cursu Spirituali* of Othlonus, a monk of Ratisbon. It seems that the accused man, having undertaken to let his beard grow again, underwent the ordeal a second time, emerging from it triumphant—thus vindicating his own innocence and the importance of preserving the distinctions between the laity and the clergy if one desires divine favour. Failing to realise the significance of this fact, the man most ungratefully neglected to keep his promise, shaved again, and was in due course punished for his wickedness. Providence made use of his personal enemies, who captured him and gouged out his eyes.

Unorthodox views of Burchardus

Burchardus, Abbot of Bellevaux, is one of the strongest exponents of the iniquity of shaving among the laity. Indeed, he appears to have been opposed to shaving altogether—a remarkable thing in a twelfth century cleric, though not altogether unique. (Apart from the doubtful testimony of later representations of the Popes, an enamelled effigy of Ulger, Bishop of Angers in the twelfth century, has been described as showing him with a moustache and a very short beard, slightly forked. There are also some other bishops of this period who were similarly represented in contemporary art). But Burchardus felt strongly enough about beards to write his great tract, the *Apologia de Barbis*. Was not David's beard, on which he dribbled, a mystery of the wisdom of man being foolishness with God? The matter was of the greatest import.

Some of the arguments of Burchardus will by now be familiar. The first consideration, he says, is that the beard distinguishes one sex from the other, man from woman, since it is the nature of men to have beards and of women to be without them. This seems clear enough, though it led the good abbé into some difficulties, because his honesty obliged him to add that it occasionally happened that men were beardless and women bearded. The question of bearded women is then discussed, but this we will leave for the moment. I am most impressed myself with the metaphysical arguments :

> *Caput nostrum Christus est, et venit spiritus*
> *sanctus a capite. Quo ? Ad barbam.*

Our head is Christ, and the Holy Spirit comes from the head. (That's *filioque*, without a doubt). Where ? To the beard. *Argal*, as the grave-digger would have remarked, *nec barbam radat*. The point is clear—on this question Burchardus sides with the Greeks, having established his Latin orthodoxy in the other matter. The beard, he continues, marks young men who are strong, strenuous, energetic and lively ; and when we wish to describe such we say *barbatus homo est*, he is a beaver. How the Paraclete reaches a woman is not made clear, except she be endowed with God's gift to man.

Visions of Beards

The pro-beard party could cite visions as readily as the protagonists of the shaven Peter. One such you will find in Migne's Latin Series (xli, 809) in the Epistle of Lucian to the Whole Church concerning the revelation of the body of Stephen, the first martyr. The good priest saw St. Stephen with a *barba prolixa*. And was not Gamaliel such a one, asks the Abbot of Bellevaux. To those whose beards grow *in mento*, religion shall grow *in mente*. Some will laugh, says Burchardus, and deride him as a barbologist ; Very well—let them, if they dare, laugh at Aaron's beard, dripping with oil ; or Ezekiel's, which he divided into three parts to show the destiny of Israel ; or at the beard of the holy woman Galla. And Ezra, who plucked out the hairs of his beard—who would laugh at that, and not rather mourn ? *At ille qui socio dicit : barbam hirci habes, male ridet, quia deridet.*

Beards at the Last Trump

But last—a point not easily to be answered—in his chapter *De claritate et gloria barbarum post hanc vitam*, concerning the splendour and glory of beards after this life, the abbé quotes from Revelations : His head and his hairs were white like wool, *candidi velut lana*. And will not beards also be white as wool ? When the righteous shall blossom like the lily, and flourish *in eternum* before God, to what shining lilies shall their beards be compared ? If in that light and glory the righteous shall glitter like the sun, if they shall be even whiter than snow, brighter than milk, then how white, how dazzling do you think beards will be ?

Beards as a protection against flies

It is indeed a solemn thought. And there is another side to the question, in a story from the life of St. Macarius, concerning two young men, one of whom was bearded and the other shaven. The shaven youth (so we are assured) was posssesed with devils, who took the outward semblance of flies. (Our fore-fathers were well aware that flies are devils, and used the *flabellum* to protect the altar and officiating priests from their presence, two deacons being detailed to swipe at any fly which approached too near, as Cabanès mentions in his chapter on the origin of the comb— *Moeurs Intimes du Passé*, Vol I.[1] Dr. Cabanès also discusses the ritual of hair combing by the priest before officiating—for there would be a circle of hair around the tonsure unless the good man was bald—the combing accompanied by prayers which resemble those used when shaving. Much could be written of the liturgical use of the comb, which is—alas—beyond my present scope.) So then, beards are part of the resurrection of the just, and shaven faces an invitation to devils. The story of the devils masquerading as *muscæ* will be found in the *Acta Sanctorum* and has suggested to me the idea that possibly beards are cultivated in the East as a protection against these incarnations of the Evil One—especially mosquitoes.

There was always, in some minds, the suspicion of effeminacy in shaving, just as others saw carnal appetites in a beard. And each party accused the other of vanity. Du Cange quotes an Old French poem about a man who *voult ses ans dissimuler*, an

[1] See also the article on the *Flabellum* in the *Catholic Encyclopedia* and Rendel Harris's interesting monograph on combs.

obvious step being to shave off his beard (*et reire ses Barbes flories*) to give himself a more youthful appearance. Caught between two such conflicting influences, the practice of laymen in the Middle Ages varied and fluctuated.

Origin of the oath by the beard

In the civil wars of King Stephen's reign—the king himself was bearded—we read of men hung up by their beards to extort money from them. Of the Holy Roman Emperors we have already noticed the beard of Otto the Great, a famous one whereby he would swear on all solemn occasions, according to the *Percy Anecdotes*. I have been reflecting on this habit of swearing by the beard, for which I have already suggested an oriental origin. The beard would have been held in the hand (hence *barbam tangere*) like the bible in court. But was not this a refinement of a yet earlier custom, which we find used by Abraham and Jacob, in Genesis xlvii, 29 and xxiv, 2 ? (*Pone manum tuam subter femur meum*, says Abraham).

Seals of later Emperors show Henry III as bearded and Henry IV with a moustache only. Barbarossa stalks through history like a legendary hero who has wandered by happy chance from pre-historic gloom into the sober chronicles of the twelfth century. Like Holgar, or Ogier, the Danish hero of the Carolingian cycle (whose beard still grows, they say, through a stone table in the Castle of Kronborg at Elsinore) Frederick sleeps in a cave of the Kyffhäuser in Thuringia. And there his great red beard grows through the stone like that of Ogier, though I find much petty quibbling on this point in the *Encyclopædia Britannica* and in back numbers of *Notes and Queries*.[1] (There were two other *Barbæ*

[1] See articles in this *Encyclopædia* on Frederick I and Frederick II, in both of which the legend is transferred to the latter, though his beard was quite un-important and could not possibly have grown through a stone table. A writer in *Notes and Queries* (July 1, 1939) with world war imminent, took it upon him to explain that the red-bearded sleeper was not a kaiser waiting for *der Tag* (we need have no fear) but none other than Good King Wenceslas, who would awaken with his knights to save Czechoslovakia. Two further letters appeared (CLXXVI, 409 and CLXXVII, 14) ; and finally on Oct. 16, 1948, the subject had shifted to Jenghis-Khan, but without any specific reference to his beard. So sleeps Arthur of Avalon, Charlemagne with his peers, Charles V (some say) and many another ; and I cannot believe they are regularly shaved.

Rossæ, both infidel admirals. These were clearly impostors, though I make no doubt that they wore beards of some kind and colour.)[1]

Fatal shave of Louis VII

But in spite of bearded emperors, the campaign against beards continued. Louis VII of France, in his wars with the Count of Champagne, captured Vitry and was held responsible by the Pope—with whom he was already on very bad terms—for the death of a number of people who perished by fire in a church. With a typical medieval *volte-face* the king, reduced to terror by his confessor, agreed to shave off his beard as a penance and to go on a crusade. These measures proved fatal to his marriage, for his wife—Eleanor of Aquitaine—reproached the young king with imitating not only the shaven habits but the celibacy of the monks.[2] On the Crusade she is said to have compensated herself for the deficiencies of her spouse, to whose shaven features she had taken a considerable dislike. (One assumes that she had never really seen his face till he removed his beard, and that the result was a shock). Nothing was ever proved regarding her alleged improprieties, discussed with some heat by Mézeray in his *Histoire de France*, but they included a supposed *affaire de coeur* with Saladin, then a youth of thirteen, hardly bearded, but presumably very precocious (though not remarkably so for an Oriental). However, evidence is lacking.

Responsibility for the Hundred Years War

Louis at least found no further satisfaction in his marriage. Eventually he obtained a divorce from his queen, who later married Henry, Duke of Normandy, taking with her the vast possessions of her family to add to the strong foot-hold which the English kings already had in France ; for Eleanor's second husband became Henry II of England. She continued to provide

[1] These men were brothers. It has been suggested that the name was a corruption of that of the elder brother, Baba-Arooj. The name Barbarossa was, however, equally applied by Christians to the younger brother, Khair-ed (or Haired) Din. There was also an Italian poet of the seventeenth century who shared this distinguished *soubriquet.*

[2] Michelet's *Histoire de France* (1835) iii, 69 and footnote.

plenty of entertainment by her numerous political intrigues, though her most famous alleged exploit, the poisoning of Henry's mistress, Rosamond Clifford is certainly apocryphal. At least it may be conjectured that Louis' shave bore some responsibility for the Hundred Years' War, which would hardly have been possible if the possessions of Eleanor had not so strengthened the English and (by their withdrawal) proportionately weakened the French crown. According to the *Percy Anecdotes* one reason why this fatal shave was urged upon Louis VII was to set an example and end the fierce beard controversy still raging in parts of France. Incidentally, Eleanor's second husband also shaved.

An interlude in the Crusades serves to show that, even when Western Europeans wore beards, they did not regard them with the sanctity which the Orient attached to them. Baldwin of Edessa—later crowned as Baldwin II, king of Jerusalem—belonged to an age when Eastern influence had made a marked effect on the Crusaders. (It is a curious fact, not unnoted by historians, that one effect of the Crusades was a good deal of fraternising between Christians and Saracens, whilst relations between the Christian powers involved became steadily worse. Apart from the standing dispute between the Greek and Latin Churches—culminating in the sack of Constantinople—there was a perpetual struggle for supremacy among the Western potentates. But Coeur-de-Lion, who quarrelled with almost all his Christian *confrères*, contemplated a marriage alliance with Saladin's family ; and Frederick II—*Stupor Mundi*—who spent most of his life quarrelling with the Papacy, lived on excellent personal terms with Saracens, whether as friends or foes.)

Pawning of a beard

This Baldwin, then, was bearded like a Greek or a Saracen. He had married the daughter of a wealthy Armenian, Gabriel of Melitene. Being hard up, he decided to approach Gabriel, and we are informed that to *extort money from his Father-in-law, he had impawned his Beard for a great summe to certaine creditors.* [1] The old man

[1] *Purchas His Pilgrimes*, Lib VIII, Cap VI, 5. T. A. Archer in *The Crusade of Richard I* (Note L.) assumed that it was Gabriel's *own* beard which was pawned. I think this was due to a misreading of the story as told by William

at once produced 30,000 Byzantines *to prevent that disgrace to his family, and on condition never to engage his Beard againe.* How was it possible, asked Gabriel, for a man to find it in his heart to pledge a thing that should be so carefully preserved (*rem tanta diligentia conservandam*), the glory of the face, the proof of manhood, the peculiar source of male authority? The Greeks and other Eastern peoples, as the Archbishop of Tyre commented, held it for the greatest shame to lose a single hair of the Beard. Their Latin imitators could never quite share the view—worthy indeed of St. Clement of Alexandria—that it was *argumentum viri, vultus gloria, hominis præcipua authoritas.* It was merely a beard. A marginal rubric to this story, as given in Purchas, is somewhat baffling : *The Westerne Church for many ages used much shaving, as in old pictures is seen Beards of price.* What this means I have no idea.[2]

Informative Sermon by Satan

Actually, whatever mystical value has attached itself to hair in the West has often had a vaguely diabolical significance. Fraser in his *Folk-lore in the Old Testament* (1918, Vol. II, 485-486) tells how Satan himself, in a sermon preached from the pulpit of North Berwick Church, comforted his many servants by assuring them that no harm could befall them

> *sa lang as their hair wes on, and sould newir latt ane teir fall fra thair ene*

This sermon may have been a model for the Pobble's aunt, who

> *said no harm Can come to your toes if your nose is warm*

The hair of the head has never been holy in Western Christendom, and the beard did not acquire holiness again until the Protestant Reformation revived Judaism in Europe. Until then the history of the beard in the West is a subtle record of rival influences,

of Tyre, in his *Historia rerum in partibus transmarinis gestarum*, Lib II, Cap. IV. Nicephorus is quite clear that it was Baldwin's beard.

[2] A later case of pawning a beard is mentioned in Septenville's *Découvertes et Conquêtes de Portugal.* This is the case of Juan de Castro, who offered to pawn his beard in order to raise some money at Goa.

fashion occasionally triumphing over the weight of religious opinion, which is predominantly anti-beard until the sixteenth century.

The beard as a subject of frequent inaccuracy

Among so many conflicting tendencies and opinions the difficulty of discovering the truth is further complicated by the carelessness of those who offer information. We have already noticed the strange errors of Mr. Hugh Ross Williamson and the graver error of the *Encyclopædia Britannica,* from which a higher standard of accuracy might have been expected. *Chamber's Encyclopædia* (1935) is not less misleading, having an article on Beards in which it is claimed that *the wearing of the beard . . . was usual amongst the gentry from the tenth to the twelfth century*—a statement which completely ignores the supremacy of the razor, particularly in northern France and among the conquerors of England in the very middle of the period to which the encyclopædist refers. Older authorities are often as irresponsible. A passage in Higden's *Polychronicon,* relating to the Irish, is Englished by one early translator as *suffrenge the hynder parts of theire hedes to groe into a grete lengthe.* One might easily be misled by such a passage if one did not refer to the original : *barbis et comis a posteriore parte capitis luxurians.* The sense of this is much more correctly rendered by Trevisa with *they useth longe berdes and long lokkes.*

According to Roger of Hoveden's *Cronica,* Richard Cœur-de-Lion let his beard grow as a disguise when crossing Germany on his way home from captivity. The disguise was apparently unsuccessful, but we may infer that Richard did not normally wear a beard—indeed that is how he is shown on seals and in his effigy at Fontevrault. Long hair continued to be worn, and in the reign of Henry III, as Sir Thomas Hardy points out (in a footnote to William of Malmesbury's *Historia Novella,* I, 4), the king felt he must intervene, this long hair being found even among the clergy. Regarding Henry's strict orders, Hardy quotes Prynne, who found in them *a memorable precedent, fit to be imitated and put in execution in our own effeminate degenerous age.* Prynne had in mind the love-locks of the contemporary Cavaliers, his enemies at that time (he himself being shorn of his very ears) ; for in the Royalists of the seventeenth century he saw *long haired ruffians, both of clergy, court, city, country, needing such a reformation and reform as this writ* (that of Henry III) *prescribes.*

The law of compensation

As to beards, one of our oldest English ballads, a satirical account of Richard, Earl of Cornwall, brother of Henry III and titular king of the Romans, declares that

> *Sire Simond de Mounfort hath swore bi ys chyn.*

This reference (from Wright's *Political Songs*) is curious. It may be merely that Simon de Montfort's chin fitted better into the rhyme than his beard. Or was it that those who had no beards to swear by had taken to swearing by their chins instead? Henry III himself wore a long beard, in spite of his objection to long hair. Indeed, by some law of compensation long beards are often found with short hair and long hair in a shaven age (e.g. the long powdered hair or wig worn in the eighteenth century—and was it mere accident that an age which abhorred a beard in front ended with a pigtail behind?)

Immaculately curled is the short beard of the effeminate king, Edward II (1284-1327), his long moustaches trained like well-bred wall plants to keep their places. The cheeks are shaved. On his last journey from Kenilworth to Berkeley Castle, the unhappy monarch was allowed no shaving water but what he could find in a ditch, whereat he wept and told Maltravers that here at least was warm water on his cheeks whether (said he) you will or not. Poor wretch, his sufferings had but begun. He survived imprisonment in a dungeon that was little better than a common sewer, only to die a horrible death, *cum veru ignito inter celanda confossus ignominiose peremptus est*, as Higden's *Polychronicon* has it—which Trevisa translates with the simple words that he died. Soon after his death there begins another great bearded age, the fourteenth century, the pattern being the long, flowing forked beard of Edward III, as it appears in his effigy at Westminster Abbey.

Face fashions not to be explained by changes in armour

Some have attempted to explain the variations as to shaving, or the length of beard, by the type of armour in use in each period, and I have been offered examples of men in our own time, who removed their beards in order to accommodate themselves to the solitary confinements of a gas mask (with the suggestion that mediæval armour must often have presented similar problems). But an examination of the styles of armour in use at different times does not support this supposition. If ever a noble knight had cause to remove his beard it was in the sixteenth century, when the head was more closely cased than ever before ; yet the sixteenth century was the great age of beards, which were somehow squeezed into beavers that swept up to the eyes, leaving barely room (one would have imagined) for a presentable chin. Indeed, the sixteenth century knight in his harness looks as though he did not possess a chin at all. But *beaver . . . the very word is like a bell, to toll me back*, etc. This, I suppose, was the origin of the modern cant word. The word which was used to describe the lower part of the helmet, protecting the face, was derived from the Old French *baviere*, a child's bib. That's very suitable. What else is a modern beaver but a bib ? From *bave*, saliva—even better : that was how King David used it. Giraldus Cambrensis discusses somewhere whether it is legitimate to eat beavers on a fast-day ; but I fear a digression.[1]   Let us return to the long beards of the fourteenth century.

One of our old monks of Glastonbury (that noble town in which I am proud to have been born) wrote a chronicle of his country. His work was continued by William Caxton, who thought good to share its records with the public *in the yere of thyncarnacion of our lord Jhu crist*,1480.

[1] In spite of my firm resolution at this point I could not resist the temptation to look up *Beaver* in Murray, and drew some prize items as a result. Spenser associated them with Griffons, Minotaurs and Centaurs as *Monstrous Beasts*, and a writer in 1528, evidently referring to the Pope, spoke of the *thre folde crowne of anti-christ hys bever ;* (and, come to think of it, the Popes did wear beards in those days). Adam Smith, in his *Wealth of Nations*, judiciously calculated *that one beaver should exchange for or be worth two deer*, but in June, 1885, the *Cornhill Magazine* remarked (somewhat proleptically) that *there might be some difficulty in lighting on a beaver nowadays except in a museum*. The Arch-Beaver of all Victorian Bores, Thomas Carlyle, found the nineteenth century possessed of a *mechanical or beaver intellect*—indeed, he reverted continually to the subject. I find also a reference to *beaver-like sagacity* and to a *Beavery* as a place where beavers are kept (very properly) under a curator. See Appendix B.

Long beards in the time of Edward III

In the XX yere of the Regne of Kyng Edward the fourthe (wrote Caxton) *Atte requeste of dyuerce gentilmen I have endeuored me to emprinte the cronicles of Englond as in this booke shall by the suffraunce of God folowe.* Of the reign of Edward III these chronicles record that the English at that time wore *long berdes*, adding a couplet which the Scots made in mockery of the English and their beards (also of their painted hoods and gay coats) from which I can only assume that Scottish *berdes* were then worn shorter. *Ye Scottes, we are told, made a byll that was upon ye chirche dores of Saynt Peters towarde Stengate, & thus sayd ye scripture in despyte of Englysshemen.*

> *Longe berdes hertles, peynted hodes witles,*
> *Gaye cotes graceles, maketh Englonde thryftles*

(Thrift being their principal virtue it will be noticed that the Caledonians could find no greater insult than to suggest that the English lacked it.) The lines were parodied by the author of a ballad, about a hundred years later, against the sartorial excesses of the clergy, though there was (of course) no reference to *longe berdes* in the case of the priests, and by that time even the laymen were shaved, for the most part. Already, in fourteenth century France, beards were worn short or not at all—hence the success of the long-bearded impostor who appeared in Paris (1392) and was accepted on his own assurance as the Patriarch of Constantinople.

But with the fourteenth century the English beard has a fine flourish before its extinction for about a hundred years, after Henry V came to the throne—he it was who set an example of the clean shave, doubtless in reaction to *that villainous, abominable misleader of youth, Falstaff, that old white-bearded Satan*, the archetype of an earlier age, and his own unprofitable youth. I will sooner, said Sir John (prophetically, of Prince Hal) have a beard grow in the palm of my hand, than he shall get one on his cheek.

The beards of Chaucer's pilgrims

Chaucer, who died in 1400, recorded an age when beards were still common, and of variable shapes and sizes. T. S. Gowing has listed these styles, including that of the Merchant (to which we have already referred). This forked beard resembled that of

Franklin whose brass effigy at Shottesbrooke is mentioned in Fairholt's Glossary (under *Beard*). Chaucer's Franklin also has a beard—white as a daisy. The Miller's beard is red as a fox, and broad as though it were a spade—a sinister beard that, as we shall see. There is the Shipman's beard, shaken by many a tempest ; the Reeve's, close trimmed ; and the Sompnour's, *pilled*—that is to say, scanty (?)—a strange picture, with his fire-red, pimply cherub face and his narrow eyes under black brows, looking *likerous as a sparrow*.

The Pardoner, of course, is shaven :

> *No berd hadde he, ne never sholdë have,*
> *As smothe it was as it were late y-shave*

But to a layman the idea of a beard as a most treasured possession still holds good in Chaucer's time. Thus, in his Knight's Tale, we read of Arcite's vow to Mars :

> And eke to this avow I wol me bind
> My Berd, my here that hangeth low adown
> That never yet felt non offensioun
> Of rasour ne of shere, I wol thee yeve.

Edward IV's feet washed every Saturday night by his barber

Yet towards the turn of the century there were signs that the beard was on the decline. That of Richard of Bordeaux hardly exists, and Henry IV wears little more—a mere token. In the fifteenth century the slight growth sometimes noticeable on male chins (e.g. in the time of Edward IV and Henry VII) hardly merits the name of a beard. A shaven monk following his rule could have made almost as good a show, if his Order laid down intervals of a fortnight ; and those whose code specified but six times a year could have done much better, and still been counted shaven men. An order of Edward IV's time, quoted by Sidney Young from the *Liber Niger Domus Regis*, among the Harleian MSS, provides for *a barbour for the kingis most highe and drad P'son*. The king appeared to have been shaved weekly, but he expected more service than mere shaving, and was prepared to pay for it. *This Barbour, we read, shall have every Satterday night if it will please the kinge to cleanse his head leggs and feete and for his shaveing two lovis one pitcher wine.*

This command performance eventually became a daily habit, and from the same source (Young's *Annals of the Barber Surgeons of London*, page 68) I learn that it was later

> ordeyned that the kings Barbor shalbe daylie by the kings upriseinge readdye and attendant in the Kings Privye Chamber there haveinge in reddynesse his Water Basons knyvess Combes scissours and such other stuffe as to his Roome doth appertaine for trymminge and dressinge of the kings heade and bearde.

We are further informed regarding the barber honoured by this appointment that he is to use himself always honestly in his conversation *withoute resortinge to the companye of vile persons or of misguided women in avoidinge such daunger as by that meanes hee might doe unto the kings most Royal person.* For such attentions the parsimonious privy purse of the first Tudor is recorded to have paid £2 12s. 0d., the reward of three months' service.

The idea of shaving as a daily habit, rather than an occasional rite, we have already observed to have been a thing unthought of in mediæval (as it was rare even in Tudor) times, though not unknown among the ancients. The Egyptians were clearly more frequent in their shaving, and Scipio Africanus (who was for this reason considered somewhat effeminate) shaved daily. But some lines of Ausonius appear to assume that Tuesday was shaving day at Rome, indicating that for most Romans it was a weekly performance ; and this was perhaps the average standard of frequency in mediæval and early Tudor times, among those who shaved at all. No more than that is implied in the statement that the fifteenth century was a shaven age.

The Legend of Bluebeard

One advantage of the practice of shaving is that the character of the face can be more clearly scrutinised when the features are not masked by a beard ; and we are fortunate in having portraits of Richard III upon whose shaven features there is no trace of the villainy imputed to him by the historians of his reign. The slanders of the Tudors and their literary hacks are denied by the sensitive features of a man whom research has vindicated, though nothing will ever destroy the legend of a monster immortalised by Shakespeare[1]. A similar legend hard to eradicate is that of Gilles de Rais, another fifteenth century ogre of romance. In spite of his *confession* (in circumstances which had made even the Maid of Orleans weaken and abjure, for a few days, the mission of her life) the crimes of Gilles were never proved. But tradition is even wider of the mark in identifying this greatly talented and much maligned man with Bluebeard, regardless of that fact that he only had one wife, who survived him ; that there is no evidence of his ever having worn a beard ; and that if he did there is no reason to suppose it would have been a blue one.

Even Brewer's *Dictionary of Phrase and Fable* (an undated edition published by Cassells, but claiming to be *thoroughly revised*) made the astonishing statement that Gilles de Rais *was accused of murdering six of his seven wives*. And Mr. Bernard Shaw could not resist the temptation of introducing him, complete with the mythical beard of blue, into *St. Joan*—regardless of the fact that beards were then very uncommon. Had Gilles worn one at all (let alone dyeing it blue) the precularity would surely have been sufficiently notable for at least one of the contemporary chroniclers to have remarked upon it. If Shaw atoned for Shakespeare's sins respecting Joan of Arc (whose reputation was indeed fortunate to have survived the Stratford mud that stuck to Richard III) we must mark up that beard on Shaw's debit account. And yet how well those dyed whiskers harmonise with the theology of hairy excrement as the symbol of inner corruption, if the story is merely regarded as a fable, a picturesque sermon in the manner of Durandus !

The hairiness of hermits

The young courtiers in the illuminated copy of the *Roman de la Rose* at the British Museum (Harleian MSS. 4425) show clean shaven faces. They belong to the end of the fifteenth century.

[1] An engraving of perhaps the best of these portraits of Richard III will be found in Francis Grose's *Antiquarian Repertory*. The best vindication of Richard —still unanswered—is Sir Clements Markham's *Richard III, His Life and Character*.

and are typical of the period. Among the few instances of beards at this time I notice one in a story by John of Glastonbury. The story relates to King Arthur, but my friend Mr. Harry Scott-Stokes, who quotes it in an entertaining little book on Glastonbury, regards the legend itself as late mediæval, and it should be taken as a reflection rather of the chronicler's own period (late fifteenth century) than of the legendary Arthurian age. In this story we are surprised to meet a venerable *priest* with a *flowing beard*—on reading of which I immediately wrote to Mr. Scott Stokes demanding an explanation. My friend replied that the priest was clearly a hermit—which indeed, the story makes clear —*and I should think,* he added, *that hermits were always hairy, though I don't suggest any connection between the two words.* Clearly shaving facilities would not have been easily accessible in an hermitage ; and in any age or civilisation there would be something vaguely improper in the idea of a hermit even wishing to shave. [1] The explanation is not, however, quite so simple in the case of a certain episode in Malory's *Morte Darthur.*

In this story (Book I, Chapter XXVI) we read that Ryons, King of North Wales, sent a message to King Arthur announcing that he had overcome eleven kings and that every one had done him homage—and that was this (he said) they gave him their beards clean flayed off, as much as there was (a pleasant touch of irony when demanding the first fruits of Arthur's adolescent chin, which was the ultimatum that followed). It appeared that Ryons had indulged the fancy of *purfling*—i.e. bordering—a mantle with the beards of kings and needed one more to have the job completed . . .

Royal reply to a villainous and lewd message

Malory himself wrote in a beardless age, but seems to have entered very fully into the spirit of a legendary epoch when beards were more valued. Arthur considered the demand of King Ryons *ye most vylaynous and lewdest message that ever man herd sent unto a kynge.* To this he added —not without a becoming sense of modesty—that his beard

[1] Nevertheless St. Peter Damian is quoted by Seghers as strongly disapproving of the long beard worn by a hermit (*Amer. Cath. Q.R.*, 1882, page 303).

was as yet too young for the purpose. *But telle thow thy kynge* (said he) *this,*

> *I owe hym none homage, ne none of myn elders, but, or it be longe to, he shall do me homage on bothe his kneys, or else he shall lese his hede by ye faith of my body, for this is ye most shamefullest message that ever I herd speke of.* [1]

Certainly, Arthur could not have put more strongly his demand for the unconditional surrender of the Beard Snatcher, and one feels every sympathy for him. It is a pity that in the next chapter he models his behaviour on a Pharaoh or a Herod, calmly ordering the death of all children born on May-day, begotten of lords and born of ladies—a lapse discreetly over-looked by Tennyson when bolstering up this legendary barbarian as a symbolic stuffed owl, vaguely identified with the Prince Consort.

Re-appearance of the false beard

We have as yet made no reference to *false* beards since Egyptian times. It may well be imagined that in every age when beards were fashionable, those whom Nature had inadequately provided would have had recourse to Art. Hence it was that (among other products of invention) the golden beards of the ancient divinities appeared once more upon the chins of the *preux chevaliers* as tokens

---

[1] Rowland, in *The Human Hair*, draws attention to other versions of this story. Rheta Gawr (Malory's King Ryons) in the account by Geoffrey of Monmouth is regarded as reducing the Kings to slavery, of which shaving is a symbol. A ballad on the subject was sung at Kenilworth before Queen Elizabeth, in 1575. Arthur in this account challenges the King of North Wales, on receipt of his insulting request, to try:

> Whether he or King Arthur shall prove the best barbor ;
> And therewith he shook his good sword Excalābor.

There is also an allusion to the incident in Drayton's *Poly-Olbion*, and Spenser adapted it in his *Faerie Queene* (Book VI). A French writer of the nineteenth century (who held that *c'est un fait digne de la plus sérieuse considération que la barbe se montra constamment auprès du berceau des empires, et le rasoir auprès de leur tombeau*) claims that one of Charlemagne's paladins had such a cloak, and that another slept on a mattress made of his enemies' beards—*et cela était mille fois plus beau que de reposer sur des lauriers.* (M. Quitard—v, Barbe in Larousse, *Dictionnaire du XIX Siècle.*)

of victory. It is curious, indeed, that this custom survived the temporary extinction of the natural beard, and that even in the shaven fifteenth century a beard should still have been thought suitable to certain occasions. The parallel with Egypt is close— the beard is extinct, but certain ceremonial occasions still demand it ; so (like the wigs worn in a Court of Law) false beards have to be donned ritualistically by those who no longer wear natural ones. (Even the Irish hero Cuchulain was once reduced to this necessity.)

Thus, in 1477, the triumphant René, Duke of Lorraine, attended the funeral of his defeated enemy, Charles of Burgundy, wearing a golden beard which reached to his waist. As the continuator of Monstrelet tells us (cited by André Favyn in his *Histoire de Navarre*) :

> *Ledict Duc de Lorraine vestu de dueil* (there is a suggestion of insincerity in the mourning) *ayant une grand barbe d'or venant iusques à la ceinture à la facon des anciens Preux, & pour signe de la victoire qu'il avoit obtenue, luy vint donner de l'eau beneiste.*

There must certainly have been a suggestion of low comedy in such a funeral.

False beards forbidden in Catalonia

In Spain the art of manufacturing false beards was already so highly developed in the fourteenth century that the products were said to the indistinguishable from those of nature. The custom of wearing such beards—different styles for different occasions, including those which required a disguise—eventually met with official disapproval in the time of Pedro IV, King of Aragon (known as *The Ceremonious*, for the strict etiquette maintained at his court, which evidently excluded false beards). The Estates of Catalonia, meeting in 1351, passed an act against these works of art—*ne quis barbam falsam seu fictam audeat deferre vel fabricare.*

It may have been part of an attempt to stop masquerades, in which false beards were so commonly in use that these popular entertainments were known as *barbatoriæ.* Fangé even traces the word back to the uncertain but very early age of Petronius (probably the time of Nero) by quoting *Hodie servus meus Barba-*

toriam fecit ; and the abbé also pointed out that the word was still in use in eighteenth century France—*des Barboires, des Barbadoueres* and *des Barbauts* were apparently different provincial renderings. Many of the clergy took a poor view of such goings-on, as Du Cange shows in his *Glossarium* (1887, Tom X, page 74 of the *Dissertations*, also under *Barbatoria*). At the Feast of Fools such gear would be in evidence, like the false noses I remember on the faces of hundreds of children, one wild night at Dubrovnik. But such false beards or false noses and other grotesque human or animal caricatures seemed (to the sober minded) *formæ adulteræ* and *species monstruosæ*—so the domain of the Abbot of Misrule was formally abolished in France (1444) and later in England, by Henry VIII, that stern chaperon of Moral Propriety.

The same in Normandy

The *parlement* of Rouen, according to a footnote in Canel's work, found it necessary to forbid the wearing of false beards in 1508 and 1513. The people were forbidden to wear *masks, noses, or beards*, because *ces gens masquez et embastonnez se rendent de maison en maison, soubz prétexte de jouer aux dez, et troublent le repos public.* Clearly the beards here indicated were not real ones, as the Rouennais could hardly have been forbidden to wear real noses. [1]

Bottom's enquiry, when contemplating the rôle of Pyramus— *What beard were I best to play it in ?*—appears to have referred to a false beard. But a false beard is not easily superimposed upon a real one, and most Elizabethans were bearded. It has therefore been suggested that Bottom's offer to discharge the part in your straw colour beard, your orange-tawny beard, your purple-in-grain beard, or your French crown colour beard, your perfect yellow, referred to different dyes. (Of this art, in which the Elizabethans were masters, we shall speak later). But in Act IV,

[1] E. L. Tilton in *Folklore* (1895) described the burning of an effigy at Pylos, when a mock priest wore a false beard which he threw on the flames. Sir James Fraser, who recalls this incident in *The Dying God*, remarks that the ceremony is believed to be a protection against all kinds of misfortune ; and I find sinister significance in the fact that in his next story, which concerns the pretence of bleeding a patient to death and bringing him to life again, Sir James calls the physician *Dr. Iron-Beard*. The doctor functioned in Swabia every Shrove Tuesday in those days, but he may no longer be practising.

Scene II, when Bottom says *good strings to your beards,* the implication appears to be that false ones were in use, in spite of the obvious difficulties. Certainly in *Twelfth Night* the clown wears a false beard to impose upon Malvolio—but clowns, like the Roman clergy, seem to have had a long tradition of shaving (and, indeed, a more consistent one).

Among false beards the most curious on record, perhaps, were those worn by the *Timmermän* of the Swedish Army. I first saw a reference to these in an article by William Sansom, and have since confirmed from the Curator of the Armémuseum at Stockholm that men marching at the head of these columns (*Timmermän*) had to wear false beards if they possessed no real ones. The practice was discontinued on June 21, 1833.

John Bulwer, writing in the middle of the seventeenth century, spoke of false beards even among Red Indians :

> In Elizabeths Island, toward the North of Virginia, the men have no Beards, but counterfeits, as they did think our mens also were, for which they would have changed with some of our men that had great Beards.

True beards on fictitious artists

Outside of the stage and the pages of fiction false beards are seldom encountered today, though they predominated over real ones at a *Bal des Barbus* held by the *Fédération nationale des artistes* in Paris (reported in *Vu,*May 24, 1949). There be many disciples of Coleman, the bearded blasphemer of *Antic Hay,* which have made themselves beavers for the kingdom of Heaven's sake, or whatever substitute they have found for the kingdom. I meet them daily in the King's Road, Chelsea, but a friend of mine remarks that the beards are real enough—it is the reality of the artists which is questionable. They face up to fiction, as Huxley once said of a film star in her private life—but not, as far as I know, to the model which Huxley himself created in Theodore Gumbril. The study is an interesting one—the transformation of the mild and melancholy pedagogue into the Complete Man, jovial, massive and Rabelaisian. So eloquent is the description of this metamorphosis that one is almost persuaded to become a Beaver, at least for long enough to know whether one could acquire such superb self-confidence and bang one's fist down on a publisher's desk, as the Complete Man did in his transactions with Mr. Boldero. [1] Did Huxley, I wonder, ever experiment himself with a beard, or even a *barbe postiche*, to know the mysteries of the manly chin ?

But to the introspective soul the glory of any beard not honestly come by must surely be transient. Gumbril himself came to look upon his ornament as a foolish pretence. He was only, he reflected, a sheep in beaver's clothing. And for those of us whom Nature has not equipped to imitate Bishop Serlo's goats, it is perhaps better not to borrow their plumes. We are not *lascivi hirci* but sheep, and may as well submit to be shorn.

[1] It is not quite clear what happens if both parties are similarly armed, *id est, barbati*. An experiment might solve the problem as to what occurs when an irresistible force meets an immovable mass.

CHAPTER VIII

MAMBRINO'S HELMET AND THE BEARD OF BESSARION

Go round about, Peer Gynt
The Boyg

I beseech you, be hairs so filthy and so greatly to be
despised that they are not worthy to come near the
Blessed Sacrament ?   Valeriano Bolzani

IN my last chapter I said something of barbers, and this may be
the best place in which to speak further of them before I become
entangled in another theological mare's nest. I am already convinced that Lear's Old Man—the most amazing of all his
elderly heroes—who discovered such a remarkable aviary in his
beard, was a theologian. It would not have happened to anyone
else.

The Annals of the Barber-Surgeons

For the history of British barbery there is no better source of
information than Sidney Young's rare and companionable volume
The Annals of the Barber-Surgeons of London, of which (alas) there is
at present no copy in the British Museum. [1] Here the reader
may find every kind of information, from the Christmas Box of
seven shillings and sixpence paid to the hangman in 1723 (whereof
more anon) to a sum paid for redeeming the Company's laundry
from pawn.

Richard le Barbour, first master of the Barbers Company, was
sworn at the Guildhall in 1308. A picture by Holbein com-
memorates the marriage of this Company with the Fellowship of
Surgeons in 1540, when they were jointly incorporated as the
Barber-Surgeons Company. All but two of the Barber-Surgeons
in the picture are clean shaven. In spite of this union two distinct
crafts were recognised : Surgeons were prohibited from parti-
cipating in the feat or craft of Barbery and barbers were only

[1] As this book goes to press the gap (a result of the Blitz) has been filled.

permitted to draw teeth in addition to their normal functions. But these distinctions were frequently overlooked.

French notaries forbidden to practice shaving

In France the barbers had to compete not only with the surgeons but—it would appear—with other professions. A decree of Philip IV makes it clear that the public notaries had been poaching :

> Item. Tabelliones seu Notarii publici auctoritate nostra, nullo vili officio vel misterio immisceant.

They are not to get mixed up in menial jobs. And among those specified as forbidden are the crafts of the carnifices and the barbitonsores, the butchers and the barbers.

Such disputes as to the functions of the professions are frequent in the history of barbery. Whilst lawyers and surgeons had to be restrained from shaving (that is, literally) their clients or patients, barbers were with difficulty prevented from performing major operations and from driving a trade as restaurateurs with their waiting customers. But they were not without lofty ideals ; and the earliest record of the fraternity tells us that the original Barbers Company of London existed primerement al honourance de Dieu et touz ses Seyntes, also to encourage the common people in well doing.

Unseemly behaviour of barbers

Their habits, however, did not always please the authorities. An order of 1307, De Barbours, forbade them to display vessels of blood in their windows en view des gentz, mais pryvement le facent porter en Thamise—the blood was to be unobtrusively taken and deposited in the Thames, the common sewer of London, and also the reservoir of the city's water supply. Richard le Barbour, in taking his oath, undertook to fine any members of the trade whom he discovered to be keeping brothels or acting unseemly in any other way. They had, in fact, exceptional opportunities for unseemly behaviour, for their diocese included the public baths, those Seminaria Venenata, or hot-beds of vice. When beards were fashionable the baths became the principal milieu of the barber's trade, especially in France, where depilation of the body hairs became fashionable at one time. Canel has some interesting notes on this in an appendix to his *Histoire de la barbe et des cheveux en Normandie*, where he quotes a quatrain by Clement Marot, apropos of the blow dealt to the barbers when Francis I re-introduced the bearded fashion in France. Further information will be found in Dr. Cabanès' *Moeurs Intimes du Passé* (Vol. II : *La Vie aux Bains*).

St. Damian's Urinal

Unauthorised practitioners were punished ; and we read of one being led through the City of London, with trumpets and fifes. He rode bareback, a urinal hung before him and another behind, just to learn him. An order of the Court of Aldermen, by the prayer of the Barbers' Company, forbade any barber or person *using barbourye* to teach any foreigner any point *that belongeth to the craft of barbourye or surge'ye*. Even men from *uppelande*—country men coming to town—were subjects of complaint. From a Londoner's standpoint they too were foreigners. The urinals used in the penitential procession of the quack were not necessarily a sign of ridicule. On the contrary, they were badges of the trade, for the patron saints of the Barber-Surgeons were Cosmo and Damian, St. Damian being represented in mediæval art with a urinal as the symbol of his tutelage of medicine. (The Medici family, originally physicians in all probability, were under the special protection of the same saints.)

Sabbath breaking by barbers was a frequent cause of scandal. An Archbishop of Canterbury[1] is found complaining about the matter, to the Lord Mayor, and in 1556 an order of the Company's Court of Assistants prohibited *any shewe of Barborye one Soundais or other holy days*. Apprentices, before being bound, had to present themselves before this Court to see if they were *cleane in p'son and Lymme and meete for the exercyseinge of the same mysterye*. In the same

---

[1] In later years clerical interference was greatly resented by the Barber Surgeons. In 1689, when it was feared that the Bishop of London might oppose an attempt of the Company to obtain the sole authority for licensing surgeons, they threatened to propose legislation to make the Bishop's licence conditional on the Company's approval.

order it was found necessary to repeat the injunction against displaying vessels of blood, a practice still obstinately followed by certain barbers *exercyseinge fleabothomye or bloud lettinge*. In 1599 one Marmaduke Jefferson was fined for hanging out his basins on May Day.

In one respect the Barber Surgeons were evidently ahead of State practice by the eighteenth century, for in 1712 a minute of the Court of Assistants records that a certain Walter Browne, *being one of the people called Quakers*, was admitted into the freedom and allowed to make a solemn affirmation in place of the oath. (According to Wharton's Law Lexicon the affirmation was not recognised till the time of George IV, so far as legal practice was concerned). The Barber-Surgeons were expected to show a high sense of resonsibility, stimulated by the public demand for a *quid pro quo* when they paid their money. There are numerous instances of patients bringing actions against the Barber-Surgeons for cures paid for but not effected ; and in one case the Court gave an order that they should deal further with the plaintiff (a Carpenter) for his health. Some, for their ignorance, were ordered never to meddle in any matter of surgery, from which we may concludethat some confusion still existed at that time (1578) as to the functions of the two branches of the profession.

Norman barbers forbidden to cure toothache

In France there was sufficient clear distinction, by the year 1684, for two *chirurgiens* to be prosecuted at Rouen for making and selling wigs. Canel tells us that they were fined and all their wig-making instruments confiscated. But two years later the surgeons of Rouen had their revenge, obtaining an injunction against the barbers to stop them concocting infallible remedies for toothache. The dispute in France had been an old one, but the surgeons had struck a death-blow at the amateur efforts of the barbers as early as 1499. The barbers had been anxious to learn *chirurgie*, but (according to Fangé) their request was met in a back-handed manner by a decree of October 18, 1499, permitting the reading and expounding of books on surgery to the barbers, but only in Latin, *cum Magistri non soleant aliter libros suos legere*. (The reader who cannot understand will not be offended.)

A digression on eccentric corpses

I am tempted, however, to digress somewhat on the subject of the surgical activities of the London Company. The surgeons learnt their anatomy by dissecting the bodies of condemned criminals, of which there was a plentiful supply, owing to the old English custom of hanging people even for the most trifling offences. Any proposal to have abolished the death penalty would have filled the Company with horror, for there was no other legal way to obtain possession of a nice fresh corpse.   On February 20, 1587, a corpse which had been taken to the Surgeons' Hall came to life—a reflection, no doubt, on the inefficient methods of hanging then in use ; though it is said that even contemporary practice is not infallible.   The man, as a result of his unpleasant experiences on the scaffold, died three days later, and his body was doubtless put to good use by the surgeons after all.   But there was no security for the surgeons, who had paid good money to the hangman, that a corpse might not revive and refuse to die a second time, in spite of all that medical and surgical skill could do to assist him.   In that case the surgeons would be out of pocket ; so we are not surprised to find a resolution in their Minutes to provide against financial loss if such a thing should ever happen again.   And happen it did, in the celebrated case of William Duell, on November 23, 1740.

I must deny myself the macabre delight of discussing the case of William Duell, also many other grim stories anent the corpses of criminals, which will be found in Sidney Young's book, by the few who can lay their hands on a copy.   Some hint of these stories may be found in the accounts books.   In 1720-21, seven shillings and sixpence was paid to the High Constable of St. Giles's Parish for assisting the beadles in recovering a body which had been taken from them by the mob.   The hangman's Christmas Box, already mentioned, was entered in the accounts as half a crown in 1717-18 ; but after the row in the parish of St. Giles (not unique by any means) the hangman was paid fifteen shillings *for the dead man's clothes* (perquisites of the executioner) *which were lost in the scuffle and for his Christmas Box.*   It was in 1723 that the Christmas Box was increased to seven shillings and six pence, business being doubtless more brisk by then, and a receipt was signed for it. But in 1743 *John Thrift, Esq., hangman*, as he is styled, being unable to sign for his *pourboire*, made his mark.

Decision not to dissect corpses in the kitchen

Reluctantly I turn from the magic casements of Sidney Young and the fairy land forlorn of Serendip. There is the acquisition by the Barber Surgeons of a monopoly of embalming, the examination of a monstrous birth, and the decision (in 1631) to build a room for dissection, in order—very reasonably—*to preserve the kitchin to its owne prop' use.* (What difficulties they must previously have experienced, what disputes there must have been with the cook as to the most urgent use of the kitchen table and the carving knife . . . ! Small wonder that in 1615 the cook had been dismissed *for a generall dislike taken against him by this howse* : he was probably unreasonable about the whole business.) Sums of two shillings are mentioned, and twice the even stranger sum of two and twopence for sending children to Virginia. A much more expensive item about the same time (early seventeenth century) is that of fourteen shillings *for two whippes for correction.* They must have had hard usage, for further sums are laid out later for their repair. Twenty-five shillings is paid for a noise of trumpets on the Lord Mayor's Day in 1622-23 ; but in 1735 the Company bought seventy-nine gallons of wine for this occasion. Such occasions called for special preparation, as the accounts for 1638 demonstrate ; for at the *Entertainment and Dynings of the Lords of the Councell in our great Parlour at the Publique Anatomye* six shillings and eightpence was paid for *the hier of two Close Stooles.* Some years later (1662-63) they paid five shillings and six pence *ffor a large Chamber pott* ; and *a wooden stand for ye Chamber Pott* is mentioned among the amenities of the Parlour in an inventory of 1711.

But I must remember that I am not writing a supplement to *Cleanliness and Godliness.* I am merely filling in the time while the shaven fifteenth century passes (and the Middle Ages with it) by some reflections on, and suggested by, the barbers who reigned in that Age. With the Renaissance the beard re-asserts itself, and by strange irony it begins in the Roman Church—almost, one might say, on the Pope's chin.

The beard of Bessarion

There are, of course, in every age, some who either have too much initiative to be bound by fashion, or are too conservative to follow its changing course.   A tapestry of the middle fifteenth century shows Henry VI and his court—all clean shaven save one, who is believed to be the Duke of Gloucester—Shakespeare's *good duke Humphrey*. He alone wears a magnificent beard, though his upper lip is shaven. An excellent reproduction of this group will be found in one of the plates illustrating Shaw's *Dresses and Decorations* (1843) Vol. II. But such beards are isolated exceptions. [1] It was to a shaven world that Bessarion came from the Byzantine Empire, destined to bring with him a new fashion. For though he became a convert of the Western Church, and accepted *filioque*, he adhered to the unorthodox reading of the famous canon—*nec barbam radat* ; and his firmness on this point seems to have had a profound influence on the Church, beginning with Pope Julius II.

Of brotherly love

Johannes Bessarion (or Basilius Bessarion) was born about 1400 A.D. at Trebizond—a name as magical as Camelot or El Dorado, Samarkand or Serendip, or even Glastonbury. He lived at a time when both the Eastern Empire and the Papacy were in difficulties—the Emperor of Constantinople being threatened by the Turks, and the Pope by a Church Council which seemed to doubt his infallibility.   The Emperor, John Palæologus, decided that the time had come to heal the Great Schism. The rival factions of the Western Church both grasped—nay, grabbed—at the olive branch, and vied with each other in their eagerness to welcome a potential ally. To Pope Eugenius IV it meant the hope of spiritual reinforcements in his struggle with the Council of Basel. The priests and prelates at Basel, on the other hand, hoped to negotiate the re-union of the Eastern and Western Churches themselves, and thus to increase their own prestige

[1] Among such exceptions there are several beards in the painting by Pinturicchio showing Aeneas Sylvius (later Pius II) being created Cardinal in 1456. But as the artist was two years old at the time his evidence is not very reliable.

vis-à-vis the Pope and the Roman curia.[1] Palæologus, who wanted allies against the Turks, found himself confronted by two Western factions, each eager to out-bid the other for his support. He negotiated with both parties, and each sent ships to fetch the Greek deputation—one fleet with orders to bring the Emperor and the Eastern patriarchs to Italy, the other with instructions to keep them out of the hands of the Papal emissaries, so that the negotiations could take place beyond the Alps and the influence of Rome. The Commander of the Papal fleet had orders to sink the rival expedition if met on the high seas, but as things turned out they did not meet, and the Roman fleet was the first to arrive. It bore the Emperor and his deputation in triumph to Italy.

With both Emperor and Pope so eager for a settlement, and the latter anxious to show himself more reasonable than the fathers at Basel, it is not remarkable that agreement was speedily reached. A mild hint from the Emperor helped his patriarchs to make up their minds ; for he indicated that if the Roman terms were not accepted by any of them, those who objected might be left to shift for themselves in a country where they had no means of livelihood. They had therefore a choice between honour and promotion, with all that the liberality of Rome could offer as a further inducement, and the unattractive prospects of penniless schismatics in a hostile country. Indeed, many of them had not much better hopes even if permitted to return to the East ; for the Turks had over-run some of the most profitable sources of their former affluence, enabling many of the patriarchs to say truthfully with St. Peter, *Silver and gold have I none.* But such apostolic poverty had little appeal to the Greek deputation, to whom Peter's successor spoke now in very different language, better suited to the spiritual modesty of both parties. One did not offer, nor did the other ask, so close a comparison with so holy an apostle.

---

[1] The Fathers at Basel discussed beards, among other matters of importance. They generally cropped up at Church Councils, and at the Council of Trent an Archbishop delivered a long oration on the beard of Aaron.

Bessarion earns his hat

Among the dignitaries of the Eastern Church whom the Emperor brought with him was Bessarion, whom John Palæologus had made Archbishop of Nicæa. He was present at the joint councils held with the Papal representatives at Ferrara and Florence, distinguishing himself by such zeal for re-union and such eagerness to accept the Roman terms that the Pope lost little time in offering him a Cardinal's hat. In accepting the hat, but retaining his oriental beard—of no mean dimensions— Bessarion broke the tradition of centuries. Here at last was a bearded priest of the Roman rite once more, and no mere nonentity, but a member of the Sacred College. For whatever else he could stomach, the good man refused to be parted from his beard. His obstinacy made history.

The re-union of Christendom in 1438 proved both illusive and transitory.[1]   The terms were repudiated by the Eastern Church, and the circumstances in which a Byzantine Emperor had sought for unity with Rome were soon to be completely altered by the collapse of the Empire itself. Historians have long discarded the view that the Renaissance was engendered by wandering Greek scholars who fled from Constantinople with their books and the hoarded wisdom of the centuries, when the city fell to the Ottomans. But the New Learning in the West certainly owed a great deal to the scholarly patriarchs who came to Italy with John VII and preferred to remain there rather than return to face the crescent moon of Islam and the fury of their own brethren, whom no Turkish peril could reconcile to the Vatican. Of these patriarchs who adopted the Roman rite and made their home where it was practised none was more distinguished as a scholar than Johannes Bessarion. It is not an exaggeration to say that his is one of the most significant personalities in the Renaissance ; and it is most appropriate that with Greek scholarship he brought the Greek beard.

[1] When the articles of re-union were formally read to the united gathering, only one of the Eastern delegates (Mark of Ephesus) protested—though another of the Eastern delegates (a brother of the Emperor) had already withdrawn from the synod. But Gibbon, in a footnote, recalls that a favourite hound of John Palæologus barked incessantly during the reading of the act of union. The phrase *not a dog barked*, may well originate from this incident.

Mishap to a bearded ambassador

As Latin Patriarch of Constantinople (a mere title bestowed by
the Pope, for Bessarion never returned there) Bishop of Frascati
and Papal Legate on various missions, Cardinal Bessarion played a
distinguished part in the Church politics of the West. It is true
that, in an age when even laymen were shaven, this bearded
Cardinal caused some scandal. For a slight breach of etiquette,
when Bessarion was sent on an embassy to Louis XI, in 1471,
the French king seized him by the beard and rough handled him
—an affront which so upset the Greek that (according to Dulaure)
his death a year later must be attributed to it. The reader who
recalls the words of William of Tyre, regarding the pawning of
Baldwin's beard (*Mos est Orientalibus, tam Græcis quam aliis nationibus,
barbam tota cura et omni sollicitudine nutrire*) will find it easy to
believe that Bessarion pined away from shame and grief.

One story, which Père Fangé recalls, is that Bessarion's beard
cost him the Papacy. According to this account he was at one
time in the running, but other cardinals objected to the idea of a
bearded Pope. *Nondum barbam rasit Bessarion,* exclaimed one of
them, Bessarion has not yet shaved off his beard, *et nostrum caput
erit ?* And he is to be our head ? A bearded cardinal was bad
enough, a bearded pontiff still unthinkable. But one of the
cardinals at least had eyed that beard with envy, and it was his
good fortune to succeed to the keys of St. Peter. Secure in the
impregnable infallibility of the Vatican Julius II grew the
flourishing beard in which Raphael painted his portrait.

The Beard at the Vatican

Julius II was Pope from 1503 to 1513. A picture in which he
appears as a cardinal shows that he was then beardless; and even
the early medals which show him as Pope make it clear that the
beard was not grown during his first years of office. The innovation, according to Spondanus, was conceived as a means of
inspiring greater respect. Beards were still rare exceptions, even
among the laity, at the time of his death; so the sight of a
bearded Pope must have startled Christendom. It was almost as
though the Supreme Pontiff himself had capitulated to the
rumbling criticism of the Lollards, who had denounced shaving

among the evil practices of Rome. Back in the fourteenth century John Wycliffe had proclaimed that the priests of Ante-Christ were known by *crowne and berdes shavynge*, and in all the portraits of Wycliffe his long beard is invariably to be seen. It had been an open challenge to Rome ; yet here was Rome wearing the same badge. The beard was an essential aspect of *terribiltà* in the self-dramatisation of Julius II, consonant with the singularly unsuitable medal which he caused to be made, showing him chasing the French with a whip.

Remarkable talents of Julius II

Pope Julius II was a della Rovere, the nephew of Sixtus IV ; and his uncle (in the best papal traditions) had made good use of the Keys to unlock the caskets of earthly treasure in the interests of his family. One had only to read the lives of the popes in the *Catholic Encyclopedia* to understand the meaning and origin of the word *nepotism*. Within a few months of his uncle's elevation to the Holy See, the young Giuliano della Rovere had (from complete obscurity) become a cardinal ; and in the succeeding years he acquired the revenues of twelve bishoprics plus the archiepiscopal See of Avignon. Julius II had been, in fact, for years the absentee landlord of countless souls and the power behind the papal throne of Innocent VIII, a man of straw whose election he had himself secured by bribery—an expedient which (I quote from the *Catholic Encyclopedia*, a work of praise-worthy frankness, on the whole) he *did not hesitate to employ* in securing his own election. A man so gifted in the arts which are most honoured by mankind deservedly enjoyed the prestige earned by his own talents. In his memory did Michelangelo design the monument at St. Pietro in Vincoli, where that monstrous Moses with his beard of fantastic length has been described as the spiritual portrait of Julius II.[1] But the world paid tribute even more

---

[1] Julius II, who had the mentality of a brigand, and so little respect for his own office that he pawned the Triple Crown, was universally disliked ; and Michelangelo, who flattered him thus in public, left us his real opinion in one of his sonnets. I refer to the one which reads :

Qua si fa elmi di calici e spade
E 'l Sangue di Christo si vend' a giumelle, etc.

profound to this bearded Pope, for it imitated the fashion which he inaugurated.

The Beard Royal an imitation of the Papal Beard

Francis I of France is described by Chambers in his *Book of Days*, as an imitator of Julius—he was certainly one of the first public figures, after the Pope, to appear in a beard, which he grew for reasons similar to those which induced Hadrian to wear one—to conceal the accidental wounds caused in a mock battle. Henry VIII followed (in 1535, according to Stow) by growing the beard without which it is impossible now to imagine him—it became so essential an aspect of his personality. From the leading kings and their courtiers the new fashion spread rapidly among all classes in the sixteenth century.

At what point is a beard nourished ?

Of most interest, however, is the vogue in clerical beards which began from this time and lasted nearly two centuries. The immediate successor of Julius II was Leo X, whose *fat, shiny, effeminate countenance with weak eyes* (I gratefully acknowledge the phrase once more to the *Catholic Encyclopedia*) is shown by Raphael, who painted him with two of his cardinals. He was clean shaven, and so was Hadrian VI, who followed him. [1] But Clement VII, the next Pope (though illegitimate, he was well qualified by a Medici father) wore a long beard, as shown in his portrait by Sebastian Luciani. Father Thurston, in his article on

Or, as J. A. Symonds rendered it :
> *Here helms and swords are made of chalices,*
> *The blood of Christ is sold so much the quart . . .*

[1] According to Eugene Müntz (*Histoire de l'Art pendant la Renaissance*) Leo X attempted to lead a reactionary movement against this innovation of his predecessor. See Vol. III, page 157, where Müntz described the amusement of Rome at the grief shown by a certain Domenico of Ancona, from whom the inflexible demands of Leo exacted the sacrifice of a beard which had been immortalised in a sonnet by Francesco Berni. Hadrian VI was also a persecutor of clerical beards. *Il reprenait sévèrement* (says Müntz) *les ecclésiastiques qui portaient la barbe longue, à la façon des soldats.* Oddly enough, Hadrian VI, the last shaven Pope for nearly two centuries, was also the last *Pontifice Barbaro*—a Dutchman, born in Utrecht.

Beards in the *Catholic Encyclopedia*, made the curious error of claiming that *to judge by the portraits of the Popes it was with Clement VII (1523) that a distinct beard began to be worn.* He must have forgotten Raphael's portrait of Julius II and the written records which refer to that scandalous growth of his.   Thurston, however, correctly points out that in the sixteenth century the phrase *barbam nutrire,* to nourish a beard, began to take on a new meaning. The prohibition against *nourishing* a beard, which had descended by such a doubtful pedigree from the supposed Fourth Council of Carthage, was actually repeated, in the last year of Julius II, by the Fifth Council of the Lateran.   With such a flourishing beard on the chin of the Holy Father himself, the injunction that a priest should not *barbam nutrire* clearly cannot have been taken to mean that he must shave.   But what exactly *did* they understand by it?

Father Thurston argues that the Church had begun to interpret the phrase as *not inconsistent with a short beard.*   But the beard of Julius II was not very short, and that of Clement VII was distinctly long.   Certainly, Clement's beard was not quite as long as it appears in the famous woodcut used by Foxe in his *Actes and Monuments.* Here the Pope, with a beard worthy of a goat, is represented as being trodden upon by Henry VIII, to whom Cranmer is appropriately presenting the Bible.   But it was none the less a long beard, as Clement's portraits make clear ; and it is difficult to see at what point a beard might be said to be *nourished.*   Paul III, who followed Clement VII, is represented with a long white beard by Titian, and similarly by Michelangelo. By the latter he is made to look so pious that it is difficult to believe he was the father of Pier Luigi ;   but even Popes and Cardinals had their little slips in those days. [1]   And the ecclesiastical by-blows could always be sure of papal patronage.   (I beg the reader's pardon,—we seem to be off again.)   Two reflections occur to me, both relating to Alexander VI, that great expert in the art of poisoning.   And I cannot even claim him as one of my bearded popes, but simply can't get him out of my head, so here we go.

[1] There are two Titians, one of which shows Paul III with his *nipoti*, looking not so pious but quite incredibly crafty.   The two young men look, if possible, even less trustworthy.

They were a wonderful family, the Farnese. Pier Luigi, the Pope's son, known to history as a murderous ruffian, was made Captain General of the Church, Duke of Parma and I know not what beside. And Pier Luigi's son—Alessandro Farnese, a grandson of Paul III—was created Cardinal at the age of fourteen. The papacy looked, for a moment, as though it was on the point of becoming hereditary, though necessarily on the wrong side of the blanket. But Paul III himself owed his good fortune largely to the fact that his sister had enjoyed the honour of being the mistress of Alexander VI ; and the white bearded patriarch was small beer indeed when compared with this eminent predecessor. It is as good an excuse as any other for dragging him into my story.

Some thoughts on a beardless Borgia

In the hey-day of the Renaissance the Church certainly did not persecute bastards or bastardy, provided that the clerical errors came of a good stock. Cardinal Rodrigo Borgia, later crowned Pope as Alexander VI, had (in the words of the *Catholic Encyclopedia*) even after his ordination to the priesthood, in 1468, continued his evil ways. . . . Towards 1470 began his relations with the Roman lady, Vanozza Catanei, the mother of his four children. Of these the most infamous was Cæsar Borgia, born in 1476. In 1480—I still follow the mild and apologetic pages of the *Catholic Encyclopedia*—Pope Innocent VIII made the child (an infant of four, mark you) eligible for orders by absolving him from the ecclesiastical irregularity that followed his birth *de episcopo cardinali et conjugata*, and conferred several benefices upon him, including the Bishopric of Pampeluna. When Papa became Pope, young Cæsar, who was not even ordained, was granted, at the age of eighteen, the Archbishopric of Valencia—a place to which he never in his life paid so much as a visit.

Special pleading in the Encyclopædia Britannica

It is a typical Renaissance story. (Protestantism inherited the system ; and for some 300 years the history of the Church of England is one, very largely, of fat benefices enjoyed often by absentees, merely as sources of revenue—the perquisites of birth or the reward of political services.) But what has struck me with some astonishment is some special pleading on behalf of Alexander VI in connection with what was perhaps his most cynical act. The place in which I noticed this attempted justification made it, in my view, most remarkable. It will probably be remembered that it was this Borgia Pope, Alexander VI, who divided half the world between Spain and Portugal, disposing of populations like so many heads of cattle. The curious reader may find in the fourteenth edition of the *Encyclopædia Britannica* a truly incredible attempt to justify this donation (as it was termed) in the article on the Papacy (Vol. 17, p. 211) written by Achille Luchaire, a former professor of Mediæval History at the Sorbonne. The professor actually found a parallel between the patenting of an invention or the copywriting of a literary work and the discovery of a country, so that the country discovered, with all its inhabitants became the property of the discoverers—the more so if they had been *conquered by arduous efforts*. There is a kind of political Berkleyanism about the argument that is fascinating—for if Europe had been discovered by the Red Indians (as it was, according to one old story, [1] we might easily have become their lawful property on the grounds that they saw us before we saw them. If they did, however, they neglected to shoot at sight ; and clearly that was the true basis of the claims recognised by the Pope—what better argument to offer a Borgia ?

Reflections on Papal Ethics abandoned with regret

Only a strong sense of duty prevents me from dissertating further on the ethics of the Popes, a truly fascinating subject. But I wish the story of Benedict IX were better known. Rodolphus Glaber mentions him (Lib. V, cap. V) *Fuerat enim eidem sedi,* says he, *ordinatus quidam puer;* a certain boy, he calls him. (He was certainly not more than twenty when made Pope.) His was perhaps the most remarkable of all papal histories, for he grew bored with his infallibility, decided (so some say) that he wanted to marry, and sold the job for a lump sum to his pious successor. But all this will not help us disentangle these papal beards. I think I was discussing the meaning of *barbam nutrire*.

[1] In 1508 according to Baring Gould in *Curious Myths*. It was only chance that Columbus beat them to it.

Father Seghers observes that all Popes were bearded from Clement VII (1523) to Clement XI (1700), who began the new shaven series that has lasted to the present day. During this period one is astonished, not only at the beards, but at the number of moustaches worn. There is Paul IV, who may be seen in Richardson's illustrations to Granger, wearing a moustache with his square beard. Clement VIII also wears a moustache with his beard—very shocking this, after all we have read about the hairs of the upper lip. And of two celebrated bearded nepotists, Alexander VII and VIII, the latter is depicted on a medal with a moustache in addition to his pointed beard. Urban VIII, whose kindness to his family, at the expense of the Church, was considered even in those days quite phenomenal (he also had the distinction of condemning Galileo) was another moustached pope —his portrait may be seen in the illustrations to Granger (Richardson's Collection) with a very square Cathedral beard, continued in a fringe to the ears, and as smart a pair of moustaches as a man could wish for. To say that the popes did not *nourish* such beards seems too much of a strain on one's credulity—or had they by then decided that *nourishing* meant using a hair restorative ?

The beard worn with the tonsure

The beard of Gregory XIV is forked, after the old Saxon fashion. (His other claim to distinction is that he tried to stop betting on the results of Papal elections.) Bearded cardinals are now numerous, but the tonsure long remains—it survived the advent of the beard, but disappeared permanently in England and some countries (among the secular clergy) when it was eventually abandoned for reasons already mentioned. But in Reginald Pole's time the English Catholic clergy are still the *shaven men*, though many of them are bearded. Pole's own beard would have merited the description *barba prolixa*, so often forbidden to the clergy even when little beards were permitted ; but (as a Cardinal) Pole also displayed the tonsure ; and it is on record that the Pope (when the decision was taken in 1536 to offer Pole his cardinal's hat) sent a barber with the Papal Chamberlain. The function of the barber was to shave the crown of Reginald's head in order that he might be ordained as a deacon—a necesssary preliminary if a layman was to be hustled into the Sacred College. But in an earlier (or later) age the barber would have been instructed to remove that uncanonical beard. [1]

Beards Protestant and Popestant

Hence the attacks on *shaven priests*, which are so often to be found in Protestant writings of the sixteenth century, do not necessarily refer to the chin. Protestant and Popestant seemed almost to compete for the honour of presenting the best beards ; and the distinguishing mark was the tonsure, so long as it lasted. It was primarily to this that Latimer would have referred in his first Sermon before Edward VI when he defined the Papist objective *to make the yomanry slavery and the cleargye shavery*. The same applies to Tyndale with his frequent comments (*Shaving is borrowed of the hethen and oylinge of the Jewes*, he says in *The Obedience of a Christian Man*. This is a curious work, by the way, worth more attention. It sets out the cheerful doctrine of absolute obedience on the part of subjects to their princes, servants to their masters, children to their parents and wives to their husbands. Knox himself was not a deadlier opponent of Women's Rights than our William Tyndale. But what is really interesting is the assumption throughout his argument that the influence of Rome is subversive of the despotic system he advocates as being ordained by God and St. Paul).

The Defence of Woman

By the year 1548 beards were common enough in England for good Bishop Hooper to speak of them as causes of idleness and vanity among such as had but forty shillings a year. In his *Declaration of the Ten Holy Commandments of Almighty God* he affirms that a man of such standing will take as long in the morning to set his beard in order as a godly craftsman would be in looming a piece of kersey. By 1560 further refinements had been added, as described in *A Lytle and bryefe treatyse called the defence of women, and*

[1] Actually the tonsure rests on much firmer ground than the shaving of the beard. The canon law still insists that all clerics are bound to wear the tonsure ; and the practice of thousands of Catholic priests, who do not do so, is an open breach of their own Church discipline with the connivance of the Holy See.

especially of Englysshe women, the work of one Edward More, who thus describes one of the services rendered to Man by Woman :

In combing of theyr berdes, in strokyng them full ofte,
In wassyng them with wassyng balles, in looking all alofte
In plaitting of them divers wayes, in bynding them in bandes,
Wherein their hole delyght always consists and stands.

The first three lines may be taken as sociological evidence ; the last, being written by a man, is not beyond suspicion.

The Beard Patriarchal

In spite of all efforts to limit their length and profusion, many beards of this time ran to great length. John Knox wagged a preposterous growth against the *Monstrous Regiment of Women.* Archbishop Cranmer, trailing dismally around with his wife in a box (such was still the prejudice against married clergy ; and she nigh died of suffocation when the box was once inverted, with the ventilation holes at the bottom) might well wear the beard patriarchal to signify the new function of the reformed priesthood. Great is the beard of the Bishop Bale, that man of bile ; long and pointed that of Thomas Bickley, Bishop of Chichester in the time of Elizabeth ; and the fashion continues well into the seventeenth century. Thomas Morton, Bishop of Durham, wore a rounded beard, with a heavy moustache. Tobias Matthews, Archbishop of York, is pictured at the age of seventy-eight, in 1624, with a fringe of beard and curled moustachios. His successor, George Mountaigne, wears a great, thick, black beard, with a moustache and heavy side-whiskers. John Prideaux, Bishop of Worcester in the time of Charles I, wears the square Cathedral beard. John Bridgeman, Bishop of Chichester, is pictured in 1623, wearing the full round beard, with side-whiskers and moustache. French protestants of this period are also bearded. But we will leave these Protestant beards for the moment and return to the Beard Catholic and Apostolic.

Beards of the Catholic Martyrs

The bearded fashion spread rapidly among the higher Catholic clergy. John Leslie, Bishop of Ross, the loyal friend of Mary,

Queen of Scots, could wag as good a beard as his enemy, John Knox. Cardinal Pietro Bembo, in the mosaic by Francesco and Valerio Zuccato at Florence, has a beard like a Jewish patriarch. But the fashion was not long confined to the higher ranks. Selecting almost at random from the supplement to Richardson's illustrations to Granger (London 1820) I notice among the Catholics a number of bearded priests who were executed in England at different times. The famous Jesuit priest, poet and martyr, Edmund Campion, wears a short pointed beard. A short beard, side-whiskers and moustache are worn by Martin Woodcocke, who was executed as a Catholic priest at Lancaster in 1646. (*If a Turkish dervise had then preached Mahomet in England* —the comment is Granger's—*he would have met with much better treatment than a Catholic priest*.) Johannes Baptista (executed 1642) and the Jesuit Henry Gernet (executed 1606) are both bearded— the latter still wearing the tonsure with his square beard and clipped moustache. Another Jesuit, Peter Wright (executed 1651) wears a small beard, like a postage stamp, with a small moustache—both fashionable at that time. Francis Bell (executed 1643) uses a similar style. I also notice that Father John van Bolland, S.J., the initiator of the *Acta Sanctorum*, wore a short beard and a moustache.

A tax on clerical beards

Nevertheless, it is with the bishops and archbishops that the fashion begins, and of them that it appears, generally speaking, to be most typical. Cardinal Guglielmo Sirleto (1514-1585) was bearded. Cardinal Allen, who divided his life between the fostering of Catholic colleges in Europe and abortive attempts to bring about the Counter-Reformation in England by foreign intervention, wore (appropriately) a two-forked beard. A vast beard was worn by Wolsey's colleague, Cardinal Campeggio. Cardinal Rossetti, three generations later, represents the height of fashion in the time of Charles I—curling moustachios and a straight, short, narrow beard, coming to a point. Some priests might tolerate, and others imitate, such innovations. But in many places a sharp struggle resulted between the bearded end of the hierarchy and the lower members. This was especially the case in

France. One reason for this fact was that in this country Francis I, who had himself done so much to reinstate the beard by growing one himself, obtained permission from the Pope to tax clerical beards. The higher clergy, being able to afford it, paid the tax and grew their beards ; the lower clergy, being unable to pay, were for the most part unable to nourish beards, but many of them nourished in place a dark, unutterable hatred for the bearded prelates who flaunted their wealth upon their chins.

Beard or Bishopric ?

A classical instance of this feud is said to have been that of Guillaume Duprat, whose alleged adventures are recalled in the Percy Anecdotes of Fashion (Vol. XIX of the *Percy Anedotes*, 1823, page 87). Duprat, the son of a well-known French Chancellor and himself the founder of the Jesuit college at Paris, was appointed Bishop of Clermont ; but the Dean and Chapter took such exception to his beard (said to be one of the finest in the kingdom) that they would not let him take possession of the benefice while he wore it ; and on his arrival they met him with shears, razors, soap and basins, prepared to remove by force the object of their loathing. Duprat with difficulty escaped from their hands (crying, *I Keep my beard and quit my bishopric*) and retired to his castle of Beauregard, where—*on dit*—he fell ill of vexation at the insult offered to his beard and swore never again to set foot in Clermont ; an oath which he kept to the letter, for of that sickness he is supposed to have died. Before his death he is said to have exchanged his bishopric with Cardinal Salviati, a nephew of Pope Leo X, so young that he had no hair on his chin (another of these infant prodigies, no doubt, who sprang miraculously from the papal families).

The legend of Guillaume Duprat discredited

Fosbroke refers to this story in his *Encyclopædia of Antiquities* ; and Cabanès in his *Curiosités de la Médecine* (Vol. I, 79-84 where he discusses shaving) appears to accept its authenticity ; he quotes from Bédollière's *Histoire de la mode en France* :

> De ce prélat tel fut le sort
> Que sa barbe causa sa mort.

T. S. Gowing also accepts the story in his *Philosophy of Beards*, adding the picturesque details that the Dean, Prevôt, Chantre and Chapter, on this celebrated occasion, solemnly closed the brass gates of the chancel and pointed to the statutes *de radendis barbis*. He also adds the information that it was on the advice of Duprat's father, the Chancellor, that Francis I instituted the tax on clerical beards.[1] But the story is none the less highly suspect, as Dulaure shows. It may have been invented by the Abbé Faydit, a misopogon who wished to discredit beards and used this account in an attack on Jean Savaron, one of the ablest scholars who ever defended the beard clerical. Guillaume Major, a doctor of the Sorbonne, in his *Défense du feu M. Savaron*, claimed that, although there was some resistance to Duprat's beard, the Bishop asked for permission to attend a synod unshaven and that this was granted. He quoted several resolutions of the chapter confirming this permission.

This account certainly appears the more likely as Duprat was appointed Bishop of Clermont in 1529 and did not die until 1560 ; so that if he died of grief at his rejection by the Chapter then Old Rowley's *unconscionable time dying* was a poor effort by comparison. The *Biographie Universelle* attempts to reconcile the dates by implying that the clash took place after the Bishop had (apparently) long been installed—an unlikely hypothesis. The *Nouvelle Biographie Générale* is discreetly silent, and both Père Fangé and Father Seghers are openly sceptical.[2] However, even the modified and less dramatic account of the Affaire Duprat given by Dr. Major indicates some difference of opinion between the Bishop and his Chapter. And undoubtedly such clashes occurred, as Henry II of France found it necessary in a letter to the clergy of Troyes (dated December 27, 1551) to intervene in a

[1] The authenticity of this story is also accepted by Barbier de Montault (*Le Costume et les Usages Ecclésiastiques*, II, Cap 20, section 4). Can it be that Duprat was inspired by his ancient predecessor, Sidonius, in his enthusiasm for beards ?

[2] Duprat attended the Council of Trent ; and one thing which I looked for in vain among all these authorities was a reference to the heated dispute at that Council, when the Fathers are said to have pulled each other by the beard. Surely so notable a beard as that of the Bishop of Clermont would not have escaped ?

similar dispute. *Dear and well beloved,* he wrote (so the passage is quoted by Edmond Martène and Ursin Durand),[1]

It is said—but we doubt it—that you make a difficulty about receiving into your church our well beloved and trusty cousin, Anthony Caraciole, your bishop, without his being first shaved, on account of some statutes which you have been accustomed to observe. Therefore we have thought fit to write you these presents to request you that you will not insist in this matter . . . as we mean to send him for a short time to some place outside the kingdom, on business that concerns us, where we would not have him go without his said beard . . .

Battle of the Beards in France

There are many similar stories. The canons of Le Mans refused to accept Cardinal Jacques D'Angennes because of his beard, and even the king's requests proved ineffective until he sent a peremptory order. Jean de Morvilliers, Bishop of Orléans, was also refused admission by the Chapter because of his long beard, in 1552. For him the same excuse was made that served in the case of Anthony Caraciole—the story that his beard was necessary as he was going into foreign parts (an assumption which, as we have observed, has always been held a valid excuse for the Latin clergy to grow beards). The letter which caused the Chapter at Orléans to revise its decision—doubtless with some regret—explained that it was the royal wish that he should be accepted

> *sans s'arreter a ce qu'il porte Barbe . . . attendu qu'elle lui etoit nécessaire pour ses fonctions d'Ambassadeur en pays étrangers*

Anti-beard bishops

Antoine de Créqui was only admitted as Bishop of Amiens on production of letters patent from Charles IX—this Bishop's law-suit with the canons of the Chapter regarding his beard was a *cause célèbre* of its time. Pierre Lescot, Sieur de Clagny, the great architect, when made a canon of Notre Dame, experienced the same opposition, for the same reason, from his fellow canons at Paris. On the other hand Canel produces a few instances of bish-

[1] *Veterum Scriptorum et Monamentorum,* etc. (1724-33).

ops about this time trying to enforce shaving among reluctant subordinates—a reversal of what were clearly the usual rôles in this conflict. In 1550 Robert Cenalis, Bishop of Avranches, ordained fines for members of the Chapter who failed to present themselves *freshly shaven* at a council. The bishop wrote convincingly, both in prose and verse, on the subject. God, he said, calls us to sheep-like ways—he drives away those who are like goats, curses them and delights in their absence :

> *Nos vocat ad mores auctor pietatis ovillos*
> *Hircinos abigit, damnat, abesse jubet.*

One of the bishop's successors, François Péricard, was evidently still in difficulties in 1600, and on the retreat. In place of an absolute prohibition of beards, we find him asking his priests either to shave or at least to keep their beards *d'une longueur modeste et convenable*—to which he adds, significantly, *sans aucunes moustaches*. Claude de Sainctes, Bishop of Evreux, in the year 1576, forbade priests in his diocese to wear beards. But eighteen years earlier the Chapter at Rouen had already withdrawn all prohibitions. Their decision was submitted for approval to their Cardinal Archbishop, who evidently decided that *nihil obstat*, for he told the Chapter that he did not find the innovation contrary to the Glory of God. Not long afterwards the Chapter received a letter from Catherine de Medici, who was evidently unaware of the revolution that had taken place, for she asked if they would allow one of her clerical clients to wear a beard as long as a finger— *luy permettre de porter barbe de la longueur d'un doigt*. The Sorbonne, however, took a sterner view ; and in 1561, having deliberated the matter, the pandits of Paris published to the world their considered opinion—they held beards to be immodest, especially long ones.

Revival of the beard in Lombardy

Similar views were held by Archbishop Gian Battista Foppa, who presided in 1656 over a Provincial Council at Benevento. The people of this city were accused of retaining the long beards of their Lombard ancestors ; and Père Fangé even suggests that they had maintained an apostolic succession of beards from the

time of Rotharis, in spite of Charlemagne's efforts to suppress
them. But already at Benevento, in 1656, it was thought impossible to enforce shaving among the clergy, and all that the
Anti-Beard Party could extort from the Council was an order
that priests should cut their moustaches sufficiently short to avoid
defiling the sacrament :

  Ut Sacerdotes a superiore labro Barbam ita tondeant ne
salutare corporis & sanguinis sacramentum sumentibus impedi-
mentum afferant.

The Misopogons in retreat

  Such is the tendency of ecclesiastical regulations, especially in
the latter half of the sixteenth century. The Jesuit historian Jean
Hardouin, in his *Conciliorum collectio regia maxima*, gives several
decisions which illustrate this trend. At Mayence and Narbonne,
in 1549 and 1551 respectively, Provincial Councils ordered all
priests to shave (at least once a month, the Council at Narbonne decided). And ten years later the Parlement of Toulouse, apparently
encroaching on ecclesiastical ground, forbade the clergy to wear
beards. But Councils held at Rheims and Bagnères in 1583 insisted only on the shaving of the upper lip. Opposition to the
beard was evidently in retreat, but it clung fiercely to the preser-
vation of the sacraments from the hairs of the moustache. There
are, of course, exceptions—even throw-backs—in this general
tendency. At Rouen, in 1581, the previous decision to permit
beards even appears to have been reversed, and shaving enforced
once more for a while. Much would depend on the individual
taste of the bishop. More typical are two decisions at Malines—
the first in 1579, condemning the beard, and the second, in 1587
ordering only that the moustache should be kept clear of the upper
lip. Once more the last bastion of the Anti-Beard Party is clearly
the argument that hair polluted the chalice.

  The validity of this argument had already been hotly disputed
by the Italian priest and theologian, Valeriano Bolzani. As the
English version of his treatise (*Pro Sacerdotum Barbis Defensio*)
expresses the matter, God is not offended with hairs, *the whiche
serve to expresse the perfecte state of man*. In a passage of which part

has already been quoted at the head of this chapter, he says in my Tudor translation :

> I beseeche you, be heares so fylthy and greatlye to be despised, that they are not worthy to come near the blessed sacrament ? But foule nayles, scabby fyngers, a fylthy face, with all the reste of the bodye besyde may do it none unreverence.

The logic of Valeriano Bolzani

But next he strikes home with an accusation of inconsistency. We have observed that shaving in the Middle Ages and the sixteenth century was not a matter of daily practice and a cheek kept smooth. It was rough, awkward, and (by our standards) infrequent. If the objection to hairs is to be sustained, Valeriano argues, out of respect for the Sacrament, then shaving should be practised daily, as was the case with the priests of Egypt[1], but not with the Christian clergy of his own time—and he writes in the early sixteenth century, after some four hundred years of very ineffective shaving had been common among the priesthood. The reason did not tally with the actual practice. Let them, suggests Valeriano, *plucke out the heares by the rootes*, or at least shave daily, if they intend to censure beards.

The circumstances which occasioned this tract were—according to the author in his epistle dedicatory, to Cardinal Ippolito de' Medici—that there was a move on foot to persuade the Pope to renew the papal ban on clerical beards. In anticipation of this step the Cardinal had warned all the priests under his personal dominion that they should forthwith shave off their beards in order that they might be the first to set a good example and do with a good will what they would otherwise be compelled to do maugre their heads. The writer, though willing to obey his superior, nevertheless sets forward the objections held by certain men outstanding (he says) in wisdom, learning and virtue. The beard was something that Valeriano took very seriously. Who would dare to maintain, he said, that it was not the ornament of man, the symbol of his probity and justice, or that it did not give him a grave, stern look ?

[1] This statement regarding the Egyptian priests was incorrect. See page 29.

Valeriano and his English translator

Valeriano's treatise was published at Rome, in 1529, with the privilege of Pope Clement VII, who had every reason to sanction a defence of beards.   It had the great good fortune to be Englished in a rare edition of 1533, of which I know of but one copy, to be found in the British Museum, in a very fine and peculiarly legible black letter type, with an introduction to the English reader.   Here the writer is presented as *Valerian a greatte clerke of Italie*, which indeed he was, though little remembered today.   Among the observations in the translator's preface it may be noted that he says of shaving in Italy, at that time, that it *is as lyttel used there as beardes be here*.   Indeed, he considers that *in no realme have they bene less accepted* than in England, and of himself he writes that he has ever used to wear a beard *and have ben many tymes challenged and rebuked for the same;* which you may think strange in the year 1533, though I shall show that his experience was by no means unique.   But of himself the translator says little which is of value.   He argues that *if it be proved no unmete thynge for a prieste to weare a bearde, who shuld both in apparell and dedes shew a sad and an honeste example, it may seme so moche the more sufferable in a laye manne.* Which of the two he was himself, the reader must therefore conjecture for himself.

This translation shall now serve us, though on the good man's own admission it is free enough.   The argument will not be unfamiliar in its inception: *I thynke*, says Valeriano (through the mouth of his contemporary and admirer) *I thynke there is no man that wyll denye, but that a bearde shall become a good and an honeste man.* To deny this, he continues, is merely to assert a prejudice in despite of reason.   If, then, it is agreed that a beard becomes a good and honest face, *a fortiori* it is argued that *it is so moche the more meter for a prieste.*

Nothing filthy or dishonest in a beard

As for shaving, this author holds it womanish, and says of Scipio Africanus that he was ever called *a softe and a feminate fellow.*   And of Octavius Augustus, who followed Scipio very diligently (says Valeriano) we learn that he *was never so moche suspected to be of a femy-*

nate mynde by the baudy versis he wrote in the baynes, as by the often use of shaving. With regard to the objection to priests wearing beards, *what fylthyness* (asks he) *is in a berde ? For truely I can fynde in it nothynge filthy nor dishonest.* And so he proceeds first to define a beard as a garment for manly cheeks, given by nature for comeliness and health, shewing that the Romans so considered it of old, counting all who lacked this garment as naked and unclad. To be shaven Valeriano holds to be womanish, which is as much as to say, a thing of scorn. To have but little beard by natural endowment, he considers a misfortune to be bewailed ; for as, says he, pearls are esteemed the most precious for their greatness, *even so of the greatness a beard taketh his praise.*

Shaven men lose their teeth

Next, as to use (for this learned clerk would not allow that the beard was only for ornament) he says that it sucketh out the abundant and gross humours of the cheeks and by that means it preserveth the teeth long from perishing—*dentes diutius a putredine conservat*—and what more could you desire ? For as our author points out, most shaven men are toothless before their time or at the least they suffer from toothache. Indeed, why should Aesculapius himself have worn so notable a beard if it were not equally notable that to do so preserved the health of the body ?

And why, asks Valeriano, should men presume to think that where a beard is there can be no goodness, no holiness, no perfect religion ? Why should the bearded priest be despoiled like one that has forsaken his faith ? That the Law of Nature ordains beardedness is beyond doubt—what say the laws of God and Man ? To this end he cites Moses and the rest, so coming to the Divine Example, of which he confidently asserts that *there be certeyn men, which so descrive the face of Christ by knowledge of their fore fathers, that they affirme, he had a longe and a yelowe berde ; neyther he is none otherwyse peynted nor carven of the grekes, the latines, nor none other nations, as it is openly knowen.* And so with the apostles, says he— all bearded and none with a greater beard than St. Paul, as he is shown in colour and carving. As to St. James the Just, he repeats a story which I have often come upon (though the source is obscure) that this apostle was much praised, *bycause he never used shavynge nor annoyntyng, nother yet washing in baynes*. His justice, one might well imagine, lay in neither bathing nor shaving.

And now Valeriano's guns are trained upon the Fourth Council of Carthage, of which I have already said enough. But I may add here as an historical oddity that it is not without interest, in considering the English translation of Valeriano's work, that it was published in 1533, openly and in London, two years after Henry VIII had declared the English Church independent of Rome ; and that this treatise nevertheless is quite explicitly, as well as implicitly, papist in its doctrine. It is, in fact, a fairly faithful English version of a tract by a Catholic writer who, though he disputes the view traditionally held among Catholics in this matter of beards (which it was all the safer to dispute at a time when both Popes and Cardinals showed such heterodox chins) nevertheless argues from the authoritity of these dignitaries —a fact surely remarkable when we find such a book construed for the consumption of English readers under such a tyranny and at such a time. Indeed, the translator, in his preface to this papistical work, did not find it necessary to mention the breach with Rome, still less to apologise for translating it, complete with a dedication to a member of the Sacred College.

Pope Joan

But I will make a good guess at the cause why such a book was suffered to be printed in London ; for though it is by a clerk of the Catholic Church it contains much that must have been meat and drink to the Anti-Papal party. Why, says he, by this habit of shaving *the people was so disguised that men and women were scant knowen asunder (difficulter vir a fæmina internosceretur)*. Here we have it—Pope Joan is about to enter the argument : *And by this it happened (if the tale be trewe that is in everye mans mouth) that a woman was chosen pope of Rome* . . . Here indeed was a scandal for Tudor England to enjoy, with veiled references to the *cathedra stercoris*, that mysterious chair which was always used at Papal elections until the time of Leo X. Jean Crespin, in his *Estat de l'Eglise dès le temps des apôtres jusqu'à 1560* (Paris 1564) claimed—not without malice—that when the Cardinals had made the great error of choosing a woman for Pope *ils ordonnèrent qu'un diacre manierait les parties honteuses de celui qui serait élu pape, par dedans une chaise percée, afin qu'on scust qu'il est masle ou non.* To which he added that nowadays the cardinals gave such proof of their virility in the engendering of bastards that nobody could have any doubt ; for which reason the custom had been discontinued. This account of the *stercoraria* (which was undoubtedly used and is still in the Vatican Museum, as far as I know) is discussed at some length by Dr. Cabanès in his *Indiscrétions de l'Histoire*, where he quotes a proverb of the late fifteenth century :

> *Nul ne pouvait jouir des saintes clefs de la Rome*
> *Sans montrer qu'il avait les marques de vray homme*[1]

Unsolved riddle of the Stercoraria

Cabanès cites also the evidence of the Byzantine writer, Laonicus Chalcondylas on this subject (*De rebus Turcicis*, Paris, 1650) where the same explanation is given, which will also be found in a work by an unknown Venetian priest. A woodcut of 1671 depicts the ceremony, the investigator pronouncing the single word *Habet* ; and a similar illustration occurs in a History of Pope Joan published in 1758. Whatever its entertainment value, the story seems to have no solid foundation, though the chair remains a mystery which no doubt occasioned the invention of the legend and perhaps of Pope Joan herself. She too, I fear, is an unhistorical character ; the nearest thing to a female Pope was the illegitimate daughter of Alexander VI, whom he once left in charge of the Holy See. As to the famous seat itself, we know that the Popes in the sixteenth century made use of such conveniences :

> *Papa Pius quintus, ventres miseratus onustos*
> *Hocce cacatorium nobile fecit opus*

But such ancient *graffiti* cannot be specifically applied to the *stercoraria,* nor can we explain its use at a papal election ; and the official explanation that it was in order to dramatise Psalm CXIII, verse 7, which was sung on these occasions (. . . *and lifteth the needy*

[1] He would, in fact, be disqualified for the priesthood, let alone the papacy, without a special dispensation. The matter is learnedly discussed by Cabanès.

out of the dunghill) is unconvincing.[1] No wonder that credulous minds accepted an explanation which had all the advantages of being scandalous, though the chair was in use before the Pope Joan legend was ever bruited, and Corio's circumstantial account (. . . *e domesticamente toccatogli li testicoli* . . .) is manifestly fabulous.

Why (argues Valeriano) all this pother and ballyhoo when a beard would prove the point, *without any such wonderment* ? For myself I doubt his logic, for there have been bearded women, of whom I shall have something to say presently; and if there were ever a Pope Joan she could as well have worn a beard as carried the keys. But Valeriano finds here another *caveat* against the razor, for he cannot discover that any such inconvenience came by the means of beards.

Beards of mourning

Finally, citing what were then modern precedents, our author recalls that the Popes Julius II and Clement VII had both set an example of bearded chins. He speaks of bearded cardinals and (what is more surprising) of *poore priestis* who were bearded. The question is—*shall we devyse to renewe weake lawes* ? For to do so, maintains Valeriano, is not only to blame the *hyghe bysshoppe, prelates and other sadde men*, but to *damne Peter and Paul and all the appostels* . . . As to those who said (and it appears that such there were) that a shaven priest was the better for removing a token of sorrow and a heavy mind—for such they esteemed the beard to be—ought not priests most of all to mourn in this miserable world, when there was no man that had any cause to laugh ? So the whole case revolved itself finally that priests should wear beards in mourning for the state of Italy, as a meet expression of sober sadness and a symbol of the fact that they have been despoiled of all else.

[1] The seat was not actually a chaise percée, but a Roman chair used in the baths—a sort of *bidet*. Du Cange is unable to say when the use of this chair began, but quotes an account of the coronation of Boniface VIII (1294) in which it is mentioned, and says there is no reference to it before the tenth century. Baronius mentions the *Stercoraria sedes, in qua creati pontifices ad frangendos elatos spiritus considerent, unde dicta* (a theory upheld by Chambers in his *Book of Days*, where he says that this seat served to remind the Pope that he was, after all, but a mortal man). The lines about Pius V are from the *Ménagiana* of Gilles Ménage (Amsterdam, 1693). Article 1183 is among the missing material from Buckle's *Common Place Book*, and refers to the *Stercoraria* (see Appendix F).

CHAPTER IX

THE AUGUSTAN AGE OF THE PHILOPOGON

> Julius II, as we have seen, innovated in this point of
> discipline by letting his beard grow. Let us bear in mind
> that the Pope is not, strictly speaking, subject to a law
> purely human, merely ecclesiastical ; Julius II, therefore,
> cannot be called a transgressor of ecclesiastical canons . . .
>
> The Most Rev. Charles J. Seghers, D.D.

Dilemma for Orthodoxy

From this wise observation, in that back number of the
American Catholic Quarterly Review to which we have so often
referred, the reader will gather something of the delicacy of the
problem which arose when Bessarion was accepted into the Latin
Church, complete with his beard, as a member of the Sacred
College. An infallible Pope had made him a Cardinal, and before
long another infallible Pope had seen fit to imitate him. The
advocates of Church Discipline were not in an easy position.

But Valeriano had anticipated correctly the reaction against
bearded clergy, and we have already seen something of the battle as
it was fought out on the soil of France. Here, as in Spain, a
strong nationalist tendency was observable within the Catholic
Church, the Gallicans aiming at an independence of papal domination almost equal to that enjoyed by the schismatic Church of
England. The shadow of the Pope's beard did not fall beyond
the Alps, and the advocates of the razor in France did not much
care if their campaign implied a criticism of the Supreme
Pontiff, or even if it were interpreted as a personal attack upon
him.

Campaign of Charles Borromeo

In Italy the situation was very different, the more so as the Holy
Father was also a powerful temporal prince in the country. We
have already noticed the circumspection of the Archbishop of
Benevento in his limited attempt to revive canonical practice.
Equally cautious was the first move of St. Charles Borromeo.

By a decree of the Provincial Council at Milan (where he was then Archbishop) he warned all priests in 1565 against nourishing beards, and reminded them that the moustache should be kept short, *ut pili, in Sacrificio Missa, Christi Domini Corpus et sanguinem sumentem non impediant*. But in 1578 Charles went further. In the age when *non nutrire* was taken to mean that one should not grow a beard like a goat (*hircorum et caprarum more*), and many Churchmen disregarded even this limitation, St. Charles dared to re-assert even in Italy the traditional doctrine of many centuries. The fourth decree by the Synod held that year at Milan quoted the Fourth Council of Carthage, the views of Gregory VII and the whole Western tradition as a preliminary to ordering all priests to shave off their beards entirely.

Borromeo's shaving orders were, of course, such as would not now be considered very rigorous. His clerics were to shave once a fortnight, or more often if necessary. A man who had not shaved for two weeks would hardly, in our own days, be considered clean shaven. Nevertheless, this was Reaction in a big way.

His rapid promotion

This Archbishop of Milan was a man of some influence and power. His mother was a Medici, and his uncle, formerly the Cardinal de' Medici, on being crowned Pope as Pius IV, had not forgotten his relatives. Charles Borromeo had been a layman at that time, which had not precluded him from becoming a titular abbot before he was fourteen. Appointed Secretary of State for the Papal dominions (before his uncle had been Pope for a couple of weeks) he had been created cardinal-deacon about a week later, together with two other kinsmen of Pius IV. Nepotic zeal went even further ; and among the burdens loaded upon the shoulders of a young layman of twenty-two had been the administration of the Archbishopric of Milan, the spiritual needs of the See being relegated to deputies responsible to a young politician and man of letters at Rome who was not yet a priest. In the history of ecclesiastical sinecures even younger men, and mere boys, had been loaded with heavier responsibilities—or, at least, with their financial emoluments ; but few have spiritually survived the test as did St. Charles Borromeo.

Three years after this shoal of honours descended upon the young man, and in spite of all advice to the contrary (the Pope himself having counselled him to marry) Charles had made an unusual decision which amounted to transforming the administration of the See of Milan into a serious job. At the age of twenty-five he had been, within three months, ordained priest and consecrated bishop. Another three months had seen him a fully fledged Archbishop, as ready to take over his spiritual responsibilities as he had previously been to pull the wires at Rome, making his puppets dance to his tune at Milan. He had first visited the See of Milan at the age of twenty-seven, and the really strange thing about this story is that from that time until he died, nineteen years later, he really did live the life of a saint, and made strenuous efforts to remove the causes of that ecclesiastical corruption of which his own early career had been a mild example. His canonisation, only twenty-six years after his death, was still slightly reminiscent of the speed with which promotion had come to him in his life on earth.

The views of this remarkable man on the subject of beards are recorded in his pastoral, De barba radenda. A successor[1] of St. Charles in the See of Milan, was his cousin Federico Borromeo ; and it is not without interest that he wore a small beard, in spite of the desperate efforts of St. Charles to abolish the beard clerical. Archbishop Federico Borromeo also shared some of the spiritual favours which the Church then lavished upon young men of good birth and property, for he was made a Cardinal at the age of twenty-three.

According to the Catholic Encyclopedia the length of clerical beards decreased during the seventeenth century—no doubt due to the change in fashions rather than to a narrowing interpretation of nutrire—but they did not disappear altogether until the close of the century, when the influence of the French Court (which was establishing a pattern of beardlessness that lasted among

[1] Ten years after the death of St. Charles. An elegy on Federico was written by the Admirable Crighton, of which a translation appears in Harrison Ainsworth's romance on this remarkable Scotsman. Seghers observes that St. Charles himself wore a beard at the beginning of his episcopate. His pogono-phobia developed later.

laymen for a century and a half) combined with the efforts of Cardinal Orsini, Archbishop of Benevento, to bring about a general reform. [1] These two influences, mentioned by the *Catholic Encyclopedia,* indicate that what was a return to mediæval tradition, in the case of the clergy, might not have been brought about if it had not coincided with a modern fashion that was almost universal and quite unconnected with clerical practice or bees in the biretta.

Protestantism and Pogonotrophy

Among those who fought for the Cause, Valeriano did not stand alone.   The Reformation produced a host of bearded Protestants, many of whom saw a Papist plot in every razor.   Rudolf Hospinian (1547-1626), a Swiss Calvinist, wrote and published in 1609 a work entitled *De Monachis : hoc est De Origine et Progressu . . .* (and so forth, for the title rumbles on like a wheelbarrow on crazy paving).   Pages 67-70 of this treatise will be found to contain a defence of beards.   In England the Reformation probably assisted the return of the beard.   In the very year that Henry VIII declared himself head of the Church (and where could England have found a more pious founder for her national religion ?) John Longland, Bishop of Lincoln, ordered a Fellow of Oriel College, Oxford, to give up wearing a beard.   But the Bishop was too stout a defender of the Royal Supremacy to continue long in such a course when the new National Pope—following the example of Julius II—was a bearded monarch.   We hear no more in England of priests persecuted for their whiskers, though most of the Protestant Martyrs under Mary Tudor were (as T. S. Gowing proudly reminds us) *burnt in their Beards.*

Literature and the Beard Question

Much pogonological lore is to be found in Tom I of the *Amphitheatrum* of Caspar Dornavius (Hanover 1619).   First (pages

---

[1] *Frustra S. Carolus hortatus est clericos,* wrote Wernz and Vidal, *Quod verba Sancti Caroli non effecerunt id pruritus imitandi mores Ludovici XIV præsertim ab anno 1680 denuo in praxim deduxit.* (*Jus Canonicum,* 1928). For Orsini's decrees see Barbier de Montault (*Le Costume,* etc., II, 20, 4).

318-328) there is the dialogue of Antony Hotoman[1]—in the main a summary of some ancient practices which we have already surveyed, with the views of ancient authorities. The form used is that of a discussion between *Pogonias* and *Misopogon*, who hurl at one another chunks from Clement of Alexandria, Plutarch, the classics, Julian the Apostate, and others, with references to the beards of the barbarous Lombards or the savagery of Cæsar's Britons, who shaved below the mouth. (Pogonias crowns his case with Aesculapius, *qui prolixa barba semper a pictoribus & poetis fingitur*.) Next follows the treatise of Valeriano, *Pro Sacerdotum Barbis*, and on pages 335-338 Christian Becman discourses *De Barbigenio Hominis*. His theses are unfortunately as barren of wit and wisdom as those of Thomas Sagittarius, whose *Exercitatio Extraordinaria de Barbigenio* (pages 338-343) adds nothing to our knowledge, though it raises some interesting questions. Why, asked this Professor of Logic and Metaphysics, did the Romans refrain from shaving at the time of the public games ? Why the beard philosophic ? Who first grew a beard ? Why were red beards held in such low esteem ?

Barbæ Maiestas

The last in this series (classified by Dornavius under *Barba*) is Johannes Barbatus, who wrote *Barbæ Maiestas, hoc est De Barbis Elegans, Brevis et Accurata Descriptio*. As may be imagined from the short title (for there is, of course, much more of it) this is largely an eulogy of beards in general. But there is also a very strong plea for the beard sacerdotal, in particular. Peter and the Apostles were bearded, claims Barbatus, proud of his beard-brotherhood with these holy men. As for the Fourth Council of Carthage, he gives yet another version of it, citing the forty-fourth canon as *Clerici neque comam nutriant neque Barbam radant*. Or rather, that is how it should read, but *lectio enim illa est corrupta*, the text has been cooked, and *radant* omitted—a thing not beyond possibility, as he shows by other and more obvious corruptions of old writings.[2] The celebrated physician, Andrew Boorde, wrote a book against beards, unfortunately lost to posterity. Nothing

[1] First published at Antwerp in 1586.

[2] The evidence for the corruption of the forty-fourth canon was also discussed by Jacques Sirmond in his edition of Sidonius (1618).

is known of it except through the reply by a man called Barnes :
The treatyse answerynge the boke of Berdes (about 1543).

It grieves me to quit the subject of clerical beards, the more so
as I fear I can never again return to it, so far as Rome is concerned.
When the Augustan Age of archiprotopapal pogonotrophy ended
(not with a bang, but a whimper, to steal a High Anglican
autobiography) it left us a Church deforested forever. We shall
never again see bearded Cardinals and Popes ; so before I pass on
to the Tudor and Stuart laity, I intend to present a fine specimen
of a bearded Cardinal, who lived in the time of Elizabeth and
James I.

John Bulwer, when mentioning the cases in which dandies of
his time enclosed their beards (we have already noticed the use
of such contrivances for the moustache) quotes an observation that
will serve as an excellent introduction to our next performer.
The quotation concerns a man of whom it is said :

That the fashion of his Beard was just for all the world like
those upon your Flemish Jugs, and that a nights he puts it in a
presse, made of two thin trenchers, scrued wonderfully close
. . . that it may come forth the next morning with even corners,
bearing in grosse the forme of a broome, narrow above and
broad beneath, his Mustachoes, Ruler-wise, straight and levell
as a line.

Greybeard Jugs

The description of the beard is that of the *Cathedral* style,
and the Flemish jugs were those famous Greybeard Jugs made by
his enemies as caricatures of Cardinal Bellarmine—canonised in
modern times as St. Robert Bellarmine. This satirical delf went
out from the Lowlands to all parts of the world, finding (it would
seem) a particularly eager welcome in Scotland, where *Greybeards*
are frequently found in literary references. The jugs were also
known at one time as *Bellarmines*, but seem to have been familiar
as Greybeards, long after their origin had been forgotten, among
people who were unlikely ever to have heard of the Cardinal.
Indeed, as Chambers points out in his *Book of Days* (Vol. I, 371-372,
where there is a useful note on these jugs) the *Greybeard* became
eventually a name merely for the vessel, from which both beard

and face had disappeared—*sic transit gloria barbæ*—a thing without a soul.

Orthodoxy of Bellarmine

A more devout Catholic than St. Robert Bellarmine it would certainly be hard to find. Writing of the papacy (*de Romano Pontifice*, IV, 5) he went so far as to state that—although the Catholic Faith teaches that every virtue is good and every vice evil (a matter, one would have thought, rather of definition than of doctrine)—yet, if the Pope should err and order vices or prohibit virtues (*si autem Papa erraret, præcipiendo vitia vel prohibendo virtutes*), the Church would be bound to believe vices to be good and virtues to be evil, unless it wished to sin against conscience :

teneretur Ecclesia credere vitia esse bona, virtutes
esse malas, nisi vellet contra conscientiam peccare

Greater faith hath no man than this, that he lay down both his virtues and his reason and believe what Papa tells him to believe.

Like Father Seghers (witness his memorable dictum on the beard of Julius II, which heads this chapter), Cardinal Bellarmine was well-equipped to cope with the intricacies of the beard situation, and able to rationalise its contradictions. For Bellarmino was a Jesuit ; and one of the great Catholic critics of the Society of Jesus in the seventeenth century remarked that a logician must be either very unfortunate or very stupid if he cannot find exceptions to every conceivable rule. That Pascal had the Jesuits in mind is clear enough ; for they were—as they still are—among the foremost controversialists and logic-choppers in the Church. Granted that all Jesuits I have ever met have had both charm and charity—major graces—I would answer with more assurance for the fact that Jesuits are wise as serpents than I would for the belief that they are harmless as doves. In the art of reconciling opposites and of finding those exceptions of which Pascal spoke (whereby most things can be justified if one has the inclination) they were famous from the beginning; and in the historic controversy of Pascal versus *Probabilism* I am on the side of Pascal every time.

Bellarmine's Beard did not trip him up

It was, then, with all the armoury of casuistry—a word with an innocuous meaning which has earned ill repute through the doubtful dealings of moral sophists—that Bellarmine, the great controversialist of his time, entered upon the question of beards. Indeed, he had need of all his training from the outset—for (like his contemporary, Cardinal Baronius, whose paradoxical position we have already observed) Bellarmine was an exponent of the propriety of priestly shaving, who nevertheless wore a beard himself. I was frankly so perplexed by this fact when I first came to consider St. Robert's contribution to the subject that I decided to consult some Jesuit scholars before being so rash as to offer an explanation myself. I was not long in obtaining very courteous replies from two learned Fathers, to the following effect.

Father James Brodrick, S.J., who gave me considerable help in tracing references and in the use of books at Farm Street Church—no small kindness to a complete stranger—offered his opinion that Bellarmine wore a beard because his health was bad. He thought that most Jesuits of that time were not bearded—an opinion which I would not be so bold as to dispute, coming from such an eminent scholar who was playing on the home field. But the statement surprised me on account of the number of bearded Jesuits I had myself noticed—if my engravings of seventeenth century characters are to be relied upon, as I think most of them are. (I see that Fairholt mentions another instance.) However, I yield to the scholarship of Father Brodrick and can accept the view that the shaven Jesuits were nevertheless considerably in the majority. We have still this beard of Bellarmine to explain. If it was a matter of health it is at least odd that it coincided with fashion. I cannot recall any priest in the eighteenth century, when beards were abhorred throughout Europe, growing one for his health.

A Beard cannot be kept secret

Probabilism might, for all I know, explain the coincidence of health and fashion weighing down all the canons, decrees and long traditions which Bellarmine himself quotes in favour of shaving. But even so neither *probabilism*, nor I, nor even Father Brodrick can explain why the Cardinal chose to damn by implication in his writings a fashion to which he himself, the whole College of Cardinals and the Popes of his time conformed. Many a preacher has condemned in public the sins he practised in private ; but a beard, if it be a sin to wear it, cannot of all things be called a secret sin. To wear it and yet to condemn it is surely asking for trouble. And another very odd thing is that neither then nor in later years did any of those who wrote against Bellarmine, either on things in general or on the matter of beards in particular, charge him with this glaring inconsistency. Like Baronius, he was often attacked for his opinions, and the accuracy of his factual statements was frequently challenged. But neither of these Cardinals appears to have been taunted with wagging a bearded chin in defence of the razor.

Probabilism and pogonotrophy

Father E. A. Ryan, S.J., of Woodstock College, Maryland, was no less willing to help than his colleague at Farm Street. His case was, firstly, that Bellarmine said very little about beards, which is true enough ; but he said enough to draw the fire of the pro-beard party. As to the Fourth Council of Carthage, St. Robert—says Father Ryan—merely quotes the forty-fourth canon without defending it. Here again I must interject to point out that, though this is true enough, Bellarmine quotes only one reading (without the *radat*), as we shall see. So that it is still remarkable that such a scholar should have preferred a version which was not only doubtful but so highly embarrassing to himself. Surely if the text was even in doubt (as the Saint must have known it was[1]) then *probabilism* or some equally convenient doctrine should have indicated that the beneficiary of that doubt should be one's own chin. Or—even more important—that of the Supreme Pontiff. However, it is time we looked at the Cardinal's actual words.

[1] Jean Savaron and the Jesuit, Jacques Sirmond (an intimate friend of Bellarmine) also Labbe, Hardouin, and the eminent lawyer and Lutheran apologist, Molinæus, all took the opposite view, some of them citing at length the palæographic evidence ; for there were many ancient copies of the forty-fourth canon in which *radat* was found—including one at Paris and one at the Vatican. Surely so eminent a scholar as Bellarmine cannot have been ignorant of the existence of these MSS ?

It is in Lib. ii of the second General Controversy of St. Robert Bellarmine, *De Membris Militantis Ecclesiæ*, that the subject of beards is discussed.   Lib. ii, *De Monachis*, will be found, with the rest of the *Secunda Controversia Generalis* in the second tome of the edition of 1601 (Bellarmine's *Disputationes*) ; and in the fortieth chapter, *De habitu & tonsura Monachorum*, this most erudite Jesuit quotes ancient authorities to prove the antiquity of the tonsure and of shaving among monks.   Among his citations he mentions the forty-fourth canon of the Fourth Council of Carthage, which, says he, *prohibit Clericos alere comam aut barbam*.   Of the objectors to Catholic tradition and usage he says that their arguments from the Old Testament have no more value than the rest of the old law, such as that relating to circumcision and to sacrifices.   The Jews were forbidden to imitate their ungodly neighbours ;   and Jeremiah laughed at the priests who shaved their heads and beards, merely because they did so in honour of wooden gods who could not reward their worshippers (*quia id faciebant in honorem Deorum ligneorum, qui non poterant remunerare cultores suos*).   But this was no longer relevant, said St. Robert.

Bellarmine with the soft pedal

Nevertheless, Cardinal Bellarmine does not appear in his most vigorous vein in this controversy.   He admits that the habit of shaving is not so old as that of the tonsure, and that most of the early Fathers advocated the latter without mentioning the former —the possible exception being Pope Anicetus, and the authority in this case a doubtful one.   The hesitation of Bellarmine to defend Catholic tradition on this point with his usual vigour is, I think, obvious by comparison with his writings on other subjects.   But his position is still perplexing.   Father Ryan points out that Bellarmine was here writing for monks, and that monastic rules did not apply to himself and other *clerici regulares*.   Yet his quotation of the forty-fourth canon applied indiscriminately to all clergy, and he chose to read it as an order not to nourish beards.   Of course, *barbam nutrire* or *alere* may not mean simply growing one, as we have already suggested—a revised interpretation with which Father Thurston explains the whole revolution begun by Bessarion and Julius II.   So thinks Father Ryan, in the present instance. The prohibition, he suggests, applies to keeping a beard in elegant condition, and he encloses in his courteous letter a small print of St. Robert to illustrate his thesis that the Cardinal's beard was *scrimpy* and *scanty*. Surely no one could say that it was nourished ?

Precise size of the beard Bellarminical

At any rate, concludes Father Ryan, *be as kind as you can to St. Robert*. I hope I shall not too greatly disappoint him. I assure the entire world that I would not have grudged Cardinal Bellarmine as great a beard as that of Vermeijen, the friend of Charles V, who kept his beard in a velvet bag because it would otherwise have tripped him as he walked. But as to the size of this beard Bellarminical, it varies, like the moon. I will discount the testimony of the Greybeard Jugs ; what the caricaturists said is not evidence. But Father Brodrick in his admirable book on Bellarmine reproduces an engraving by Valden of Liége, dated some time before 1620, where St. Robert appears with a Cathedral Beard. This broad, square-cut style was so called because—so Randle Holme tells us—*bishops and grave men of the church, anciently did weare such beards*. The word *anciently* should not be taken too literally : the style is characteristic only of the bearded period in the sixteenth and seventeenth centuries. Bellarmine leaves us, in fact, exactly where we found ourselves in the last chapter, completely unable to fathom the meaning which those who wore such beards could possibly have attached to the word *nutrire*.

The Beard as a Mask for Treason

While cardinals and popes were growing beards which they undertook not to *nourish*, the beard was making great progress also among the laity. But laymen, too, had some prejudice to overcome. Once more, in France, we shall notice a discrepancy between the court fashion set by Francis I and attempts made—with his sanction—to keep the beards of lesser folk in check. Cabanès (*Curiosités de la Médicine*, Vol. I) says that in 1525 the people were forbidden to wear long beards *qui . . . semblent cacher quelque dessein pernicieux contre le repos de l'Etat*. It is a curious reason, the first of its kind—that the beard is a manner of mask to hide pernicious designs against the peace of the State, which designs (presumably) would be so plainly written on a man's face that without a beard he would soon be detected.

An Edict of Beards, in 1523, had already forbidden French magistrates and lawyers, even litigants, to appear in court with long beards. In 1536 Francis Oliver, *Maître des Requêtes* was refused admission into the Paris *Parlement* on account of his long beard; and Gentien Hervet (*De Radenda Barba Oratio*) even speaks of a bearded plaintiff at Toulouse, who was told by the *Parlement* that he should have justice when he shaved. A similar story is told by Dulaure of an advocate at the Parlement of Paris, who was ordered by the First President, Pierre Lizet, to cut off his beard immediately, or the court would not listen to him. Dulaure even claims, on the authority of Regnault d'Orléans (*Pogonologie, etc., Rennes,* 1589) that a certain magistrate at that time ordered all the millers of his district to remove their beards.

Inconsistency of Francis I

Canel speaks of similar efforts to check the Beard Movement in Normandy, where judges at Rouen were forbidden to wear beards in 1540, because *ce n'est pas là habits de juges*. Each year the Rouen Parlement renewed its orders to all its members to shave their beards and to let their hair grow. Incredible as it may seem, Francis I is found forbidding magistrates in 1540 to wear *barbes . . . et autres habits dissolus*. The way in which this bearded monarch abused and persecuted beards, both lay and clerical, is as strange as the defence of shaving by bearded Bellarmine.

Bearded Men and Orphans

Similar opposition was experienced in England. In the Guildhall Records Office, there is a curious Order of the Court of Aldermen, made in the year 1543.[1] It bears all the marks of

[1] Letter Book Q.87; 10 July, 35 Henry VIII. The Order is quoted by Sidney Young as *An Acte Agaynst Bearded Men,* and it is described as an Act (i.e., of the Common Council) in the margin of this MS., also of another MS. copy at the Guildhall. It is nevertheless not actually an Act but an Order of the Court of Aldermen, as stated above. In either case it would, of course, have applied only to the City of London; but the second copy at the Guildhall will be found under Repertory 10 folio 343b of the Court of Aldermen, leaving no doubt as to its actual character.

having been inspired by the Barber-Surgeons, fearful of losing their customers. As the Order is of some length, I have modernised the English.

Item, for divers and sundry considerations and causes moving this Court, it is this day ordered & decreed & established by the same that from henceforward there shall be no citizen or other inhabitant of this City using or having a great beard (*greate berde*) of more notable prolixity or length than other the said Citizens of this City do now use or have heretofore of late years used to wear, either be inhabited, permitted or suffered to receive or take any orphanage into his hands and custody, albeit that he would find never so good sureties for the same. . . . And it is also assented and agreed that no person having any such beard shall be admitted by redemption into the liberties and freedom of this City as long as he shall wear any such beard (*were eny such berde*).

The curious use of the word inhabited (*inhabited, permitted or suffered*) may be noticed—it is not to be found in any dictionary that I have consulted, though I understand from better scholars than myself that this use is not uncommon in sixteenth century legal documents. What will perhaps strike the reader as most curious is that long-bearded men are considered unsuitable to have the custody of orphans, or (which is more probable) that the denial of this right was regarded as a punishment. Doubtless the wardship of an orphan, if he had enough property left to him, could be quite a profitable undertaking. One is reminded of an Arab proverb which says that *the barber practises on the orphan's head*.[1] The Court of Aldermen, for those divers and sundry considerations and causes which they did not think fit to specify, decided that nobody should practise on the orphan's head unless he paid tribute to the Barber-Surgeons.

A project of the Peruque Makers

The barbers were certainly not above bringing a little influence

[1] But not in these islands. Witness the evidence of an Account Book of 1680 : *To Jamie Gray to buy a sheep head and soap to learne him to barbarize*, oo. 3. 6. (*Notes and Queries*, 11th S., IX, 386).

to bear when their interests were threatened. Many years later, when the peruke makers—who practised a mystery or feat closely allied to barbery and were included in their Company eventually —found that there was a decline in the eighteenth century wearing of wigs, they wanted to petition the king on the subject, in 1764, as Sidney Young tells us (*Annals of the Barber-Surgeons*, page 166) :

> We most humbly hope not to be too bold in wishing Perukes may soon be as much in fashion as the wearing of hair is at present, which will increase the revenue, give happiness to the indigent and distressed Peruke Makers and increase the many unmerited Favours We as a Company have received from Royal Hands.

What exactly the king was supposed to do about it, short of ordering his subjects to cut off their hair so as to provide employment for the indigent and distressed Peruke Makers, I do not know. But in 1764 the Barbers were perhaps too respectable to descend to such tricks; their Court of Assistants considered the proposed petition, but rejected it.

We must return to the Tudors. Mrs. Charles Ashdown, in her *British Costume during XIX Centuries*, remarks that the fashion of wearing a beard appears to have been introduced by the king (i.e. Henry VIII) to which she curiously adds that *among continental nations the old fashion of being clean shaven was retained, thus affording us another example of the strong individuality of the king*. This is a typical historical bungle—facts adjusted to fit a theory.[1] We have already noticed the progress of the beard in other countries, in spite of opposition to it. In England there was the same opposition and the same obstinacy eventually wore it down. But Valeriano Bolzani's English translator was probably right in saying that the English (when he wrote in 1533) were less addicated to beards than any other nation.

Beards penalised at Lincoln's Inn

The Burghmote books of Canterbury mention fines paid in

[1] Even more extraordinary is a statement in *The History of the Surgeons' Company*, by Dr. Cecil Wall (1937) that *in the Tudor period beards went out of fashion* (page 18). Rees's *Cyclopædia* has some similar historical howlers about beards, which are hard to explain.

1542 by the Sheriff and another person for wearing beards—three shillings and fourpence by the Sheriff and one shilling and eight-pence by his fellow delinquent. In the same year we find an order that no fellow of Lincoln's Inn who wore a beard should dine at the Great Table, as Dillon mentions in his glossary (article on Beards in Vol. II of *Costume in England*, by F. W. Fairholt). In 1550 there is another order at Lincoln's Inn, this time forbidding members to wear beards of more than two weeks' growth. If found guilty more than twice, the offender is to be expelled—though it is not clear how a fortnight's growth was then assessed. Three years later the authorities at Lincoln's Inn were still fighting what was evidently a losing battle : those who wore beards were now to incur fines and loss of commons. But these desperate efforts proved ineffective and the statutes were soon repealed. [1]

Henry VIII had died in 1547. Beards were already flourishing in the time of Edward VI, good specimens being worn by the Protector Somerset and his brother, the Lord High Admiral, that rollicking ruffian who was the first lover of the Princess Elizabeth, at the cost of his head. By 1555 beards were common enough in London for the Court of Assistants of the Barber-Surgeons (in a Minute of October 1) to order that no one should shave, wash a beard, or trim any man with any instrument or to make clean teeth upon Sundays. This was in the time of Mary Tudor, during whose brief reign an effort was made to prevent Com-moners from wearing a beard of more than three weeks' growth, under a penalty of forty shillings.

As late as 1558, in the first year of Elizabeth's reign, an attempt was made to tax beards according to the age and social standing of their proprietors. Once more many bearded men had to consider whether they could afford three shillings and fourpence. But the following year all orders penalising beards were repealed. The way appeared to be clear at last for that great crop of beards which, in its infinite variety, was to characterise the age of Shakespeare.

[1] Nares, in his *Glossary of Shakespeare*, deals with these measures, quoting contemporary authorities.

A shock to the City of London

Edward Clodd, in the *Encyclopædia of Religion and Ethics* (v. Beard) says that Stow in his *Survey of London* mentions the beard of a Lord Mayor of London as a matter as scandal as late as 1563. This Lord Mayor was Sir Thomas Lodge, an enterprising merchant who appears to have been among those responsible for originating the African slave trade. (Among other activities, he claimed that, by procuring human skulls as drinking vessels for men suffering from lead poisoning, he had cured them—he was truly a versatile genius.) Of Sir Thomas's beard Stow is reported to have said that he was the first that ever ventured thus to deform his office, and that the City hardly supported the shock.[1] One might have thought that there were things about the Lord Mayor more outrageous than his beard ; but I have no doubt that it was a matter of deeply-rooted custom and tradition. (I doubt if, even today, we have advanced very much in this respect. Like those Barber-Surgeons who were not shocked at hanging, but outraged by a good corpse sitting up on the kitchen table, most of my English contemporaries can stomach the thought of ritual murder, but would be pained if the judge forgot his wig or adjusted the Black Cap at a jaunty angle over one ear.)

Toothpicks parked in beard

The frontispiece to Saxton's *Atlas of England and Wales* (1579) shows the allegorical figures of *Geography* and *Astromony* with vast and bushy beards. Such, perchance, was the beard of Gaspard de Coligny, the Huguenot admiral (son of a *renegado* Cardinal, who was married in all his scarlet robes). According to Brantôme,

---

[1] There is an unsolved mystery here, for among Richardson's illustrations to Granger there is a portrait of Sir Thomas Lee as Lord Mayor of London in 1558. He wears a thick and bushy beard with long *handle-bar* moustaches. I do not know whether this portrait is reliable ; but if it is Stow made a curious mistake considering that he was living in London at the time, and should surely have known about this earlier Sir Thomas (whose name is more commonly spelt Leigh) and that Lodge's beard was not such an innovation as he suggests. But the mystery is all the greater because I cannot find the reference quoted by Edward Clodd in either of the editions of Stow's *Survey* that I have consulted. I hesitate to suggest that Clodd *invented* the great scandal of 1563, which would be even harder to explain than the carelessness of Stow if he is correctly quoted.

Coligny used his beard as a sort of pin-cushion in which to park his toothpicks, when not in use. In France, as we have seen, the beard fought a long battle for its existence, but obtained a complete triumph before its ultimate decline. There was a slight set-back, during the reign of Henry III (who was shaven himself) but even some of the King's *mignons* at that time were bearded, in spite of their elaborate imitation of feminine habits—satirised by d'Aubigny, who also lampooned shaving. (They used a night mask of flour, cheese and white of egg to preserve their complexions, like the famous *Poppæana Pinguia*, Poppy's Paint, invented by Nero's wife. Those who were bearded set their beards with coloured wax. They also plucked their eye-brows, and went to bed wearing gloves soaked in ointment.) The bearded fashion in France, which had begun as a court vogue in the time of Francis I, opposed by grave and elderly men, was to end as a characteristic of the elderly and grave, derided by the courtiers of the late seventeenth century, who made increasing inroads with the razor until the last vestige of beard and moustache had disappeared. Fangé records that magistrates and prelates eventually clung longest to their beards—among them that Bishop Jean Pierre Camus, whose use of the beard in his sermons I have already mentioned.

French beard styles

The variety of sixteenth century beards is imposing. In France Aubril wrote in his *Essai sur la Barbe et sur l'art de se raser* (Paris 1860) of *barbes pointues, carrées, rondes, en éventail, en queue d'hirondelle, en feuille d'artichaut*, also of *barbes à la Ligue* and *barbes en Satyre*,[1] all of which flourished in the time of Henry IV. And he assures us, on the authority of Saint-Foix, that men spent as much time on their beards as the most painstaking coquettes upon their toilet, brushing them, perfuming them and enclosing them for the night in those *bigotelles* which we have already noticed.

In Germany we have a similar history. Max von Boehn, in *Die Mode*, mentions the opposition to beards, the new fashion being attacked by Geiler von Kaisersberg and others as effeminate—a curious conception, but a true echo of Bishop Serlo. Magdeburg

[1] I cannot resist the observation that the original bearded Silenoi were *horse-dæmons*. The Rolleston Riddle seems inescapable.

was at that time ruled by Protestant Archbishops—temporal
princes with an ecclesiastical title. (Eventually, in 1648, this
Archbishopric became an hereditary Duchy, without any notice-
able difference or any appreciable loss to the kingdom of Heaven.)
Sigismund, who was Archbishop in 1564, in that year banned
beards, but the tide of fashion could not long be stemmed.
Typical figures of other countries show the same vogue : Tycho
Brahe (1546-1601) wore a short beard with a very long moustache.
Grotius, a generation later, wears a moustache and square beard.
But Spain, before all European countries, seems to have led the
fashion. Indeed, the Spaniards even appear to have forestalled
Pope Julius II ; for a woodcut of 1493, on the title page of an
Italian book, shows Ferdinand of Castile with a pointed beard.

Discovery of the New World and the Old Beard

This Italian book is a rare translation by Giuliano Datis of the
first letter of Christopher Columbus, describing the discovery of
the West Indies—*La lettera dellisole che ha trouato nuouamente il Re
dispagnan,* done into *ottava rima* and published at Florence in the
year of the discoverer's return. In the woodcut the Spanish king
is shown, seated upon his throne in the foreground of a scene
which includes those *doom-burdened caravels* of Columbus, also the
inhabitants of the New World. The pointed beard of the king is,
however, all that really concerns me in this book. The woodcut
shows at one stroke that Spain discovered the beard even before
Christophero Colombo discovered America : in both matters the
Spaniards clearly had the lead. It is almost impossible to imagine
a conquistador or a Devonshire pirate of the Spanish main without
a beard : if they had not existed it would have been necessary to
have invented them.

Indeed, they enjoyed a respect almost distinct from that due to
the wearer—witness the beard of Sir Thomas More, which had
not committed treason and was so carefully saved from the
headsman's axe. In like predicament Sir Walter Raleigh refused
to have his beard trimmed while he was waiting to learn his fate
—there was a law-suit pending, he said, betwixt himself and the
King, respecting this head, so until the matter was settled the
beard should not be touched. And the Master Butler of Pem-

broke Hall, in *Pierce Penilesse* had *a Beard that is a better Gentleman than all thy whole body*.

Beard of the Gentleman Adventurer

Note well that it is the king of Spain's *beard* that Drake singes at Cadiz—he does not tweak his nose or kick him in the pants. The metaphor is geographically eclectic. Even in 1744, when Zachary Grey was annotating *Hudibras*, he could comment that it was deemed as dishonourable to be pulled by the beard, in Spain, as to be *kicked on the seat of honour in England* (though what beards the Spaniards had to pull when Dr. Grey was writing I cannot imagine). *To beard* has always expressed offer of insult with an implication of courage, e.g. in bearding the lion in his den. Repton compares the French phrase *faire la Barbe à quelqu'un* and the Italian (*fa la barba ad uno*) with the use of this metaphor as found in Spenser and Shakespeare.[1] In *The Honest Whore* the insult of cutting off a man's beard is regarded as worse than cuckolding him.

It is the Spaniard who sets the fashions of the sixteenth century—who else but the successful swashbuckler?—and the jaunty morion he borrowed from the Moors crowned a head which we all recognise today as that of the Gentleman Adventurer. The moustache is well trimmed, the beard clipped to a short point and compelled—if necessary with the aid of starch—to ride like a bow-sprit on the chin, a pirate's challenge to the Universe.

But while such becomes the standard, variety survives. Long curling moustaches, for example (without a beard) have always been the chosen badge of villainy ; and to this rule the Elizabethans were no exception. In *Arden of Feversham* a knave (one Jack Fitten) is thus described :

> His chin was bare, but on his upper lip
> A mutchado, which he wound about his ear.

[1] The Italian also has *A far questo tu non ci hai barba*, meaning you haven't the guts to do it. Sebastian Cobbarruvius tells of a Jew who planned to avenge himself on a dead Spaniard by plucking his beard. The dead man sat up and the intruder, not unnaturally, fled. Compare the story on page 140 (footnote). The *Cads beard*, sometimes mentioned in Elizabethan literature, did not signify what the words would mean today. *Cad* is probably a corruption of Cadiz, and further evidence of Spanish influence.

Who would suspect such a man of harbouring honest intentions ? Indeed, there is, as we have already suggested, always something sinister to be said about a moustache, and a long one is especially liable to suspicion. Stubbes, in his *Anatomy of Abuses*, describing the fops of his time, noted with disgust *how their mowchatowes must be preserved and laid out, from one cheke to another, yea, almost from one eare to another*. (They were then turned up like horns, he said.) And *monstrous muchaches* were among the terrifying phenomena encountered by one of Hakluyt's Elizabethans in his voyages.

Monstrous Moustaches

Another traveller, of an earlier period, (Josafa Barbaro, whose travels in the fifteenth century were published in English about a hundred years later) makes it clear that even in a shaven age the moustache was an object of greater horror than the beard proper. William Thomas's translation of the *Travels of Josafa Barbaro into Tana and Persia* describes the traveller's horror at the people of Georgia. The men here, it appears,

> have very fylthie apparill and most vile customes. They go with their heades rounded and shaven, leaving only a little heare, aftre the maner of our abbotts . . . *and they suffer their mostacchi to growe a quarter of a yarde longer than theirbe ardes.* [1]

(In case the term should be unfamiliar, a marginal note explains that *Mostacchi is the berde of the upper lyppe*.)

Monstrous moustaches were therefore avoided by most men in Tudor times, and even beards of great length became a subject of ridicule towards the end of the sixteenth century. The fashion moved in the same circle that we have observed in France, though even as late as 1587 Harrison (in his *Description of England*) noticed that many old men wore no beards at all. For us, in the present day, the beard is still mentioned figuratively as an attribute of old age, merely because we have passed from a bearded epoch (that of the late Victorians) into a shaven one. But as an emblem of age, the beard is already outdated—our own old men of today are, for the most part, shaven ; and the few beards one sees are

[1] Not impossible, if Dickens is to be credited. He said the moustaches of the Hungarian general Haynau were about half a yard long.

generally to be found on young men. So we are already approaching, perhaps, a situation similar to that described by Harrison, when the clean shave may once more become the mark of the elderly and conservative.

The beard in modern America

But as yet we have only a mere handful of beards to show—they are the exception even in Chelsea ; and it is not many years since a writer in the *New Statesman and Nation*[1] said that a bearded man in America enjoyed all the privileges of a bearded woman in a circus. This article was concerned with the possible return of the beard in the United States (which he regarded as the most clean-shaven country in the world) grounding his speculations on the retrogressive tendencies—much more pronounced today—of feminine fashions, which were already observable.

The beard, however, was far more common among the young gallants of the period described by Harrison. It was not merely the Elizabethan equivalent (if such there were) of the parlour bolshevik, the Chelsea artist, the minor poet or the young man whose beard is his only hope of distinction, who displayed this challenge. Respectable old age long frowned upon a vast crop of whiskers, viewing with equal distaste the gold and jewelled ear-rings worn (says Harrison) by certain *lustie courtiers and by gentlemen of courage*. The ear-rings and the beards were indices of the same desire for *panache* that now swept the country, permanent stage props of Tamburlaine, Dr. Faustus and the swaggering *terribiltà* of the sea-dogs and the tavern wits. They were essential ornaments of a flamboyant age.

Rauber's beard

The long beards of the first sixteenth century vintage included that of Juan Mayo—already briefly mentioned—of whom Jan Wierix left a record in the *Pictorum aliquot Celebrium Germaniæ Inferioris Effigies*. There was also the German, Andreas Eberhard Rauber von Talberg, who was a member of the Imperial Council of

---

[1] Ernest Boyd, writing on *Beards in America*, N.S. & N., August 31, 1935. This writer considered that all shaven men look alike. Most of us have the same feeling about beards ; and I am reminded that all Chinese look the same to Europeans and *vice versa*. It is a matter purely of what we are used to see.

War in the time of Maximilian II. He went habitually on foot, the better to display his beard, which is said to have fallen to the ground with enough to spare for the end to reach up again to his belt and be wound around his staff. As he is also said to have been very tall, we may assume the total length to have been some eight or nine feet. [1]

The chief authority for the life and beard of Rauber is Baron von Valvasor's *Topographia Archiducatus Carinthiæ* ; but a sufficiently remarkable digest, relating especially to the knight's physical strength, will be found in Bayle's *General Dictionary*. A footnote to the English edition of 1739 describes the contest in which Rauber is said to have exchanged buffets at Gratz with a gigantic Jew—*baptizatus,* but not *barbazatus,* for his own beard was evidently of some length, as the story makes clear. However, neither the beard nor the muscles of the Hebrew equalled those of Rauber, who (having received from his antagonist's fist a blow that made him take to his bed for a week) upon his recovery claimed the return blow to which he was entitled. He took the precaution of twisting the Jew's beard twice round his left hand, and then, with his right, struck him such a wallop that (so my English Bayle reads) *not only his beard, but also his under jaw, came off in his hand, by which means the Jew soon after lost his life*—a very felicitous example of eighteenth century moderation in the use of words.

Beard of Hans Steininger

Pagenstecher in *De Barba Prognosticum* claimed that at Hardenberg the burgomasters were chosen for the size of their beards and their feet—the one, no doubt, regarded as an index of wisdom and the other of stability. This custom doubtless began with a period when long beards were fashionable. That of Hans Steininger, a burgomaster of Braunau, seems to have survived the unfortunate accident in 1567, when he tripped over it and fell down a flight of stairs, breaking his neck. Being removed from an owner who had no further use for it, the beard became

[1] There is said to be a portrait of Rauber in J.A. ab Auersvald, *De veterum arte luctandi,* 1720. (See *Notes and Queries,* 11th S., XI, 262) but I have not seen this likeness.

eventually the property of the museum of Braunau, in Austria, where it is credibly claimed to be still on show and to measure eight feet nine inches.

Killingworth's famous beard

Among English beards of note was that of George Killingworth. A contributor to *Notes and Queries* (September 16, 1939) to whom I am indebted for the information regarding the fate of Steininger's beard, supplied a memorandum written on the back of a King's Bench Roll (K.B. 27, 252, m. 66.) regarding Killingworth. Dated August 1586, the memorandum speaks of *one Mr. Kyllyngworth lying in Temestrete* from whose beard the writer had seen one hair that measured *threscore and sixtene enches by measure of a carpenters Rule, the rest of his berd muche longer then hym selfe.* Killingworth, then aged eighty-eight, had sworn that the *Emperore of Russye with two more emperors hadd his berd in there handes in Russye all at one tyme.*

Who the other emperors can have been I cannot imagine, but not everyone has had his beard fondled by three emperors at a time, and the matter was well worth such a grave record. The occasion appeared to have been that of Richard Chancellor's second voyage to Muscovy, when the Czar Ivan Vassilevitch (whose *terribiltà* was remarkable even for his period, and became eventually inseparable from his name) entertained Chancellor and his companions very royally at Moscow. It was then, as we know, that Ivan took Killingworth's beard in his hands and *pleasantly delivered it to the Metropolitane, who seeming to blesse it, sayd in Russe this is Gods gift.*

The Gull's Hornbook does not deal so reverently with long beards. *Those selfsame critical saturnists,* says Dekker, *whose hair is shorter than their eye-brows, take a pride to have their hoary beards hang slavering like a dozen of fox-tails down so low as their middle.* But right through the Elizabethan age, and after, there were those who affected long beards, and even made their length a point of pride. We may note that (like the burgomasters of Hardenberg) Beaumont and Fletcher's King of the Beggars is chosen for his beard, the longest and largest in the company. It is compared to *Beggar's Bush*

Of which this is the thing, that but the type.

Beard of the Rev. More

Such a beard was that of the Rev. J. More, of Norwich, of whom James Granger wrote (in his *Biographical History of England*) that he was one of the worthiest clergymen in the reign of Elizabeth, and that he carried *the longest and largest beard of any Englishman of his time.* [1] This More explained by saying that he so wore it that no act of his life might be unworthy of the gravity of his appearance. We must assume from this statement that the vicar's use of his beard was not that to which a character in Lyly's *Mother Bombie* referred when he said, *my beard is as good as a handkerchief* (which sounds worse today than it did when written).

William Harrison provides a further account of styles and fashions—of which some are shaven from the chin (says he) like those of the Turks, not a few cut short like to the beard of the Marques Otto, [2] some made round like a rubbing brush, other with a *pique de vant* (O fine fashion !) or now and then suffered to grow long. . . . This *pique* (or pike) *devant* was the same as the *stiletto* or *bodkin*. Hence in Lyly's *Mydas* : *I will have it so sharp pointed that it may stab . . . like a Poynardo.* As to the uses of such modes :

> . . . if a man have a lean and streight face, a Marquese Otto's cut will make it broad and large ; if it be platter-like, a long

[1] In addition to the long beards already mentioned, Dickens in *Household Words* (No. 177) refers to that of a Venetian magnate *of whom Sismondi relates that if he did not lift it up he would trip over it in walking. Still worse was the beard of the carpenter depicted in the Prince's Court at Eidam ; who, because it was nine feet long, was obliged when at work to sling it about him in a bag.* But there is no knowing what we might all achieve with a little effort ; for it has been calculated that a man by the age of 80 normally grows about 27 feet of beard, of which I have now shaved away nearly half—a solemn thought. Another beard of great length was that of St. Nicephorus, which reached to his feet. It is mentioned in Maundrell's *Journey from Aleppo to Jerusalem* (1732). Among modern beards the record was claimed on behalf of that worn by Mr. Richard Latter of Tunbridge Wells, who died in 1915. His beard was said to have measured 16 feet (see *Notes and Queries*, 11th S., XI, 326).

[2] A corruption from the French *marquisotte*. (Randle Cotgrave gives *Barbe faite à la marquisotte.*) This was the supposed Turkish (i.e., Persian ?) fashion, the chin being shaved, but long moustaches worn. Murray has several variations of this word.

slender beard will make it seem the narrower ; if he be weesel becked, then much haire left on the cheekes will make the owner look big like a bowdled hen, and so grim as a goose . . .

Dialogue in a Barber's Shop

I owe to Jack Lindsay, and through him to a certain John Eliot, one of the many pictures of barbering in the days before some nostalgic Jacobean wrote his bitter jibe :

Rex erat Elizabeth, nunc est Regina Jacobus.

The *Orthoepia Gallica* of John Eliot is a series of dialogues and monologues relating to practical matters, such as a traveller might be supposed to include in his programme, with parallel texts in French and English. The dialogues are spirited and often boisterous, well deserving their rescue by Mr. Lindsay when he re-published parts of the English text in 1928, in his Fanfrolico Press—using the title *The Parlement of Prattlers*. The original work was published in 1593, and the author—a Catholic and a Francophil —seems to have disappeared from all records after leaving us this delectable document. My own quotations are from the sections relating to the barber's shop and illustrate the many functions of the barber-surgeon.

John : What doth the gentle Barber ?
Barber : Welcome, Sir.
John : I come to trim my beard and my haire.
Barber : Sit you downe there : you shall be trimd by and by.
John : Will you wash me, for I have great hast.
Barber : Stay a little, I have almost done with this gentleman.
    (*To 'prentice*) Come give me some cleane cloathes.
John : What sayth your Almanacke Barber ?
Barber : That the moone is just in the eclipse of monie.
John : When is it good to bleed ?
Barber : When there are any crownes to be gotten.
John : You are as courteous as the Divell.
Barber : I ask nothing else alwaies : but health and a purseful
    of monie, for my paramour a pretty conie, and
    Paradice at the end of my daies. You have your
    beard tangled and knotty.

John : Undo my lockes with this combe. Rub not so hard.
        Rub softly.

Barber : *(to 'prentice)* : A Pomander and some soape, ho.   Hold
        up this bason.

John : Wash me gently.

Barber : Shall I cut your haire. Will you have your beard
        shaven ? Shall I wash your neck, brest and stomacke ?
        Shall I picke your teeth. Boy, where be my Cizars.
        Give my this Ivorie combe.   Sharpen a little the rasor.
        Shall I cut your mustaches ? An eare-picker and a
        tooth-picker, ho. You are almost trimmed. Take
        this glasse and behold your selfe.

John : I am well. Santie deare, I looke with a fierce and
        fellon lookes. There's to drinke, Adiew.

Using Mr. Lindsay's arrangement of the text, I have adopted
the names and stage directions which he supplied in order to
follow the speeches more easily, for Eliot left the change of voice
and the person addressed entirely to the intelligence of his readers,
which can no longer be assumed. The multiplicity of the
barber's functions will be noticed : he is willing to bleed his
customer, to wash his stomach or to pick his teeth and ears. The
final remarks of the client are too ambiguous for us to be certain
whether he was satisfied or not.

For the styles of beards worn we have a wealth of authorities.
Stubbes counted among the abuses he anatomised the monstrous
manners which the barbers had invented of cutting, trimming,
shaving and washing. They had, said he

one manner of cut called the French cut, another the Spanish
cut ; one the new cut, another the old ; one the gentleman's
cut, another the common cut ; one cut of the court, another
of the country ; with infinite and like vanities, which I
overpasse. They have also other kinds of cuts innumerable;
and therefore when you come to be trimmed they will ask you
whether you will be cut to look terrible to your enemy, or
amiable to your friend ; grim and stern in countenance, or
pleasant and demure. . . .

Regrettable necessity for barbers

Nevertheless the old curmudgeon granted that (*these nisities set apart*) *barbers are verie necessarie, for otherwise men should grow verie ougglesom and deformed, and their haire would in processe of time over-growe their faces rather like monsters than comelie sober Christians.* [1]

But this chapter has gone on long enough ; and I propose to take a deep breath before entering the taverns with the Lucianic wits, or even setting foot in the barber's shop with such company. Did not even Dekker say that a whole dictionary could not afford more words than we could hear in dialogues from the Doctors of that Chair ?

[1] The Elizabethan beard was always well trimmed ; hence the significant vow of Pericles, Prince of Tyre, who let his beard grow until his daughter should find a husband. On her marriage day he says :

> *This ornament, that makes me look so dismal,*
> *Will I, my lov'd Marina, clip to form;*
> *And what these fourteen years no razor touched*
> *To grace thy marriage day, I'll beautify.*

W. A. Clouston, in an interesting essay on beards (see his *Flowers from a Persian Garden*) mentions this as an example of the beard as a mark of mourning. Clouston also notes that in *Woodstock* Sir Henry Lee grows a beard in mourning for Charles I—evidently based on Scott's family history. (See p. 57 of this book—also p. 50 re Caesar.)

CHAPTER X

THE BEARD ROMANTIC AND THE SCANDAL OF WHISKERS

O Egregium virorum ornamentum ! O laudabile naturæ
decus !   J. F. W. Pagenstecher

Greek freedom and Greek Beards expired together.
                                          T. S. Gowing

Velvet Breeches at the Barber's Shop

Writing in the days before his melancholy and splenetic repentance (when he was to feel the mockery of his reward in this world, which was cold poverty, and the terror of a warmer welcome in the life to come) Robert Greene could describe the vanities of his time with a wealth of current cant and jargon probably unknown to Stubbes, who was a mere spectator. The description of beard trimming in the *Quip for an Upstart Courtier* brings the Elizabethan barber's shop to life instantly as the customer is asked

> whether he will have his peak cut short and sharp ; amiable like an *inamorato* ; or broade pendant, like a spade, to be terrible like a warrior and a soldado ? Whether he will have his crates cut lowe like a juniper-bush, or his suberche taken away with a rasor ? If it be his pleesure to have his appendices primde, or his moustaches fostered, to turn about his eares like the brances of a vine ; or cut downe to the lip with the Italian lashe, to make him look like a half-faced bawby in bras ?

The *inamorato* suggests the Italianate Englishman, that Devil Incarnate. Greene's *suberche* is a variant of *subbosco* (or *subosco*) meaning the hair on the lower part of the face. Murray recalls Gabriel Harvey, with *the clippings of your thishonorable moustachyoes and subboscoes* ; and a reference as late as 1654 is to be found in Gayton's *Pleasant Notes upon Don Quixote*, a neglected and entertaining work from which Murray quotes : *The boscoes and suboscoes* (I mean) *the dewlapes and the jawy part of the face*.   The word is derived from the Italian *bosco*, a wood.   *Bosky*, which was among the pre-fabs of poetic diction, is regarded by Mr. Ivor Brown (*A Word in Your Ear*) as something of a loss through its association with bad company.   Certainly a Bosky Beard, though perhaps tautologous, looks well enough to my eye.

The choice of Cloth-Breeches

However, we must return to Mr. Greene.   Such is the variety of styles which his barber offers to *Velvett-Breeches*.   But when he turns to poor *Cloth-Breeches* he offers no such range :

You either (says Greene to the barber) cutte his beard at your owne pleasure, or else in disdaine, ask him if he will be trim'd with Christ's cut, round like the halfe of a Holland cheese.

(Despite the jibe this round cut[1] was favoured by such a valiant officer as John Smith, Admiral of New England.)

The numerous styles are a favourite topic with the wits.   A barber in Lyly's *Mydas* (Act III, scene 2) instructs a boy in *the phrasis of our eloquent occupation* :

How, sir, will you be trimmed ?   Will you have your beard like a spade or a bodkin ?   A pent-house on your upper lip, or an alley on your chin ? . . . Your moustachios sharpe at the ends, like shoe-maker's awles, or hanging down to your mouth like goate's flakes ?

Ballad of the Beard

Most of these passages will be familiar to readers of Elizabethan literature and are quoted by some of my predecessors in pogonology.   Repton cites also an old ballad from a miscellany entitled *Le Prince d'Armour* (1660) indicating the function and habitat of the various styles.   Of the *Stiletto Beard* (the cut affected by the Earl of Southampton) the ballad says :

[1] Compare the *Merry Wives* (I, 4, 20).   Shakespearian references to beard styles are too numerous to quote more than a few of them : see any Shakespeare Concordance.

The Steeletto beard,
O, it makes me afeard,
It is so sharp beneath ;
For he that doth place
A dagger in's face,
What wears he in his sheath ?

The *stiletto* (or *bodkin*[1]) was, as some portraits show, favoured by martial men. It is also referred to as a *Pisa* (i.e., dagger), but not to be confused with the *Needle Beard*, mentioned in this same Ballad. Randle Holme describes the *Basket Hilt*—a rough affair. But (to return to beards military) so, even more explicitly in the ballad, was the *spade*, perhaps derived from *spada* (a sword) like the suit in cards, for in *Piers Penilesse* it is described as *sharp*.

The Soldier's beard
Doth march in shear'd
In figure like a *Spade*,
With which he'll make
His enemies quake
And think their graves are made.

The forked beard also came into use once more, that ancient Saxon emblem—though other nations wore it also, as Repton's sketches show (they include various styles of forked beard, as worn by Theodore Beza, the Duke of Alva, the historian Petrus Martyr Anglerius and John Foxe, the martyrologist. (The sketches at the end of *Some Account of the Beard and the Moustachio* are among the interesting features of this rare work, though it is unfortunate that there is a certain carelessness about this pioneer effort, which needs to be studied with caution). The *swallow-taile* is mentioned by Nashe—a style which will be found in Aubril's list of French fashions in the last chapter. It is, however, insufficiently described to identify it from two possible examples given by Repton in his sketches. Indeed, there are other cuts of the period which might be so described. Yet another style was the *sugar loaf*, as worn by the Protector Somerset, the first Protestant

[1] The *Bodkin* was mentioned by Skelton as early as 1529 and had a longer life than many styles.

ruler of England (a title which Henry VIII would certainly have rejected). It is curious that no one has yet attempted, as far as I know, to write a life of Somerset, other than the brief account of him in the *Dictionary of National Biography* : few more fascinating and enigmatic subjects could be found for a biographer.

Much Ado About Beards

While many wore *The beards of Hercules and frowning Mars* (often, according to Bassanio, as a disguise, their livers being white as milk) others still shaved, sometimes for amorous reasons. *He looks younger than he did*, said Leonato of Benedick, *for the loss of a beard*—tastes varied, and we had already learnt that Beatrice could not endure a husband with a beard on his face. [1] Perhaps such tastes among women became more fashionable in Stuart times, and gradually affected male habits. But the beard took a hundred years to disappear entirely after its peak period in Elizabethan England.

Archbishop Laud (according to a note quoted by Repton from Southey's *Book of the Church*) when advised to flee to Holland from those who sought his head, seems to have had a greater fear of the Anabaptists who—so he said—would come and pluck him by the beard. [2] Elaborate attention to the beard continued among those who still wore it in the seventeenth century, though their number decreased. Of one old gentleman, *a Turky Merchant* (meaning one who traded with the Levant, and not one who practised a seasonal trade at Christmas) we are told that his valet spent some hours every morning in starching his Beard and curling his whiskers (possibly in ringlets) during which time a gentleman, whom he maintained as a companion, always read to him upon some useful subject. The reference (quoted from *Pylades and Corinna*) will be found in Dr. Zachary Grey's edition of *Hudibras* (Part II, Canto I) and Grey also confirms the fact that some of these beard fanciers had *Pasteboard Cases to put over them in the night, lest they should turn upon them and rumple them in their sleep*. (These devices we have already observed in Bulwer's reference to Greybeards—the beard

[1] See Appendix J.

[2] Not from any antipathy to the beard as such, clearly, for Anabaptists were conscientious in cultivating it.

protectors being referred to in the *Anthropometamorphosis* as *cases invented to preserve their formality.*) Vanity even demanded special *beard combs*—mentioned by Thomas Heywood in *The English Traveller*, 1633. Beard brushes are mentioned in *The Wizard* (1640), also by Dekker (*Match Me in London*), and as late as 1656, in a work cited by Repton.[1] Perfumes and powdered orris root were also widely used.

But the long, full beard, already the butt of ridicule at the end of the sixteenth century, is completely *démodé* in the early seventeenth. Repton quotes Lyly in *Mydas* (1592) with his *dozen of beards to stuffe two dozen of cushions*, also Dekker in the *Gull's Horn Book*, where such beards are described as fit *to stuff breeches and tennis balls*. The idea of shorn beards for stuffing tennis balls is common.   (It will be found again in *Much Ado About Nothing.*) Further derisive remarks on profusion of beard will be noted in *Coriolanus* and *The Honest Whore*. In the one we read of beards deserving *not so honourable a grave as to stuff a botcher's cushion, or to be entombed in an ass's pack-saddle* ; in the other their use is again proposed to stuff breeches—a comment on nether fashions.

Beards become Smaller

The Italian painters in the *Ritratti de' alcuni Celebri Pittori* (1625) are shown with no more than a *soupçon* of a *subbosco*—a mere tuft the size of a postage stamp below the lips, and a short, curled moustache. It was the beginning of a mode that was to lead to the slow extinction of the beard, in spite even of clerical patronage. Indeed, Cardinal Federico Borromeo (1564-1631) himself wore this mere token of a beard, as though to typify the changes of his times (a half-way step in the reaction which his great cousin and predecessor in the archbishopric of Milan had laboured to bring about). Henry Hutton, in 1619, notes the continuance of the *beard precisely cut i' th' peake;* but already, in 1601, Rare Ben Jonson, even a closer observer of fashion than Shakespeare, had noticed the

[1] In *The Wizard* a man is described as turning his head and (*under colour of spitting*) brushing his beard, with a *beard-brush ever in his hand*. Beard-brushes are also referred to in *The Queen of Corinth* (produced in 1616) ; and John Davies in *The Scourge of Folly* (about 1611) refers to *quils, irons and instruments* for the beard. Luis Muñoz in his *Vida y virtudes del V.P.M.Fr. Luis de Granada* speaks of *pulidas escobillas de barba*—beard-brushes again.

pencil on your chin.[1]   This appears to refer to the Roman T. style, where a short, straight moustache was worn with a straight and very narrow beard. A variant of this was worn later by Taylor, the so-called Water Poet—the narrow beard being twisted —but perhaps because it was his own affectation Taylor does not mention it in his list of beard cuts (in *Superbiæ Flagellum*). This screw style does not appear to have been given a name and is not listed in *The Ballad of the Beard*, though the Roman T. is mentioned. About the time of James I beard fashions showed a tendency to stylisation according to the profession of the wearer.

Puritans and the moustache

Francis M. Kelly in his *Historic Costume* notes the decline of the beard and moustache after 1620, while the tendency among men of fashion was to wear the hair of the head longer, with *love-locks*, plaited or tied with ribbons.   The pointed beard dwindles to what was known in a later century as an *imperial*, or disappears altogether.   After 1640 anything larger is rare except among men of middle age and older men, some of whom still cling to the fashion of relatively long beards and short hair.   The moustache disappears almost entirely in typical Puritan portraits—though it is surprising to observe how many of the Parliamentary leaders did not conform to the stylised Roundhead pattern, but wore their hair long.[2]   With Charles II the moustache returns to fashion— a thin line of hair that anticipates the modern film star, a mere token of virility that appears to argue *I could if I would*. (Charles himself shaved his upper lip during his tour of the Hollow Oaks of England, but grew his moustache again later.) In Germany the beard did not pass so easily, or without a struggle. Bulwer's *Anthropometamorphosis* (as re-published in 1653 from the original

[1] In *Cynthia's Revels*.   There is also an allusion here to the inversion of the moustache, which may refer to the fashion of turning up the ends, or to an upward twist or curl affected by some Elizabethans. Fairholt mentions an example of the twisted moustache in an effigy of 1587 at Lullingstone Church, Kent.

[2] Some, however, felt strongly on this matter. See, for example, *The Loathesomeness of Long Haire*, by T. Hall (1654) in the Thomason Collection. Percy Scholes has some interesting observations on this subject in *The Puritans and Music*.

edition of 1650) includes a woodcut of a German wearing a long beard, upon which the author remarks that he finds these people a little too indulgent in this matter *insomuch as some of them have been seen to have their Beards so long, that they would reach unto their feet, which they have worn trussed up in their bosomes.* In spite of the dubious character of Bulwer's syntax, there can be no doubt in fact that the beards, not the feet, of the Germans were indicated.

Bulwer a champion of the beard

But the *Nationall Gallant* of England, in Bulwer's prefatory verses, is not so adorned.

> What scoffers have we here? men sore affear'd
> Of Manhood's ensigne, who abhorr a beard.
> Here the luxuriant Chin quite downe is mowne,
> The ranke Mustachio's into whiskers grown.
> The upper Lip of Hair's now dispossest,
> Which nourish't here the honour'd Chin invest.
> Now rooted out by thy malicious care,
> All the cloath'd parts about thy mouth are bare.

It will be observed that Bulwer was strongly opposed to this practice. He quotes with disapproval the habits of the Maldive Islanders, which we have already observed in considering Moslem customs, and these habits put the author in mind of the opinions expressed by Scaliger, to which we have briefly alluded in our first chapter. As rendered into English by the author of *Anthropometamorphosis* these opinions may now be considered in more detail, for Bulwer is about to confute them. Julius Cæsar Scaliger maintained (says he)

That the encrease of these haires placed about the mouth, hanging down very long, (being as a hedge about the mouth) did hinder the ingresse, and egresse of those things for whose sake Nature had formed the mouth, whose office was commestion, or assumption of solid aliment, the potation of the same aliment, but liquid, expuition and locution, and sometimes respiration.

Neither a lawyer nor a physician could have put the matter at greater length, with more precision or less lucidity. The function of the mouth being thus stated by Bulwer out of Scaliger, he proceeds with the same nicety to render the case of his *Advocatus Diaboli* against *fungus facialis communis*, the common beard and moustache :

> To the which Offices the Lips could not be prompt and ready, besieged with such long and propendent Mustachoes, as the Senses teach us ; for although we endeavour to prevent these Mustacho-haires while we eat, yet they descend, and entring together with the meat into the mouth are bitten with the teeth, whose peeces we are compelled either to spit out, or sometimes imprudently to devour : and if we drink, these haires swim in our drinke, moystened with whose sprinkling dew they drop down upon the beard of the Chin and Cloaths, which is an unseemly sight.

To this Scaliger added that whiskers are a hindrance to spitting and a disturbance to elocution, and that the weight of mustachios *may also offend the upper Lip and render it unfit for a more easie motion.* Thus Scaliger *apud* Bulwer.

The opinion of John Bulwer himself was that these were vain cavils, since all hairs could become disserviceable, but (being subject to trimming) might be regulated at one's pleasure and arbitrement. Hence Nature had called to her service *the humane Intellect as a companion to trim and keep this Fabrique for her service.* As to the clean shave such as we now use, he found it rightly reputed among our ancestors to be *piacular and monstrous* that men should in any way resemble women ; so that shaving he terms a *shameful metamorphosis,* asking how much more ignominious is it, in smoothness of Face, to resemble that impotent Sex ? To shave, says he, is an Act not only of indecency, but of injustice, and ingratitude against God and Nature, repugnant to Scripture— citing the usual passages, whereon *Rabbi Moyses Maimonides hath made very subtile and precise glosses.*

Heresies of strange peoples

I will leave the Rabbi to more careful scholars, for I am weary of Leviticus XIX and XXI. The reader may find in Bulwer a vast amount of doubtful information about peculiar people and their ways with the beard : the Huns whose faces were ironed by their mothers in infancy to prevent the hairs from growing ; the *Bramas*, who plucked out the hair with pincers, as also did the *Tovopinambaultians*, the people of Java and the *Chiribichenses* (*who call our men wild Beasts for that they endeavour to preserve their Beards*). Then the inhabitants of Good Hope, who, having eradicated the hair of the chin, painted it with divers colours ; and many more strange peoples, including those of whom Bulwer speaks on no less authority than Sir John Mandeville : *In the Kingdome of Mancy in great India there men have Beards as it were Cats.*

Bulwer held that we cannot *without the high crime of impiety leave off or eradicate our Beard, or with Depilators burn up and depopulate the Genitall matter thereof*, because the beard is part of the Divine Image. Therefore he says that haters of the beard were rightly included in Barclay's *Ship of Fooles* (though I marvel that so learned a man as Bulwer included Julian the Apostate among his Beard-haters, merely because of the title of Julian's treatise, which Bulwer cannot have read). The *Ship of Fools* to which Bulwer referred was a free translation from a German work, widely read at the time.

Many other writers on the beard who belong to the period 1500-1700 have already been mentioned in our last chapter, when discussing the great ecclesiastical controversy. But a few remain to be mentioned. We almost overlooked the Dutch physician Junius (Adriaan de Jonghe) who came out very strongly against shaving[1] in his book *De Coma Commentarium*, a sixteenth century work. (See Chapter II *de rasura capillorum*, etc.) *Servilis mihi habetur rasura*, he wrote—he found shaving servile, ridiculous and fit for morons (*ridicula ac morionum propria*). Indeed, he, like Bulwer later, found rank impiety in the removal of the beard. Barthius (*De Barba*, 1671) also belongs to this period.

The Mouse-eaten Beard in Heraldry

Randle Holme can hardly be considered as a writer on beards, but we have already quoted one of his heraldic definitions that closely concerns us, and others will be found equally informative.

[1] He was among the first to use medical arguments in favour of the beard.

Thus, of the *pick-devant* [1] in heraldry we read that *a full face with a sharp-pointed beard is termed in blazon, a man's face with a pick-a-devant (or sharp-pointed) beard*. A stranger category is the *mouse-eaten beard* which Holme describes, *when the beard groweth scatteringly, not together, but here a tuft and there a tuft*.

Marcus Antonius Ulmus also deserves mention among the barbologists of this period. His *Physiologia Barbæ Humanæ* was published in 1603. To him we owe a most careful classification (*Crispiberbes, Rariberbes*, und so weiter) also a very astonishing statement which somewhat amplifies Donne's epigram :

> Thy sinnes and haires may no man equal call
> For as thy sinnes increase, thy haires doe fall [2]

We have already mentioned John Taylor, but may spend another useful minute with the Water Poet (as courtesy still styles him) because of his careful enumeration of beard styles. Some were like brushes, he said (I will spare the reader his doggerel) and all the shapes listed by Greene appear to have been observed in 1621 by the author of *Superbiæ Flagellum*, plus the Roman T. (or hammer cut, as worn by John Bulwer, and already described) and other styles which were typically Jacobean. In Massinger and Fletcher's *Queen of Corinth* we read that *your T. Beard is in fashion*—that is to say, in 1616, when the play was first produced. By the time it was published, in 1647, bearded men were less common in England.

The beard of Hudibras

Hudibras was therefore almost an antique with his Tile Beard :

[1] Some interesting notes on the variations of this word will be found in Murray, with gay quotations from Nashe and others.

[2] The claim of Ulmus, which may be considered as a commentary on this is : *Coitus etiam diminuit Pilos superciliorum, capillos capitis et pilos palpebrarum, et multiplicat Pilos Barbæ. (De fine Barbæ Humanæ,* p. 203.) This view was widely held—see the Extra Series, Early English Text Society, vol. X, 308 (footnote). Martin Schurig, in his *Spermatologia* (1720) tells of an octogenarian who had lost both hair and beard, but grew new crops on marrying a young woman. A more likely theory about beards was that of Gentien Hervet, who claimed that shaving would cause toothache. (Hervet wrote three treatises on beards, one for, one against, and one for liberty of conscience.)

His tawny beard was th'equal grace
Both of his wisdom and his face,
In cut and Dye so like a Tile
A sudden view it would beguile . . .

It is true that beards, and even some of a good size (like that of
the Marquis of Clanricarde) continued to be worn by many
throughout the period of the Civil War, the Commonwealth and
the Protectorate. Before their final extinction at the end of the
century there was even a temporary vogue in small beards, and
even more of a fashion in small moustaches under the later
Stuarts. But between 1640 and 1660 there are more clean-shaven
faces (especially among the Parliamentarians) than at any time
since the days of Henry VIII,[1] and it is easy to understand that
a beard could already, at that time, have become the object of
offensive comments if it were of a size and shape long since
discarded.

This Tile Beard of Hudibras may have been triangular, for some
English tiles were so shaped. The description is, in fact, very
inadequate. Such styles are still worn in early Stuart times,
though slowly giving place to slighter beards. But what makes
Hudibras an object of ridicule is his oath—in the manner of the
ancients (Nazarites, Romans and Teutons) not to cut the said
beard until he should see the triumph of his party :

'twas to stand fast
As long as monarchy should last

Puritan vows, as alleged by Zachary Grey
We have the assurance of Dr. Zachary Grey that many of the
Parliamentarians did actually take such oaths though these were
clearly exceptions to the general rule in that party. One such was
commemorated in some anonymous verses of the same period :

[1] *The Ballad of the Beard*, already quoted, though published in 1660, has the
air of having been written somewhat earlier. Its flavour is distinctly Jacobean,
and some of the styles listed in it were no longer common during Cromwell's
Protectorate. Of the older styles the *stiletto* was still in common use, e.g., as
worn by Prynne.

This worthy knight was one that swore
He would not cut his beard
Till this ungodly nation was
From kings and bishops cleared;

Which holy vow he firmly kept
And most devoutly wore
A grisly meteor on his face
Till they were both no more.
(*The Cobler and the Vicar of Bray*.)

In the same spirit grew the beard canonic of Hudibras (*In holy orders, by strict vow*) losing, we may be sure, whatever shape it originally possessed. The knight's own reference to *Philip Nye's Thanksgiving Beard* is a reminder that one of the Assembly of Divines—which Parliament had set up to discuss the explosive problem of England's religion—wore a beard so remarkable that it earned for itself a special poem by the author of *Hudibras*. The beard of Hudibras himself grew upon a mere figment of fancy. It was a beard fictitious, but destined to greater fame than any that flourished on solid and material chin ; though it became so unrecognisable that the knight's Lady could not be sure of her man when she found him in the local Bocardo :

Not by your individual whiskers
But by your dialect and discourse

(a pleasant freak of free rhyming) did the Widow identify her Hudibras.

Quoth she—Those need not be asham'd
For being honourably maim'd
If he that is in battle conquer'd
Have any title to his own beard,
Though yours be sorely lugg'd and torn,
It does your visage more adorn,
Than if 'twere prun'd, and starch'd, and lander'd,
And cut square by the Russian standard.

The last line seems to me to dispose of the idea that the Tile Beard was square or oblong, as some suppose ; for the Tile Beard of Hudibras is directly contrasted with the square cut affected at that time in Moscow. I think it came to a point so long as it came to anything at all, despite all illustrations that witness to the contrary.

Influence of French fashions

France dominates the tastes of the seventeenth century, as Spain did those of the sixteenth. Elegance is what matters increasingly. The trim little moustache and small, pointed beard (diminishing to the *royale* of Louis XIII, and so to nothing in the long reign of his successor) are kept in order with the aid of cosmetics and the elaborate gadgets we have already seen.[1] But as beards shortened there must have been a decreasing need for the beard combs and beard brushes, for those *bigotelles* and the similar stables once used for the beard. The long-locked Cavaliers of Charles I and the Restoration dandies imitated every phase of French foppery, even to the pomade and perfumed wax of the French court. Not so the true Roundheads, or the crop-headed Pilgrims of New England.

Wigs versus whiskers

But in France the beard had been doomed from the day when a whim of Louis XIII caused him to play barber among his courtiers, shaving from their chins the last, small, pointed beard that fashion allowed. That was in 1628. The beards grew again, but not for long ; and when the French court finally abandoned the *royale* the rest of Europe soon followed. Wigs originated similarly, when Louis XIII began to lose his hair. The *Roi Soleil* had a fine head of hair—perhaps his only natural endowment— but he too eventually abandoned it for a peruke, following the fashion of his own nobles. For a time we see false hair on the head and real hair on the face ; but the two go ill together, and it may have been the wig, as much as anything, which eventually killed the last vestige of beard and moustache.[2] After the end

[1] That the fashion of starching beards came originally from France is indicated in some verses by Inigo Jones in *The Odcombian Banquet* (1611).

[2] It is not my business here to follow the attitude of the Church towards wigs ; but I notice a scholion on p. 113 of the *Jus Canonicum*, Tom II (Wernz and Vidal, 1928) which very definitely forbids the wearing of a wig by a priest

of the seventeenth century, for a hundred and fifty years, faces were to remain smooth.   With a few curious exceptions, we may say in general that not even moustaches remained—they were a privilege of the Swiss Guards, the grenadiers and some cavalry troops in certain parts of Europe.   There is an engraving in Frances Grose's *Military Antiquities* which shows what purports to be an *Antient Dragon*, who is undoubtedly wearing a beard. But as Captain Grose did not specify the date and has clothed his figure in a mixture of fashions there is little to be gained from following an antiquarian's fancy.   According to Repton the East India Company even attempted to interfere with the mustachios of its Sepoys, but in all my long studies of the innumerable and intolerable wrongs done to India by John Company and the British Government after it, I never remember finding evidence of this particular injury, for which (unfortunately) Repton did not give any reference.

The illusion of perpetual youth

The moustache for civilians (and for most soldiers) was killed when the Roi Soleil shaved off his own in 1680.   There have been few men more vain than Louis XIV, perhaps as a compensation for his total lack of any single quality worthy of admiration.   He desired always to appear young, and the mode in his time was a slavish imitation of this foolish fantasy of perpetual youth.   Hence when (at the age of forty-two) the king found some white hairs in his shred of moustache, the offensive truth was erased.   G. F. R. Molé's strange idea (in his *Histoire des Modes Françaises*) that the moustache disappeared at the end of the seventeenth century because of *une certaine poudre, connue sous le nom de tabac* has no apparent foundation.   He seems to have invented it, like his extraordinary ideas about the Greek clergy shaving and reproaching the Western priests for wearing beards.

Indecency of whiskers

In the time of Judge Jeffreys large beards were rare enough to

while celebrating the mass : *Qui gestat comam fictam, certe operto capite non celebrat Missam.* (Yes, the information is entirely gratuitous.) The Early Fathers condemned wigs altogether.

be a matter of comment. *If your conscience be as large as your beard,*
fellow, said the Judge to one of his victims, *it must be a swinging one.*
To which his Lordship received the reply, so they say, *If con-*
sciences be measured by beards I am afraid your Lordship has none at all.
Whiskers soon became indefinably indecent, as may be observed
in *Tristram Shandy* (Book V, Chapter I) though it must be admitted
that Sterne could give such a twist to any word if he was in the
mood for it. Nevertheless there is evidence to confirm this
view, as we may briefly observe from two examples of persecution.

The first, I regret to say, is the strong disapproval shown by his
fellow Quakers, in America, of Joshua Evans, a very worthy
Friend who wore a beard in the eighteenth century. The
Friends of West Jersey countenanced a good deal that must have
seemed very odd to them in Joshua's behaviour—his vegetarianism,
his clothes (like John Woolman's) of undyed fabric and his
objection to leather from beasts that had died a violent death,
but when he permitted his beard to grow, many of his friends became
uneasy, apprehending he was running beyond the notions of truth into
unprofitable imaginations. The story will be found in Comly's
Friends' Miscellany, where we are informed that a special committee was appointed to visit Joshua *on account of his wearing his*
beard and other singularities. A good Friend, John Hunt, who
served on this committee, recorded that *they left him with his*
beard on, much as they found him, none having power, or a razor to cut it
off. At Yearly Meeting the seats in Joshua's vicinity were avoided
by all his former friends, save one ; and pogonophobia was so
strong in the Society that a certificate to travel in the ministry was
several times refused this good man, solely on account of his
beard.

In defence of a Quaker beard

Joshua seems to have floored the deputation which visited him,
firing a broadside of biblical pogonology. Among those deeply
impressed was the John Hunt mentioned above, to whom is
attributed an unsigned letter written at the height of the controversy. *I suppose,* said the writer of this letter, *our friend*
Joshua's beard is the chief obstruction. . . . To hinder him in his religious
services on account of his beard . . . I cannot see to be right. Many

scriptural quotations follow—the writer had evidently been at some pains to dig them up, or perhaps noted them from Joshua's own *apologia pro barba sua*. And the Protestant martyrs (*whom William Penn mentions with great respect*—a good debating point, that) were also bearded. Says Joshua's champion :

> Now whether wearing the beard only is a reason sufficient, is a scruple with me, especially when I look back to former years, and consider how the Lord hath owned many worthies with their beards on, and also with them off ; as appears plainly from Holy Scripture, and likewise the worthy martyrs, as before hinted. We read of one formerly that wore a garment of goat skins and camel's hair, and a leather girdle about his loins. It's likely he made, or would now make, as singular an appearance as Joshua does . . .

Triumph of Joshua Evans

Indeed, *from some accounts*, the argument concludes, *the holy pattern here mentioned, did wear his beard*—a cautious statement on the beard of Our Lord. I am happy to record that Joshua triumphed eventually over all prejudice. Thanks to pressure from younger Friends he was eventually *liberated*, as the Quaker saying is, for his concern to travel in the ministry, *after thirteen or fourteen years struggle*. Of his subsequent success, in the last years of his life, his own account shall bear witness regarding a typical meeting :

> The wearing of my beard, I believe hath been of great use in the cause I am engaged to promote ; for I apprehend thousands have come to meetings, where I have been, that otherwise I should not have seen ; many being induced, in great measure, to come on account of my singular appearance. . . . At this place a number of gay people were observed to weep . . .

Obiit 1798, deeply lamented, his funeral attended by many Negroes and Indians (for he had been a good friend to both, a promoter of peace and a pioneer opponent of slavery). Joshua's own account, in his Journal, of the reasons which led him to grow a beard shows that it was no mere fad but a matter of principle :

After my mind was brought into deep thoughtfulness on the subject (he wrote) I was induced to conclude, that the practice of shaving was hardly introduced by the pure dictates of truth . . . I also considered it probable that the author of all pride produced a desire for shaving at first . . .

Great offence was taken by a number of my fellow-members ; bitter reflections were uttered and false reports spread. But there was a remnant who sympathised with me in my trials. . . . These were not offended at the simplicity of my beard ; although they did not see their way to forego custom, by refraining to shave their own. They also stood by me in many solid conferences which were held on this account.

Strange case of Benjamin Lay

No one who reads this saga can doubt that the wearing of a beard at this time was considered a very serious breach of propriety. Another Quaker, Benjamin Lay, who was born in 1677, half a century before Joshua Evans, and lived till 1759, was also bearded but does not seem to have endured much hardship on this account—perhaps because his views and behaviour on other matters so disturbed his fellow Friends that they disowned him ; and his beard may have seemed (by comparison) a small matter.

He lived in a cottage built by himself (half a cave), and was eccentric, particularly in the nature of his efforts to convert the American Quakers with regard to slavery—an institution to which, like Joshua, he was vehemently opposed. On one occasion he gave histrionic effect to a discourse on this subject, by concealing a bladder under his coat, which he stabbed with a sword in the peroration of his prophetic oration. The bladder being filled with a red fluid[1]   Benjamin's continual warning that the

[1] There are two accounts of this bladder incident (at Burlington, New Jersey). One in the Journal of John Hunt (Comly's *Miscellany*, Vol. IV) says that the bladder was filled with real blood, and that Benjamin *ran the sword through the bladder and sprinkled the blood on divers Friends, and declared that so the sword would be sheathed in the bowels of the nation if they did not leave off oppressing the Negroes.* Roberts Vaux in his *Memoirs of the Lives of Benjamin Lay and Ralph Sandiford* (Philadelphia, 1815) says that the liquid was poke-berry (Phytolacca decandra). This poke-berry version is very much more likely, as Benjamin

blood of the slaves would be on the heads of the Christian slave-owners was thus given dramatic realism.

My second example of persecution is also an American one, this time in the nineteenth century, and as late as 1830—the date being important, in view of what we shall note later regarding the changing fashions which followed. Quite clearly the people of Fitchburg (Mass.) were still living by strictly eighteenth century standars of decency when Joseph Palmer arrived, complete with a magnificent beard, to live in their village.[1]

Persecution of Joseph Palmer

The persecution of Palmer was much more rigorous than that of Joshua Evans. He was reviled as a Jew—an index both of anti-Semitism and of the continued association of beards with Hebrews. He was regarded as indecent, sneered at and even stoned by small boys. The local pastor remonstrated with him, but Palmer relied as ably as Joshua Evans, with chunks of Holy Writ. Eventually an attempt was made to refuse him the communion in Church, the officiating clergyman deliberately by-passing his bearded parishioner. Palmer's counter-move, in helping himself from the communion table, brought matters to a head; and four days later he was assaulted by four men who attempted to shave him forcibly. He routed them with the aid of a jack-knife, wounding two of them, and soon found himself in court, charged with *unprovoked assault*.

was a strict vegetarian. He took similar action of a spectacular character on various occasions, wore eccentric clothes, lived often on acorns, chestnuts and potatoes, and being a hunch-back dwarf withal, he was altogether so odd that his beard must have been regarded merely as one of his many extravagances. He nevertheless entertained many well-known contemporaries in his cave and counted among his friends Benjamin Franklin, who published his book *All Slavekeepers that keep the Innocent in Bondage,* etc. Benjamin was born in England, but the most active part of his life was spent in America, where he died and was too soon forgotten.

[1] It was, none the less, a curious error or misprint in *Life* (January 13, 1947) whereby Palmer was described as being born *75 years too soon to wear whiskers with impunity*. He lived to see such a crop as had not been viewed since the days of Drake.

His beard not un-American

Having been fined on this outrageous charge, Palmer refused to pay, and was put in the county jail. From here, by means of smuggled letters, he conducted a press campaign against his persecutors. Public opinion rallied, and it was soon evident that a growing number of Palmer's fellow citizens declined to regard the nourishment of a beard as an un-American activity. That Palmer was, in fact, imprisoned for wearing one, was clear enough. Authority tried its usual line of retreat, and the prisoner was told he could return home. But a question of principle was involved, and until vindicated he declined to budge.

The Bearded Prisoner of Worcester became a legend in the land, until he was forcibly ejected from the gaol. His fame was eventually perpetuated on his tombstone, where his bearded head was carved, and may be seen to this day (I am told) at North Leominster, near Fitchburg. Below the effigy are the words *Persecuted for wearing the beard*. The story of Joseph Palmer has recently been told by Stewart H. Holbrook, in *Lost Men of American History*, from which this brief résumé of Palmer's career has been culled.

Such was mob reaction to the bearded individualist during the great era of shaving, though some who defied the conventions were more fortunate. Max von Boehn in *Die Mode* mentions three eighteenth century rebels. There was Johann Christian Edelmann (1698-1767), well-known in his time for his deistic theology and his *esprit fort*, who is said to have occasioned more commotion by his long beard than he did by his unorthodox opinions. There was also Gabriel André Donath, who used curling papers for his long beard when resident in Dresden, about 1735. The sculptor Balthasar Permoser not only grew a beard but defended it in a brochure entitled *Der auf dem Throne der Ehren Erhobene Bart*, published anonymously at Frankfort in 1714. William Hone in his *Every-Day Book* mentions also Edward Wortley Montague (1713-1776), *the worthy son of his mother*, who wore a beard among his many eccentricities.

An apostle of Rousseau among the Arabs

Lord George Gordon—chiefly remembered for the Gordon Riots—having been a violent protagonist of Protestantism and flirted for a while with Quakerism, became a Jewish convert when a prisoner at Newgate ; where (to emphasise this change of faith) he grew a beard, in which beard and gaol he died (1793) after holding a popular *salon* at Newgate for some years.   Another enthusiast was a certain disciple of Rousseau, known as Arphaxad Tinnagelli (whether baptismally I doubt) who also adopted a beard, in this instance as part of the necessary equipment for converting the Arabs to the principles of Jean Jacques. He learnt Arabic, and wrote a new catechism which began :

Who is God ?   The Truth.
Who is his Prophet ?   J. J. Rousseau.

But in spite of all the trouble taken by Arphaxad he left no lasting results of his mission in Arabia.

Much wiser was the Swiss painter, Jean Etienne Liotard, who—having travelled widely—brought Oriental habits home with him from Constantinople, dressing as a Turk and wearing a most presentable beard.   This artist seems to have been one of the first to realise that he belonged to a privileged profession—the affectations that are censured in other men being indulged and even encouraged to this very day among this peculiar caste.   Liotard met with neither stones nor abuse ; on the contrary, he painted the Princess of Wales in 1753 and enjoyed a great vogue among persons of fashion.   He was perhaps the originator of the Artist's Beard as a distinctive part of a uniform still observable. Certainly it cannot be mere coincidence that among the pioneer beards of the early nineteenth century were those of the French Romantics—a literary and artistic clique which we shall presently consider—and in England the beards of two artists, James Ward and Samuel Palmer (no relative of Joseph).

Gospel of James Ward

Ward considered himself a better painter (especially of animals, but also of anything else) than his contemporary George Morland : a judgment with which many critics today are likely to agree.   But he spent much of his time as an engraver.   There is no notice of him in the *Encyclopædia Britannica*, which is scandalous, and little else apart from a rather unreliable biography (1904) and an article in the *Connoisseur* by Reginald Grunday (1909). He was vigorous, both as a painter and as a controversialist, but lost to the gallery of fame by public neglect, too much temperament and a form of religious mania which led him to associate himself with Edward Irving and the Catholic Apostolic Church. Among his literary productions was a pamphlet against docking the tails of horses[1] and another (doubtless by analogous reasoning) against shaving.

There is no copy of this pamphlet at the British Museum; but one was recently found among papers in the possession of Ward's descendants, and I had the pleasure of introducing a reading of it on the B.B.C. Third Programme. Ward's *Defence of the Beard* was primarily scriptural, and showed that a man must grow a beard *unless he was indifferent as to offending the Creator and good taste*. His grand-daughter, Henrietta Ward (*Memories of Ninety Years*, 1924) described James as well below average height, wearing a long beard in the days when everyone shaved.

Ward's dates were 1769-1859. A younger artist of the same taste was Samuel Palmer (1805-1881) who might, with a little patience, have grown his beard with the rest of the mid-Victorians, but anticipated the privilege at the age of twenty-four. In a letter to his future father-in-law, John Linnell, he made the significant statement, in May 1829 :

The artists have at last an opportunity to wear the beard unmolested. I understand from the papers that it is become the height of fashion.

The second statement would be classified today as wish-fulfilment, for even in Paris beards were in a very small minority at that time. But the first statement indicates that—perhaps inspired by Liotard—artists had long been seeking courage to grow beards.

Habits of the Only Bearded Peer

Another pioneer was Matthew Robinson-Morris, Lord Rokeby, an eighteenth century eccentric, who lived largely on beef-tea and

[1] It is curious that another eighteenth century eccentric, Martin Van Butchell, also wore a beard (which reached his waist) and objected to docking horses. He was a quack doctor of whom an account will be found in Henry Lemoine's *Eccentric Magazine* (1812). There appears to be a connection between shaving and the docking and cropping of animals.

abhorred fires. (He had a bath constructed to be heated by the sun, and spent most of his time in it.) Rokeby cultivated Whig politics and the only beard in the House of Lords. That some of the Lower Orders wore beards, even in the eighteenth century, is clear. Black George, for example, in *Tom Jones* is described as bearded. But in the same novel the Beard of The Man on the Hill (who is a gentleman) is reckoned among his strange whimsicalities.

Many who forbore to wear a beard themselves admired the fashion and some even advocated a return to it. There is perhaps a touch of this nostalgia in Cowper's ironical lines, describing the activities of Capability Brown, the iconoclastic apostle of Improvement who was then employed in ruining the stately homes of England :

> The omnipotent magician, Brown, appears.
> Down falls the venerable pile, the abode
> Of our forefathers, a grave whiskered race,
> But tasteless . . .

Earlier in the century Sir Roger de Coverley had been made the mouth piece for a lament in which the shaven faces of his time were compared unfavourably with the beards of antiquity. The whole passage was lifted—I fear without acknowledgment—by Fangé.[1] There was also a sermon preached in defence of the beard by a certain Joseph Jacob, about 1700.

Crime of Père Fangé

Dom Fangé was himself an eighteenth century victim of the same nostalgia. Published anonymously, in 1774, his book

[1] Compare Fangé's *Mémoires*, page 175, with Sir Roger's reflections at Westminster Abbey, in *The Spectator*, No. 331—*I love to see your Abrahams, your Isaacs, and your Jacobs, as we have them in old pieces of tapestry, with beards below their girdles*, etc. The *Spectator's* comments on this are of some interest, showing how soon the Elizabethan beard had been forgotten. He thought that the last effort made by the Beard *seems to have been in Queen Mary's days as the curious reader may find*; and he himself *could find but few beards worth taking notice of in the reign of King James the first.* Perhaps he meant long ones. The *Spectator's* own fear was that the revival of the beard in such an age of luxury would cause large sums to be spent by the beaux on false ones of the lightest colours and the most immoderate lengths. *We are not certain*, he added, *that the ladies would not come into the mode.*

recalls, not without a pang, an age when a priest *ut tunc moris erat, Barbam quasi in signum religionis, enutriset.* Dulaure, writing a little later, was even more emphatic than Fangé in expressing his partiality. His *Pogonologie* was written to recall to men's minds their ancient dignity, *and that superiority of their sex, which has been lost in Europe ever since the fabulous days of chivalry . . . restoring, in some respects, the sovereign power to the lawful master, and taking it away from the usurper.* He believed—a little prematurely—that the fashion of long beards was on the point of being renewed, and he hoped it would end some disagreeable customs, including that of snuff-taking, against which he fulminated very forcibly. This revival, he wrote (in 1786, mark you), was nearer than people realised. Dulaure returned to the subject frequently in his *Histoire physique, civile et morale des environs de Paris.*

Another defender of the beard in the eighteenth century was the Jesuit Father, François Oudin, who wrote his *Recherches sur la Barbe* in the *Mercure de France* (March and April 1765) on different ways of wearing a beard, and refuted Baronius on the subject of the clergy.[1] Béroalde's *Moyen de Parvenir* has some observations on the subject, and suggests that priests shave out of vanity. (It is a curious fact that, according to Dulaure, all monks in Portugal, of whatever order, were compelled by law to grow beards in 1784, i.e. at a time when shaving was still universal). Vanetti's belated reply to Van Helmont belongs to this period (it appeared in 1759) and just after the turn of the century I find that one Saggio occupied himself in *Di Storia sulle Vicende della Barba, con un' Appendice sopra i Mostacchi* (1801). These are but a few of the works that belong to this period.[2]

Admirable prejudices of Pagenstecher

But from such a list let not the great name of Pagenstecher be omitted, the first of these formidable philopogons, who rumbled of revolt in 1708 with *De Barba Prognosticum, Historico-Politico-*

[1] See Michaut, *Mélanges Historiques* (II, 329).

[2] I have since come across the work of Robert Sharrock, Archdeacon of Westminster. In a political treatise replying to Hobbes Ὑπόθεσις ἠθικ'ή, *de officiis secundum Naturæ Jus,* 1660) he contrived to work in a section *De Habitu Crinis Dissertatio Singularis.* The critic of *Leviathan* was one of the most learned men of his time in physics, horticulture, etc.

Juridicium. He was indeed *Vir Excellentissimus, Nobilissimus, Clarissimus,* as one of his admirers describes him, in some of the laudatory verses which preface the first edition :

> *Hoc tua de Cathedra vox generosa docet . . .*

Indeed, a Daniel, and (like all true philopogons) one with a hearty contempt for the beardless sex. I owe to him an older version of our saying, *A woman, a dog and a walnut tree . . .*

> *Nux, asinus, mulier, simili sunt lege legati*
> *Hac tria nil recte faciunt si verbera desunt.*

It is the same principle—*The more you beat 'em, the better they be.*

A second and a third edition appeared of this excellent work, each prefaced by new tributes in verse, including that encomium by one, J. H. Schwabe, which is quoted at the beginning of my own book—where the writer sang not arms and the man, but the beard which is greater than either. I leave this monumental work with regret ; but before this chapter closes I have something to say of Eastern fashions, and particularly with respect to Russia.

We have observed the sanctity of the beard as a mark of the aristocracy in ancient Assyria and of free men in Turkey. We have noticed its removal under the tyranny of Alexander and of the Incas. We have marked instances, too, in which shaving has been a badge of slavery. It must nevertheless be admitted that in Rome, at one time (when shaving was *de rigueur* among the Optimates, philosophers alone claiming exemption) the beard— by a reversal of fortune—became for a while the token of servitude wherever it did not specifically denote Cynicism, Stoicism, Sophism or membership of some accepted high-brow clique. The connection between beards and freedom is nevertheless a long one, particularly in the East.

Mohammed's bail

According to Fraser (who gives as his authority Janssen's *Coûtumes des Arabes au pays de Moab*) the Moabite Arabs at the beginning of this century still regarded shaving as a serious punishment, a slightly milder alternative to the death penalty. Conforming to the canons of sympathetic magic, as Sir James points out, the possession of a man's hair should be sufficient hostage for his conduct ; and the Moslems, who to this day keep a single hair of Mohammed's beard enshrined in the Mosque of the Companion at Cairawan, may be considered to hold ample security for the Prophet's good behaviour[1]. Few True Believers, however, have cared to take such risks. Honour, freedom and safety alike indicate that it is safest to keep the beard where it belongs.

Pranks of a Byzantine Emperor

Eastern Christians share this opinion. Doubtless it was with calculated malice that the Emperor Constantine Copronymus (so called because it was alleged that he had misbehaved himself in the font, on the occasion of his baptism) when confronted with the hostility of the monks in the eighth century, took a number of them and set fire to their beards. What better way to show one's loathing and contempt for those who opposed the policy of one's family ?[2] But though Copronymus loathed the images in the Churches, he did not despise the beard. On the contrary, his action was designed as the greatest injury and insult by one who appreciated its significance ; for without reverence there can be no blasphemy. The Pope broke with the Byzantine Tyrant, not because of the beards—he would have been glad enough to remove the lot—but because of the icons. From that moment the Papacy looked towards the rising power of the Franks, the breach widened between East and West ; and the Eastern Church went its own bearded way.

A shaven bishop the Abomination of Desolation

Hence it was that the advent of the Crusaders was not regarded by their fellow Christians of Constantinople with enthusiasm.

[1] The *aussuri sharif* (sacred relic) was enshrined in 1135, the mosque being built specially for this purpose. For the uses of sympathetic magic in harming an adversary by doing damage to any detached part of him (e.g., excrement) see Martin Schurig's *Chylologia*, in the chapter *De Stercoris humani usu magico seu sympathetico*, also Francis Barrett's *Magus*.

[2] Constantine V (Copronymus), Emperor from 740-775, was the son of Leo III, known as the Iconoclast. Their attempt to abolish the adoration of icons brought them into a bitter feud with the Eastern Church.

Filioque and *radat* lay between the two Churches like drawn swords, and the Crusaders were eventually deflected into a Holy War with their Christian brethren. In 1204 the captured capital of the Greeks was looted by the soldiers of the Cross as effectively as ever pagan hordes had sacked Rome. (Indeed, even the Vandals compared favourably with the Crusaders on this occasion ; and perhaps the only true comparison would be the sack of Rome, in later years, by the army of that pious and Catholic Emperor, Charles V. Certainly the Turks conducted themselves better, when the Eastern capital finally fell to them.) Baldwin, Earl of Flanders, was set up as Emperor of Byzantium, and a Latin Patriarch appointed—a shaven bishop from the West in whom the Greek historian, Nicetas Choniates, saw *the abomination of desolation predicted by the Prophet Daniel.* The clergy who followed the Greek rite could not even bear the sight of a beardless effigy in the niche of a Latin church—a saint without a beard might as well have shaved off his halo.

It is true that many Crusaders came to imitate the Greeks to some extent in pogonotrophy. When Baldwin, Count of Edessa—in a story already recalled—pawned his beard, he showed a realisation of its value. The assumption clearly was, not that the pawnbroker hoped to sell it for a vast sum, but that it was worth far more to the owner than to the creditor, like Antonio's flesh, which Uncle Shylock cannot have hoped to retail on the open market. Hence even a Frank would not, surely, forfeit *rem tanta diligentia conservandam, argumentum viri, vultus gloriam, hominis præcipuam auctoritatem.* (The hyperbole, you will remember, is chargeable to Baldwin's father-in-law.) Such was the influence of the East even on Frankish adherents of *filioque* who made their home *in partibus orientalibus.* They tended to grow beards and learnt a little at least concerning the esoteric beard cult in which the Jew, the Moslem and the Eastern Christian have mystical unity.[1]

---

[1] Even a Latin Bishop, Luitprand, grew a beard (*prolixa contra morem barba*) when sent to Constantinople, in 962, as the ambassador of the Holy Roman Emperor. But he drew the line at wearing his hair long, and bitterly denounced this Byzantine custom.

Beard Cult in Russia

It is not, then, surprising that in Russia, under the influence of the Orthodox Church, beards were universal and greatly reverenced. A note to Zachary Grey's *Hudibras*, with regard to a passage already quoted, explains that the Russian nobility, in the seventeenth century, *accounting it a grace to be somewhat gross and burly . . . nourish and spread their beards to have them long and broad—* this from an account in Purchas. Abraham Rees in his *Cyclopædia* quotes the Novgorodian Code that the fine for plucking a single hair from a Russian beard was four times that for cutting off a finger ; if so Russian law was at one time far more rigorous in this matter than that of Alfred the Great or Frederick Barbarossa.

How the Czar blew his nose

We have noticed the delight with which Ivan the Terrible handled the beard of George Killingworth. But the ambassadors who came from the West in the time of Peter the Great were smooth of cheek ; and the story goes that to one the Czar expressed his resentment at the insult.[1] *Had my royal master measured wisdom by the beard*, the emissary is reported to have replied, *he would have sent a goat*. Perhaps some such incident influenced the Muscovite. Perhaps it was merely part of his mania for Westernisation and Progress. Or perhaps there is a clue to what subsequently occurred in the correspondence of that enchanting social commentator, Charlotte Elizabeth of Bavaria, Duchess of Orléans. In one of those intimate letters to her aunt, Charlotte Elizabeth took exception to the fact that the Czar of all the Russias blew his nose with his fingers. *Quand on se mouche avec les doigts*, she complained, *comme fait mon héros le czaar (sic), on ne doit pas porter des moustaches, car le résidu reste en suspension et cela n'est guère appétissant, surtout à table.* I cannot believe that the *subosco* entirely escaped the fate of the moustachio.

It is possible that Peter discovered this, or that the lady dropped him a hint. He may have thought it out—should all

[1] According to Pagenstecher one of the bearded Roman emperors refused to receive the ambassadors of the Veneti because they were clean shaven. In some ages and in certain countries it was evidently regarded as a mark of disrespect.

Russians be provided with handkerchiefs, or would it be cheaper to make them all shave ? (Even Charlotte Elizabeth, in deploring imperial manners, had said that *Cela économise des mouchoirs.*) Whatever the reason, [1] Peter the Great decided in 1698 to abolish beards in Russia. He first shaved the principle *boyars* with his own hands and later issued a *ukase*. All were to shave under heavy penalties, graded according to rank ;   but the priests were let off with a small beard tax (no more than that paid by the serfs) of one copeck.

On the Russian gentry the razor fell like a thunderbolt. Each time a beard passed the gates of a city a hundred roubles had to be paid, the receipt being a copper disk, the *borodováia* (i.e. *the bearded*), showing a bearded head on one side. Various amendments to this law were later made, but it was not rescinded by Peter's successors, and beards were persecuted in Russia for sixty years, until the time of Catherine II. Though no general law against beards was ever subsequently promulgated in Russia (so far as I know—but it's a wise man who will speak with certainty of what may be happening at this moment behind the Iron Curtain)[2] the Czar Nicholas I in 1845 decreed that Jews in Russia should remove their side-whiskers, and forcible means were employed to this end.[3]

Massacre of the Russian Beards

The effect of Peter's edict has been compared by Dulaure to the Massacre of St. Bartholomew's Day. He speaks of the lawless violence used against those who resisted, the reluctant sighs of those who complied. Many kept their shorn glory to be

[1] The Russian soldiers (according to Rowland in *The Human Hair*) were told that they were to shave in order to distinguish them from the bearded Turks in battle. Rowland says that when the Russians later fought the Swedes, who shaved, the Russian soldiers naturally felt that they should grow beards again.

[2] I have seen it stated that the Soviet Government has revived, to some extent, the mission of Peter I.

[3] See article in the *Jewish Encyclopedia* on the *Pelot*, i.e., the side-whiskers worn by Jews, especially in Russia and Poland. See also Appendix D.

buried with them[1]—a custom comparable to that of some Moslems with the combings of their beards, as already observed.

Dean Stanley, in his classic *The Eastern Church*, explains and describes the magnitude of this revolution. Had not the Patriarch Michael Cœrularius in his *Edictum Synodale* laid it down, in the eleventh century, that the beard was one of the primary differences between the Greek and Latin Churches ? Had not a Council of Moscow, in the seventeenth century, pronounced that *to shave the beard is a sin which even the blood of martyrs cannot expiate ?* The beard, sanctified in Leviticus, was part of the image of God in which man was made. Our Saviour himself wore one . . . Deep-rooted conservatism is sometimes a useful ally when liberty is at stake ; and even Peter, in his later amendments, showed an inclination to yield a little to the die-hard obstinacy of the peasants. In the end he may be said to have failed, just as he failed to convert the *moujiks* to smoking tobacco. *Not that which goeth into the mouth, but that which cometh out of the mouth defileth a man*, they had told him when it was a question of smoking.[2] It would have been useless for the Imperial Reformer to point out that beards were analogous to the latter category, and should be removed by similar reasoning.

Peter will be remembered as the greatest persecutor of the beard in the eighteenth century, or any other time ; and beards still tremble at the memory of his name. [3]

[1] According to Dean Stanley, the explanation in the case of the Russians was that they feared they would not be recognised at the gates of Heaven if they did not wear their beards. How it was proposed to re-adjust these to their chins, in the confusion of the last Trump, has not been explained.

[2] See Matthew XV, 11, and Stanley's *Eastern Church*, Lecture XII.

[3] His reforms appear to have had a lasting effect on the Russian Civil Service, unless I misunderstand a passage in *Crime and Punishment*.

CHAPTER XI

THE NINETEENTH CENTURY : HAIL AND FAREWELL

For the place, no man can deny the face to be one of the outward parts of the body which hath an honest appearance.

ANTHROPOMETAMORPHOSIS

La guerre des mentons contre les barbes éclata. Pendant douze grands mois, on ne s'entendit plus dans la presse. Toutes les questions, question de Grèce, question des Balkans, question de Naples, question d'Orient, question d'Espagne, disparurent, dans une nuée de brochures et de feuilletons, sous la question de la barbe.

Victor Hugo

Let me stroake my beard thrice like a Germin, before I speak a wise word.

PAPPE WITH AN HATCHET

ETIENNE DE SILHOUETTE was a French Minister, before the Revolution, whose name became immortalised—some say because the taxes he proposed would have left only a bare minimum to his victims, others contending that he was in office for so brief a period that no more than a outline was seen of him. The *silhouettes* of the eighteenth century and the early nineteenth were admirably suited to the fashions of those times. Shaven faces make clear outlines. There they sit, with their powdered hair—real or false—looking like Hollywood caricatures of themselves, and never a beard in sight, bare *minima* of reality. [1]

Decline of the Wig

Wigs in their hey-day had even caused a currency crisis in France, owing to the vast sums sent abroad for the purchase of German hair ; but the industry gradually declined, and the guillotine even produced a slump in prices as the hair of decapi-

[1] In spite of the antithesis which we shall notice (*perruques* v. *barbes*) it is noteworthy that Sterne classed great wigs and long beards together under the *Magna Carta* of stupidity.

tated aristocrats, Girondists and others flooded the market. Both wigs and powder were associated in France with the old régime. Had there not been riots at Caen, in Normandy, as early as 1715 (of which Canel gives details) on account of the amount of good flour being used as hair powder—the bread of the poor being sacrificed to the fads of the idle rich?

Among the most powerful influences upon the fashion in beards, as in other things, the example of the Court has always been considerable, though not always decisive. The beard grown by George III during his insanity, under the Regency, was not imitated by his subjects. (*O Lord, shave the King* is attributed to one of his chaplains.) But for the most part vox populi is as happy to echo a lunatic as any other oracle, provided he be crowned. *Cuius rex eius religio*, or (as as old French saying has it):

> Communément la subjecte Province
> Forme ses moeurs au moule de son Prince.

But now it is the Republic which sets the pace. A short hair-cut becomes fashionable in France, and despite all prejudice gradually replaces the older styles in other countries[1]. The stage is, as it were, set for the entry of the beard; and yet it takes half a century to arrive.

La barbe and la perruque

The first Earl of Eldon, when appointed Lord Chancellor in 1801, asked the king (George III) if he might dispense with the heavy wig, and gave as a reason the fact that a judge in the time of James I did not wear one. The king (who at the time was

---

[1] The *queue* or pig-tail will be remembered as one of the last styles in which hair was worn long, and it was considered a mark of Republicanism at one time to remove it. For example, in 1799, when the *Christian Army of the Holy Faith* (a muster consisting largely of brigands and convicts, led by the Cardinal Fabrizio Ruffo) entered Naples, which had been held for a time by the Republicans, the Christian Army massacred all inhabitants whom they found without pig-tails. It was this reign of terror which was actively supported by the glorious Horatio Nelson, who arrived on the scene with a British fleet, and added to his reputation by breaking faith with the Republicans after their capitulation. They were arrested after being promised a safe-conduct, and the commander of the Republican fleet was hanged at the yard-arm on Nelson's flag-ship.

comparatively sane and completely shaven) replied that he could be excused the wig if he undertook to grow a beard, as King James's judges could be cited as a precedent for that, also. Eldon stuck to the wig.   The story is interesting as an illustration of the accepted antithesis between *la barbe* and *la perruque*.   Hence it was not remarkable that some of the Montagnards, in 1793, considered the growth of a beard as a proper accompaniment to wearing their own hair, short andunpowdered, and—in a word—to their revolutionary principles.

Aubril speaks of the beard of Jourdan (known as *Coupe-Tête*) having attained *des proportions démesurées*. But on most faces the Revolution inspired little more than a slight extension of the hair on either side—those side-whiskers or *favoris* which can hardly be regarded as political emblems at this stage, as they soon became common to all parties and most countries.[1]   Indeed, a few young bloods in England had anticipated this fashion in the seventeen-sixties, a fact which is made clear in a booklet by one John Clubbe, Rector of Whatfield in Suffolk, entitled *A Letter of Free Advice to a Young Clergyman*, published in 1765. After telling his young clergyman to wear a full wig (and not, he says, one that scarce covers your ears) because he must otherwise appear ridiculous, the Rev. Clubbe next gives a warning against wearing one's own hair till age has made it venerable ; and finally he says :

Neither come into that *Jewish* fashion of wearing a skirting of beard round the face; in *them* it may be proper enough, but with us Openness of Countenance is a Characteristic of an ingenuous Mind.

The Jewish Pe'ot

It was this Jewish *Pe'ot* that later offended the Czar Nicholas I— or perhaps his edict against it was vaguely connected with Francophobia and an association with Republicanism, as Aubril suggests. (In that case the Czar was badly out of date in his information, but it is not impossible).   Actually the fashion was

[1] They may have been of Spanish origin, and the Peninsula War undoubtedly stimulated the fashion in England. The influence of the Netherlands is also probable.

to become characteristically English, since it was in England that side-whiskers eventually attained their greatest distinction, in the elongated form of *Dundrearies* : these derived their name from a character in Sothern's play, *Our American Cousin*, and were affected mainly by the well-to-do. In France the *favori* became at the same time a mark of the Royalist—the Republicans and Buonapartists having in the meanwhile evolved their own characteristic emblems. By the end of the first decade of the nineteenth century side-whiskers were therefore well established.

Meanwhile the moustache was coming slowly into favour. Admired by the Prince Regent on the wooden faces of his German soldiers, it was grown, at Prinny's command, by his own regiment, though the Worcestershire Militia claim to have been the first English regiment to wear moustaches, in 1798[1]. Wellington, in one of his despatches of 1811, wrote : *Almost all the Artillerymen wore mustachios, which I think is contrary to your orders.* Such complaints soon became frequent—evidently the British army intended to adopt the moustache as its emblem ; and on the French side, too, moustaches increased in number among the veterans of the Napoleonic wars.

Quandary of a Cavalry Officer

In *The Life and Letters of Dr. Samuel Butler* (1896) by his grandson, the author of *Erewhon*, there is some mention of the changing fashions in the British army. This will be found in a letter (Vol. I, page 150) by one Marmaduke Lawson, who commanded a company in 1818, and mentioned that *next year we are ordered to be all provided not only with whiskers,*[2] *but with moustaches.* For this reason the writer's mother had docked his allowance of an item of

[1] As already observed, there had been an uninterrupted apostolic succession of moustaches in certain Continental regiments. An odd comment on this is afforded by an incident which marked the birth of Ludwig I of Bavaria in 1786. *The troops*, we are informed, *cut off their moustaches in his honour.* Perhaps this was another case of imitating royalty. (See *The Ludwigs of Bavaria* by Henry Channon.)

[2] Evidently side-whiskers—beards were still forbidden except, apparently, in the 19th Lancers in 1820-21. (See *Notes and Queries*, 11th S. IV, 458.) Even in the French Army beards were then worn only by Sapeurs. For further information see *Notes and Queries*, 14th Series, CLIX, 316, 355 and CLX, 64.

five shillings for shaving (a monthly sum, one supposes) *alleging that a soldier had no business with a razor—a beard was as much part of his armour as his helmet or his shield.* What troubled Marmaduke, it would appear, was the uncooperative attitude of Nature, whose poor efforts he proposed to supplement with Macassar. A plate showing English Cavalry Uniforms, 1821-1822, in Captain Gronow's *Reminiscences and Recollections* (New York, 1900, Vol II, page 192) depicts all but one of the cavalrymen wearing moustaches, the odd man having perhaps experienced the same difficulties as those discovered by Marmaduke.

The origin of the beard proper in the nineteenth century is generally assigned to the French Romantics and Republicans of the eighteen-thirties. A story which appears to contradict this, and even to give the original nineteenth century beard a very different political colour, is told by Canel. He claims that the officers who fled to Cherbourg with Charles X in 1830 grew beards as a sign of mourning—a story for which he gives no evidence, and I can find none independently. But I suspect that his source of information was Guernon Ranville, a Legitimist who accompanied the king in his flight, and a man who had a special interest in the matter, if Canel himself is to be credited on another point. There exists a book entitled *Essai sur la culture des Cheveux, suivi de quelques reflexions sur l'art de la coiffure*, purporting to have been the work of a certain hairdresser, M. Duflos, and published at Paris in 1812. This book is catalogued under the name of L. J. Duflos in the British Museum Library, but I have studied it and it is—though brief and frivolous—clearly the work of a scholar. And in the pages of Canel's *Histoire de la Barbe et des Cheveux en Normandie* (which I found uncut in the British Museum Reading Room) it is categorically stated that the work attributed to the hairdresser was, in fact, written by Guernon Ranville, later a Minister of State.

It seems probable that Canel received both pieces of information from Ranville himself, as he could have spoken from personal knowledge in each case—a supposition which might account for Canel's reluctance to reveal the source of his information. I favour Guernon Ranville's candidature for the authorship of the essay, myself, because his name indicates a hereditary interest in mustachios.

Liberty, Equality and Pogonotrophy

If, however, the beard appeared for a moment as a token of royalist grief, it was soon to be seen as a sign of republican jubilation. Indeed, according to T. S. Gowing (who claimed that *with every attempt at freedom on the Continent the Beard re-appears*) the beard had already proved *one of the most effective standards in the war for freedom when Germany rose againts Napoleon*. Mr. Gowing even held that the beard *has made many a perjured continental monarch quake and tremble in his capital*. So thought many French romantics in and after the year 1830.

In 1828 a certain Monsieur and Madame Stop had written a *Manuel complet de la toilette* stating without qualifications that

> La barbe est l'attribut de la virilité. Elle est sans contredit une des parties les plus essentielles de la toilette, et occupe le rang le plus élevé dans la catégorie des soins que l'on doit apporter à son visage.

Nevertheless the beard was not quick to sprout on the chins of all the Romantics and Republicans who were now to be considered its principal champions. Portraits show Alexandre Dumas as beardless in 1827 and still beardless in 1855. So is Eugène Delacroix in 1834, and Chopin in 1838—even Gautier in the same year. Balzac in 1842 has only a moustache. Lamartine in 1841 has side-whiskers, but earlier and later pictures show him without even these. Side-whiskers were all that Alfred de Vigny could show in 1830, or Berlioz in 1832. Prosper Mérimée in a self-portrait appears with a scanty *barbe chinoise*. Alfred de Musset's self-caricature of 1833 shows him beardless, though in 1841 he appears with a full beard. As late as 1860 a large number of the Romantics were beardless, as Aubril shows, giving a formidable list.

The Beard Romantic

One can only assume, in view of the evidence, that the beard was worn principally by the Fan Public rather than by those whom they admired. (It is significant that, with all the extravagance of dress in which many Romantics indulged, their acknowledged leader, Victor Hugo, was always immaculately respectable.)[1]   Nevertheless Louis Maigron, in *Le Romantisme et la Mode*, speaks of long hair and beards as distinctive indices of Young France at this time.   At the first nights of *Hernani* and *Antony* there were (he says) *Barbes assyriennes et cheveux mérovingiens*. Maxime Du Camp remembered them (young men *à longs cheveux portant toute leur barbe—ce qui était contraire aux bons usages*).   Such was the artist Petrus Borel, among the first to wear a long beard, *au moment où personne ne la portrait ainsi*[2].   The long beards and *cheveux flottants* were supposed to be a mediæval revival—those who wore them having but a vague conception of the Middle Ages, when custom was often so hostile to the beard.

Testimony against white linen

One of Maigron's illustrations, from the Hartmann Collection, entitled *Au bal des Romantiques* shows some very seedy beavers dancing.   It is possible that many of the Romantics grew beards as a substitute for clean linen, for the principles of some included an abhorrence of the expanse of shirt collar which marked classical (and therefore reactionary) tastes.   To exhibit any white linen at the neck therefore marked a man as *un profane, un retardataire, un hottentot, un épicier, un bourgeois, un philistin et—pour tout dire en un mot—un classique*.   The vast *cravate*, commonly of black, took the place of this Bourgeois-Hottentot fashion, so far as Young France was concerned.[3]   But doubtless a full beard must have served the same purpose.

At the famous Battle of Hernani (February 1830), when the rival factions fought for life and honour at the first night of a

[1] In all matters : he never grew a beard until it had become fashionable.

[2] Gautier couples the name of Eugène Devéria with that of Borel as the first two men in France to wear beards.   The periodic adoption by artists of this ornament, from the time of Liotard, has already been noticed.   To wear the full beard required at that time, according to Gautier, a truly heroic courage, *sang froid* and contempt for the crowd.   Gautier describes a ball given in 1830 where one could see *virgules à la Jules Mazarin* and *des moustaches civiles*—mild innovations.   This can hardly be the ball mentioned below.

[3] A certain Dr. Véron was so famous for his extravagance in this matter that a letter was addressed to him : *Monsieur Véron, dans sa cravate, Paris*.   Other emblems included the famous red waistcoat in which Gautier marshalled the organised cohorts of the Romantics (400 in number) at the *Bataille d'Hernani*.

theatrical production, Théophile Gautier (*Histoire du romantisme*) remembered the beards which appeared on the side of Romance. Similarly, at the first night of *Antony* there were seen *des royales pointues, des cheveux mérovingiens*. Before long Elias Regnault could record mediæval beards as a common sight—you could see that of Henry III, too, he said, in a railway carriage. Styles included *barbes de bouc, de chêvre, barbes à la turque, à la mauresque, à la mouche, au papillon, aux ailes de pigeon, etc.,* in addition to the full beards of Young France. Those who could not produce true beards wore false ones.

Calumnies against the beard

Between the *Barbe* and the *Perruque*[1] there was deadly war, as Victor Hugo later recalled :

Il y eut des duels de plume et des duels d'épée . . . La Barbe fut décrétée laide, sotte, sale, immonde, infecte, repoussante, ridicule, antinationale, juive, affreuse, abominable, hideuse, et ce qui était alors le dernier degré de l'injure, romantique !

It is unfortunate that Victor Hugo in this passage—which should be compared with the description of the wickedness of white linen in order to appreciate the warmth of this controversy—did not specify any duels fought on the beard question. One must suspect him in this of slight exaggeration. (The passage which precedes it, placed at the head of this chapter, is not without the same suggestion of hyperbole.) But Hugo could genuinely recall the solemn profession of faith made by Théophile Gautier during the last years of the Bourbon Restoration, in which he proclaimed the Gospel of the Beard.

Among the cruelties practised by the Duc de Modène on his estates, he is said to have cut off the moustaches and side whiskers of all whose passports were not in order. It is curious that about this time even the Sultan began to suspect beards of harbouring sedition, for a writer in *Blackwood's Magazine* (October,

---

[1] M. Quitard, quoted under *Barbe* in Larousse, *Dic. du XIX Siècle*, wrote *Honneur à ces incomparables jeunes gens, qui ont si bien préludé à la restauration de la barbe par la guerre contre les perruques !* (This was written in 1838.)

1833) recorded that in Turkey an Imperial decree had banned them. [1]

The seditious moustache

Even the moustache acquired sudden significance in the political world. In August 1830, the people of Brussels, fired by a performance of Auber's opera, *La Muette de Portici* (which eulogised the revolt of Masaniello in Naples, three hundred years ago) marched through the streets singing the popular number *Amour Sacré de la Patrie* and wearing false moustaches as emblems of national revolt. The Dutch rulers certainly regarded the moustache as seditious, and where their troops gained ground the moustaches disappeared as miraculously as they had come into being, though some of the Hollanders nevertheless claimed to have gathered enough to stuff mattresses for the military hospitals. In Paris, too, false moustaches had appeared suddenly in the previous month, as badges of revolt. Dickens in *Household Words* (August 13, 1853) claimed that the moustache was regarded as a mark of aristocracy in Germany prior to 1848, but that after the revolutions of that year the German people *took to the obliteration of the vain mark of distinction by growing hair on their own chins and upper lips*. This use of the moustache as an emblem of defiance is evidently connected with its similar use in Holland by the *Gheuses* (as recorded by Strada in a passage already quoted) in the sixteenth century.

Persecution of beards and moustaches

Charles Mackay in his *Memoirs of Extraordinary Popular Delusions* (1841), where he records the use of the moustache in the revolutions of 1830, mentions that German newspapers in August 1838 had reported an ordinance by the King of Bavaria, forbidding citizens to wear moustaches. Offenders were to be arrested and forcibly shaved. Mackay quoted from a French paper that the order has been universally obeyed. Alexander Rowland, writing

[1] Apparently unaware of the gathering storm of Paris, the same writer, speaking of beards, remarked that *no one but a Turk or a Jew is to be seen so heretical . . . as to prefer nature to art*. This writer's ignorance of the history of the Beard in mediæval and Tudor times is astonishing.

in 1853 (*The Human Hair*, etc.) reported a recent decree of the Austrian Emperor forbidding all state functionaries to wear beards ; and at the moment when he wrote (April 1853) Rowland claimed that in Naples men were being *dragged daily into the barber's shops by the police, and their beards trimmed according to the political creed of the authorities.* The subject is mentioned later by T. W. Belcher, in a work to which I shall presently refer. It was not long, he wrote (in 1864) since Francis II of Naples had forbidden beards by a royal decree *because they savoured too much of the revolutionary principle of Garibaldi.* It is worth noting that the first nineteenth century beard in the House of Commons was worn by a Radical, G. F. Muntz, in 1840. In France the persecution of the beard in academic circles continued even under the Second Empire. (The notable case of The Beard of Professor Sarcey is discussed by Maurice Rat in *Le Figaro Littéraire*, July 30, 1949.) According to Lewis Gannett, in a recent article, similar persecution has been experienced in our own time by a bearded student at New York University.

Mr. James Laver considers that by 1837 all the Romantic fashions in France had disappeared—except the beard. As political styles crystallised, Maxime Du Camp could note that the supporters of Louis Philippe wore simply *favoris*, the Buonapartists wearing a moustache and pointed *impériale*. The Republicans, together with artists, literary men and those who claimed to represent Young France, favoured the full beard. According to R. W. Proctor, in *The Barber's Shop*, edition of 1883, the political significance of whiskers in France was still observable even then, though the distinctive styles had changed with the growing popularity of the beard. He speaks of the moustache at that time as signifying either royalism or Buonapartism—*the Legitimists of the older branch having adopted a square cut, in contradiction to the Imperial which is stiff and pointed.*

An Irish Legend

As late as 1909, when the bearded vogue of the middle and late Victorians had come and gone, a writer in the *Encyclopædia of Religion and Ethics* (Edward Clodd, writing on Beards) could record that it was within the memory of the middle-aged that the wearing of beards rendered the individual liable to assault and insult, and that it met with opposition and prohibition from employers of labour and persons in authority—evidently by association with political radicalism and *La Vie Bohème*, from which the Victorian Renaissance traced its shady pedigree. Probably the last appearance of the beard political was in Ireland, about the year 1916, when patriots with Gælic *foaming like porter on their beards* (the words are, I believe, George Moore's) appeared in the streets of Dublin, and sympathisers grew beards—so I am told—to disguise by multitude the active rebels whose uniform was worn on the chin. I have heard this story flatly contradicted in Dublin, and merely throw it in because some who claim to remember the *Troubles* equally vehemently insist upon its truth. I am content that it should remain a legend, like the long beard of Charlemagne, more beautiful than prosaic truth.

The Bearded Socialist

The beards of Blanqui, Marx and the patriarchs of socialism may have had some connection with this venerable association between beards and radical opinions, though these pioneers were so soon followed by an almost universal fashion of beardedness that it is hard to distinguish the beard political from the beard *à la mode* after about 1860. The bearded socialist is nevertheless to be marked as a type, and I believe that Mr. Shaw once wrote a letter to *The Nation* drawing attention to the advantages of whiskers in political controversy. The beards of William Morris, Edward Carpenter, Hyndman, Olivier and others will immediately spring to the reader's mind—and, of course, the goat-like growth of Sidney Webb (I think the only beard in a Labour Cabinet), also the white whiskers of G.B.S. himself.[1] I recalled this when surveying a row of Labour Cabinet Ministers in the press not long since. They looked so like a mixture of Belsen guards and Belsen victims that I reflected on the value of Nature's kindly disguise, which the Labour Party had recklessly abandoned when discarding its principles. It is true that a late Labour M.P. (William Bruce) had the largest moustache in Parliament, but

[1] At the time of writing a Labour M.P., Benn Levy, still preserves the bearded tradition in the House.

socialists have moved with the times in beards as in other matters. Mr. St. John Ervine, writing of H. G. Wells (who wore no more than a shaggy moustache) says that *he frequently derided Marx's beard.*

Apostolic succession of bearded vegetarians

The Bearded Vegetarian may be said to belong to the same combine, Shaw, Carpenter and others holding shares in both companies. Thoreau, Tolstoi, Wagner, Garibaldi, Musonius Rufus and Henry S. Salt, not to mention the bearded vegetarian mentioned in Chapter V of this book and Nebuchadnezzar, also Julian the Apostate, are a few examples. Charles Forward's *History of the Vegetarian Movement* is abundantly illustrated with photographs of vegetarian pioneers, the overwhelming majority of the males being bearded. I think this is the true answer to Professor Rolleston's outrageous attempt to associate the wearing of beards with the eating of horseflesh, but I still have a thought on this, which I will share with you presently. The reader will perhaps have noted the connection of the beard with vegetarianism in the case histories of Joshua Evans and Benjamin Lay ; and I think some claim for antiquity can be made out in the names of Seneca, Tertullian, Clement of Alexandria and the Essenes. Apostolic succession or continuity could probably be traced through Bearded Vegetarians of many centuries, such as Cornaro and Sir Thomas More. Indeed, I have a mind to stake a claim for St. John Chrysostom, too. It was therefore not remarkable that beards continued to flourish on many vegetarian chins long after they had been abandoned by creophagous jaws. For some reason a beard (Vandyke style)[1] was also worn by many physicians about the year 1900, when the beard had become démodé—another curious survival which did not last long, in spite of royal encouragement and example, when Edward VII was crowned in 1901 (the first bearded monarch in England for over 200 years, if

[1] The Vandyke was mentioned by the *Westmister Gazette* of June 25, 1894, as being worn by *everyone* (we know what such statements are worth) with the comment that *a few years ago the Vandyke beard was unknown.* Actually the moustache was at that time the most common fashion, and the mark of every successful *masher.*

we omit the beard grown by the third George during his insanity).
His father had been a leader of the bearded fashion, though at the
time of his marriage he had only reached the moustache stage.

From such highly specialised or functional beards I must
return to the growth and bibliography of the common beard in the
nineteenth century. Of pogonologists Repton is the next of any
distinction. John Adey Repton, F.S.A. was the son of Humphrey Repton, well known in his time as a landscape gardener and
the disciple of Capability Brown. Repton *père* boasted *artistical
knowledge*, which, with the horrifying formula of his period, he
claimed to combine with *good taste and good sense*. The works of
such specialists, who persuaded the English gentry to spend vast
sums on ruining the countryside, were briefly referred to by
Cowper in a poem from which I have already quoted.

The work of Repton

Repton *fils* was trained as an architect. After supplementing
his father's improvements by tasteful tinkerings with stately
homes, he turned his attention to archæology, and in 1839 he
circulated privately a small octavo entitled *Some Account of the Beard
and Moustachio, chiefly from the Sixteenth to the Eighteenth Century*.
This book had its origin in a paper read to the Society of Anti-
quaries, and only one hundred copies were printed. It is a
valuable guide to facial flora in Britain, and is accompanied
by two plates showing the styles worn at different periods. To
this essay I am indebted for some significant information showing
the rising prestige of the beard, as early as 1818, for in that year
the Rev. George D'Oyly and Richard Mant, Protestant Bishop of
Killaloe, published an edition of the Bible with explanatory notes,
and commented as follows on Isaiah VII :

> The hairs of the head (said they) are those of highest order in
> the state ; those of the feet, or lower parts, are the common
> people ; the *beard*, the king, the high-priest . . .

Repton wrote simply as an antiquarian. The first vigorous
plea for a revival of the beard in nineteenth century England
appears to have been that of Alexander Rowland in *The Human
Hair* (1853), a work which has come into my hands, through the

kindness of a hairdresser, just as I am finishing this book. Rowland and Sons manufactured preparations for the hair, skin, teeth, etc. They gave two new words to our vocabulary—*Macassar*, a proprietary brand of hair oil, and *Anti-Macassar*, the protective device whereby house-wives endeavoured to keep their chair-backs clean. Rowland *fils* was manifestly a scholar and a man of strong opinions, as his book proves. Many subsequent writers, including T. S. Gowing, evidently used his researches, though without acknowledgments. To me he is chiefly valuable for his wide study of contemporary periodicals from which he quotes extensively, though unfortunately in many cases he does not date his sources.

A Methodist plea for the beard

It appears that, when Rowland wrote, the *London Methodist Quarterly Review* had recently advocated the beard for ministers of the gospel, as a prophylactic against bronchitis. *The fact that the Creator planted a beard upon the face of the human male*, said the Methodist writer, *indicates, in a mode not to be misunderstood, that the distinctive appendage was bestowed for the purpose of being worn.* Rowland also records a plea for the beard by Dr. Dixon, described as a leading physician of New York, in his influential publication, *The Scalpel*. Letters had appeared in the *Montreal Herald*, various other doctors had advocated beardedness for hygienic reasons, and the great sanitarian reformer, Edwin Chadwick, had lent his support to the agitation. A correspondent in *The Globe* (August 28, 1852) claimed that the beard was the only muffler used by Russians at 35 degrees below zero. The *Edinburgh News* published an article recommending the specific value of beards for masons. In Spain *El Siglo Medico* took the matter up in 1861 (viii, 686-687) and the same year two articles appeared in the *Medical and Surgical Reporter* of Philadelphia (1861, v, 234-6 and 262). Even earlier the *Boston Medical and Surgical Journal* (1844, 353-356) had carried an article on *The growth of the beard historically considered*; but in 1861 we are reading of *The Beard Question*. Among many entries which will be found in Poole's Index to Periodical Literature (1802-1881) articles on the beard are noticed in the *Westminster Review* (Vol. 62), *The Living Age* (Vol. 42), *The*

Eclectic Magazine (Vol. 3), *Bentley's Miscellany* (Vol. 11), *The Penny Magazine* (Vol. 3), *Once a Week* (Vol. 16), *The Irish Quarterly Review* (Vols. 8 and 9), *All the Year Round* (Vol. 23), *St. James's* (Vol. 48) and *Every Saturday* (Vol. 11)—a very mixed assortment of English and American periodicals. [1]

The sum of man's suffering

Insistence on the value of the beard to a man's health was strongly stressed, as the reader will have observed. A typical title is that chosen by a certain A. M. Adams : *Is Shaving Injurious to Health ? A Plea for the Beard.* [2] *Tait's Magazine* (November, 1852) added a playful appeal, and the *Naval and Military Gazette* (March 12, 1853) advocated moustaches for all soldiers. *The United Services Gazette* urged that the abolition of shaving tackle would lighten the soldier's knapsack (and make room, no doubt, for the Field-marshal's Baton). An Article in the *United Service Magazine* (September and October, 1851) had already protested against the daily torture of shaving—*that sum of suffering . . . which Byron declared quite made up for what the other sex endured in parturition.* Finally, the *Agra Messenger* pleaded for equality between British and Indian soldiers, since (apart from the cavalry) British regiments were not permitted to indulge in any of the freedom granted to Seopy faces. (A recent and interesting comment on the Indian troops is to be found in the magazine of

[1] A writer in *Notes and Queries* (9th S. II, 198) adds Dr. Doran's *Habits and Men* (1854) to the Beard literature of this period.

[2] *Edinburgh Medical Journal*, 1861 (VII, 566-573). Rowland quotes *Ree's Cyclopædia* (by which I suppose he means the *Cyclopædia* of Abraham Rees, though I cannot find the quotation in the article on Beards). As quoted, the *Cyclopædia* went so far as to maintain that shaving *has been supposed with much apparent reason, to weaken the understanding, by diverting the blood from the brain to the surface of the head.* Shaving was also held, on the same authority, to weaken a man physically. Curiously enough Rees was the last nonconformist minister to officiate in a wig, sufficient reason in itself for the fact that he never wore a beard on his own chin. Cabanès in his *Curiosités de la Médicine* (Vol. 1, 79-84) quotes many other authorities of this period who held shaving to be injurious to health. Apart from that his chapter on beards is disappointing for such a *savant*. An American correspondent points out that thousands of shaven men die for every one with a beard, judging by newspaper portraits, and that Insurance companies should consider this fact.

the Royal Zoological Society of Scotland—January 1949—where
Lt.-Col. C. H. Stockley has an article on *The Drinking Habits of
Wild Animals*. He finds that long haired animals require more
water, and says that in India the same is believed of bearded men.
Sikhs, he remarks, *always need more water than their beardless com-
rades of the Indian Army*. The *Agra Messenger* had not, I think,
considered this aspect of the case.)

Douglas Jerrold, in the *Weekly News*, came out for the whole
hog, without compromise—the beard, the whole beard and
nothing but the beard. Charles Dickens, in *Household Words*
(August 3, 1853) admitted that he shaved, but poured heavy scorn
upon the custom to which he conformed, praising the portent of
nostrils that *dilate over a beard curling visibly with anger*. As for Mr.
Rowland himself, he marshalled every possible argument. A
bearded man, he maintained, would not fawn or cringe to anyone.
And the appalling waste of time ! Had not the poet Campbell
(Thomas, as I suppose) calculated that in seventy years—deducting,
one presumes, those of childhood—enough time was spent in the
daily shave to learn seven languages ? Had not Southey tested and
corroborated the assertion ? Only prejudice could account for
such stupidity—a prejudice less excusable than that of those
American Indians, who abhor beards because of their own
inability to grow presentable specimens.

Shaving and the compost heap

Alexander Rowland was not always very accurate in his facts.
He believed that shaving was a *servile imitation of the first George*,
and that *prior to the reign of George I such a practice was unknown*.
But in spite of many such errors *The Human Hair* is packed with
useful information and may have helped to bring about the great
revolution for which Europe had been preparing ever since 1830.
I am grateful to Rowland, above all, for some illuminating
comments on the value of our clippings and shavings, which I
have marked for a footnote to any future edition of *Cleanliness and
Godliness*. It appears that by throwing away or destroying the
surplus hair of our heads and faces we deprive the soil of very good
manure, assessed by Mr. Rowland in 1853 at 3,000 tons annually
in Great Britain and Ireland alone.

When Rowland wrote the state of affairs may be judged to some extent by military and naval regulations. In the American army the beard was permitted, provided it was kept short. But the comments quoted from the Services Magazines will have made it clear that the British soldier was severely hampered by Red Tape. In the British navy both moustaches and *unseemly tufts of hair under the chin* were *streng verboten*. The position among British civilians in 1852 is illustrated by a discussion in *Friends in Council* (Sir A. Helps) from which it appears that the average professional man at that time regarded it as something requiring more than mortal courage to let his beard grow.

Revolution of the eighteen sixties

Fourteen years later a writer in *Fraser's Magazine* (A. K. H. Boyd in March, 1866) quoted Helps and remarked upon the progress: half the men under forty in Scotland were then bearded, he considered. Many of the Scottish clergy wore beards, and even more of the clergy in England. *Chambers's Journal* helped the campaign with a long article in 1857 (June 13), mostly lifted from Repton, and another on November 15, 1862. In America, or at least in New York, beards had already become sufficiently common by 1850 for a writer (John Waters) to make them the subject of three articles in the *Knickerbocker* (April, May and June), though Mr. Waters regarded with distaste the many *greasy Citizens* whom he observed with whiskers.

Between 1850 and 1870 the side-whisker, creeping like *the little sorrel while all men slept* down the cheeks of our forefathers, grew into the mutton chop or the *Piccadilly Weeper*, that presents so outstanding an appearance in old portraits. Leaving bare the chin itself, these strange growths hung upon either side of it, giving to the face an expression of permanent injury and grievance. That most delightful of essayists, F. J. Hudleston (the late librarian at the War Office), once made a wild guess that the term *sideburn*, often used to describe this strange experiment in topiary, was derived by some peculiar manifestation of Grimm's Law from the name of the American General, A. E. Burnside. Certainly portraits of the General show the sideburns clearly enough. But I was surprised to discover that some authorities seriously gives this derivation, as the reader may find by consulting *The Mode in Hats and Headdress* by R. Turner Wilcox (New York, 1945).

In the British Army the *Queen's Regulations* up to the time of the Crimean War forbade the growth of these side-whiskers below the level of the mouth ; and as late as the eighteen sixties an Admiralty order still decreed shaving in the British Navy. But during the war army regulations evidently broke down, and the return of Bearded Veterans from the Crimea in 1855 heralded a New Deal. The heavy outlay of the propagandists at last began to show dividends.

The beards of Erin

Richard Caulfield, an antiquarian of Cork, made his contribution in *Notes and Queries* (February 9, 1861). Discussing the *Beard Controversy* (as it had then become) he recommended Robert Sharrock's learned treatise of the seventeenth century.[1] It was written in Latin, and there were probably not more than three copies available in the United Kingdom, but that would never trouble an antiquarian. And a few years later a similar effort was made by a doctor of medicine, one Belcher, whose paper on *The Hygienic Aspect of Pogonotrophy* was published with other lectures in *Tractatus Medici* (Dublin 1864). Beginning with the usual summary of ancient history—to which he added topical references regarding the beards of the bards of Tara and that of St. Patrick— he reminded his countrymen that the Irish Saint, Finn Barr, bore a name that signified *Grey Beard*. With a wise appeal to national sentiment he proceeded next to recall the cruel Act of 1446, whereby the Irish were directed *not to suffer their beards to grow on their upper lips ;* indeed he had heard it asserted that this cruel law was still on the statute book.[2]

---

[1] See page 252.

[2] This was very typical. A letter of Henry VIII to the people of Galway town (April 28, 1536) forbade the wearing of any clothes but those *shaped after the English fashion.* Soon after follows an Act (28 Henry VIII, Cap. XV) specifying that no Irish garments should be worn and banning Irish hair styles.   In 1571 the Lord President of Munster proclaimed an ordinance at Limerick whereby the inhabitants of cities and corporate towns were ordered not to *suffer their hair to grow glib.* See H. F. McClintock in *Old Irish and Highland Dress* (Dundalk, 1943).

Dr. Belcher hailed joyfully the return of the beard and the moustache. Already in 1861 an article in the *Temple Bar Magazine* (iii, 247) had noted with satisfaction that the beard had ceased to be a mark of artists, literary celebrities and those who delighted to live *en Bohème*. It added to the gravity even of the most solemn statesman (solemn but not serious, as Chesterton said of their descendants ; and it is still true). These now carried the fashionable *cache-sottises* or (as the *Temple Bar* writer called it) *this imposing feature of a man's countenance*. In short, it was already respectable. The Prince Consort himself was leading the fashion with whiskers below the chin.

The beard praised as a mask

Dr. Belcher commended the beard because it

makes a countenance, which would without it appear weak, appear full of reflection, force and decision. It serves to conceal the thoughts . . . saving the man from those betrayals which would pull down his dignity and render him often an unequal combatant in the competitive struggle of every-day life.

This is of great import. The Victorian beard was clearly a mask behind which weak flesh could pretend to Rugged Individualism, and Paterfamilias conceal the fact that he was terrified of his wife or the next-door-bull-pup. Like T. S. Gowing, Dr. Belcher dismisses the idea that it is unfair for women and children not to be provided with the same protection. He does not even discuss whether they have an equal need to save their faces (obviously it is only man who must appear courageous at all costs, even when his lips and knees are trembling) ; but as to the matter of warmth : *Women and children were intended to live chiefly in houses*, he says. [1] Nature and Dr. Belcher had so decreed. But as for the hardy male—*Who knows how many men contract fatal chest diseases on night guards, who might have escaped if bearded ?*

[1] Charles Dickens in *Household Words* (No. 177) took the same view : *Man is born to work out of doors . . . woman was created for duties of another kind. . . .* In his commentary on Gallen, Gasper Hoffmann maintained the same view. Women, he said, *mores habent non æque laudabiles*. See also pages 22-23.

Its absence a sign of moral weakness

T. S. Gowing's *Philosophy of Beards* is undated, and is generally assigned to the year 1880. But internal evidence makes it clear that it was written during the Crimean War, before beards became common. According to Mr. Gowing :

> The absence of Beard is usually a sign of physical and moral weakness ; and in degenerate tribes wholly without, there is a conscious want of manly dignity . . . such tribes have to be sought for by the physiologist and ethnologist : the historian is never called upon to do honour to their deeds . . .

Mr. Gowing evidently did not agree that the nation is happy which has no history. He also held that it was *impossible to view a series of bearded portraits . . . without feeling that they possess dignity, gravity, freedom, vigour and completeness.* Old men, particularly, should be bearded, in order to conceal the record of their lives, which he assumed to be invariably evil.

During the Crimean War it was fashionable to admire the Turks, which Mr. Gowing could do with enthusiasm. It was a pity that the Russians were also bearded ; but at least this offered a good target for insult, and Mr. Gowing could recall with relish the truly Oriental manner in which a Shah of Persia had expressed his anti-Russian sentiments : *I spit on their beards,* he had said to a British ambassador.

The horrors of Sunday shaving

Indirect support for the Beard Party came from certain Sabbatarians, who felt strongly on the subject of Sunday shaving, as the following quotation makes clear :

> While the bells of our churches are pealing their welcome to the House of God ; while thousands of devout, albeit close-shaved, Christians are wending their way demurely to the sanctuary, where the bread of life is to be dispensed and the glad tidings of salvation are to be proclaimed for the refreshment of God's people—lo ! in every by-street a shaving-shop stands open, and through the glazed door you see, what ? a human face, soaped and lathered to the eyes, with another

immortal being standing at his side, one hand grasping his victim's nose, and the other defying the commandment of God with the uplifted steel . . .

> Shaving, a Breach of the Sabbath and a Hindrance to the Spread of the Gospel, by Theologos. (London, 1860.)

The important question as to whether a person ought to devote as much time and attention to the toilet and to the care of his person on the Sabbath, as he would do upon other days of the week, had very properly concerned the authorities ever since the time of Moses. However, as the Jews did not shave, the question of barbering did not trouble the delicate consciences of Caiaphas and the Pharisees. But in later ages the problem was a real one for those who wished (as who does not ?) to look their best in church, and to those who hoped to add to their incomes on a Sunday morning. On the general issue of cleanliness, Fangé cites the Council of Orléans (A.D. 538), Canon 28, a Synod of Paris (755), and a Decretal of Pope Alexander III in 1160, to show that the Church officially approved the employment of a reasonable amount of time on Sundays, in order to make one's self presentable. The barbers, says Fangé, claimed that these decisions beatified their labours ; but they were mistaken. Ecclesiastical authority has always damned the sabbath-breaking barber. [1]

Methodists declare against it

We have already had some glimpses of this tradition in surveying the Barber-Surgeons. Did not Henry Chichele, Archbishop of Canterbury, forbid the barbers in 1414 to open their houses or shops (domos vel shoppas) and that sub poena excommunicationis majoris, on pain of major excommunication, pro exercitio artis eorum, die dominico ? In the eighteenth century, when shaving was universal and religion highly formalised, such scruples were easily laid aside. But with the nineteenth century beards and non-conformity are in partnership. Indeed, the Methodists did not wait for the beard, but struck as early as September, 1807, when their conference at Liverpool (according to the Methodist Magazine for that month) virtually excommunicated the sabbath-

[1] See Appendix H.

breaking barbers as effectively as ever Rome had done. But the scandal continued, and many references to Sunday shaving will be found in Proctor's *Barber's Shop*, of 1883.

We may now add to our collection of beard cuts the *barbe à la Souvaroff*, where the moustache meets the sidewhiskers, but the chin is bare (a style long affected by the British army) ; the *fer à cheval*, short and divided to resemble a horse-shoe ; the *collier*, a fringe of whiskers leaving the upper and lower lips shaven (our *Varmer Joiles*, in fact) ; the *cotelettes* or mutton chops, where the side-whiskers spread towards the mouth ; the *pattes de lapin*, which are little more than a slight extension of the hair in front of the ears and the *bouc*, or goatee. (This last was sufficiently noticeable in America, by 1856, for an Englishwoman to comment upon it among the eccentricities she observed in that country). A fan-shaped beard, described as the *Masonic* is mentioned in some retrospective articles that appeared in the *Hairdresser's Weekly Journal* in 1935 and 1936. In the *Rules and Technical Handbook* of the London Academy of Gentleman's Hairdressing (undated, but evidently by the same hand and published in the nineteen twenties) I find an imposing list of styles in addition to these—the *Belgrave*, the *Boulanger*, the *Francis-Joseph*, the *St. James*, the *Natal*, *Le Markis* (yes, *sic*) and likewise *Le Counte*. America could add to this list the *Horace Greeley* (similar to the French *Collier*) and the *Uncle Sam*, which was Nature's best effort to imitate the false beards of the Pharaohs.

Abe Lincoln's beard

The beard was so important in America by 1860 that Abraham Lincoln occupied valuable time during the presidential elections of that year by staying at home in order to grow one, evidently regarding it as a valuable asset at the White House—a beard was becoming almost as necessary as a Bible to a rising demagogue, and Lincoln was a shrewd observer.

G. M. Trevelyan, in his *English Social History*, remarks that after the Crimean War the beard returned, with the habit of smoking, to that well-bred society from which both had long been banished. Thus did Britain begin its age of *muscular Christianity*, and in spite of the Queen's well-known objection to tobacco the typical mid-Victorian of all classes was the man with a beard and a pipe, tokens of his manliness and of his Low-Church, Latitudinarian or respectable non-conformist conformity. This alliance is of interest and recalls once more the fact that Montaigne considered a moustache as an admirable reservoir of sweet scents, which it retained in suitable juxtaposition to his nostrils. The stern Aubril, however, in his *Essai sur la Barbe*, is more concerned with the problem of stale or unpleasant odours, and at the end of his first chapter he lays down an axiom that the use of tobacco is not compatible with long beards. The British evidently did not agree.

It is interesting that when Millais began to grow a beard, about 1854, Holman Hunt wrote encouragingly on the subject from Cairo, but expressed some doubts in his own case because he found that a clean chin was still regarded in the East as typically English, and compelled *cringing obedience*—which Hunt valued.

Disputed case of Mr. Grace

I will pass over such questions as to whether an Australian fast bowler put a ball right through the celebrated and prolific beard of W. G. Grace in a Test Match. The Victorian beard had but a short life : common enough from about 1860 it was already disappearing by 1890, when the young *Fin de Siècle* æsthetes made a conscientious point of leading the return to the razor, just as many of their spiritual brethren (both before and since) have been pioneers of the beard. Those whose first memories were of the present century grew up to regard the beard as a sign of age or a property of Father Christmas. In France *barbe* even came to mean a bore ; and *cela me barbe* is today a way of saying that something is disagreeable. Both beards and moustaches shortened towards the end of the century, before the virtual disappearance of the beard in England.

Decline and Fall of the Moustache

Among the few who have retained the beard in our own time have been the officers and ratings of the British Navy, where (since mid-Victorian times) a man may grow both moustache and beard, but not the one without the other. The British Army, on the

other hand, has not taken kindly to beards, in spite of the
civilian revolution for which the army of the Crimea was responsible. Following a *Brains Trust* broadcast on March 14,
1949, when reasons for growing beards were discussed, a correspondent wrote to the *Radio Times* with two instances of beards
grown by army officers in Kitchener's time—and with impunity.
One was grown to keep the owner's head above water when
swimming. (For other exceptions see *Notes and Queries,* 11th Series,
297 and 386.) In 1914 the military moustache was nevertheless
so well established that British army regulations insisted upon
its growth—or, at least, upon the fact that the upper lip should
not be shaved. The distinction is important, because the
withdrawal of this order, soon after the outbreak of the war,
is said to have been due to the predicament of an Eminent
Person, who found himself as ill-equipped as Marmaduke
Lawson to produce *The manly growth that fringed his upper lip*
(Tennyson, I believe). The matter became optional, and there
was no noticeable increase in the number of moustaches. Indeed,
such as existed shrank in size, the *Guardee* (which had long charac-
terised sergeant majors) being shortened to a mere toothbrush—a
casualty of the conditions prevailing in trench warfare. The
specially designed *moustache-cup* soon became démodé and will
shortly be a collector's rarity.

Of the Indian Summer between the two world wars I suppose
one clear nostalgic memory will always be the films of Charlie
Chaplin in the 'twenties. Here the toothbrush moustache
reached its peak of absurdity; and it is curious to reflect that the
much imitated Chaplin moustache, two short smudges below
the nose, was another example of Nature imitating Art, for the
moustache of Mr. Chaplin was a false one. Among those who
copied this preposterous style was a certain Herr Hitler, [1] who
achieved the incredible feat of persuading the German people to
take his paranoia seriously, in spite of his vaudeville appearance.
Side-whiskers appeared tentatively in the 'twenties, but soon
became associated with louts and the type now known as a *spiv.*

Memories of famous beards still linger with us. That of

[1] Described in the *Encyclopædia Britannica* (14th Edition, article on Bavaria) as
a good demagogue but no politician.

President Kruger comes to my mind—as familiar in the Boer War as Hitler's moustache or that of Kaiser Wilhelm II in the caricatures of later periods. Partridge in *Slang Today and Yesterday* notes *Kruger's Ticklers* as the name of a small brush, and one of my own contemporaries remembers buying licorice sweets known as *Kruger's Whiskers* in Brixham, as late as 1930.

Beards in the second World War

The second World War produced an ephemeral crop of the genuine article, such as the temporary revival of the *collier* in the Maginot Line (for reasons similar to those which had made French soldiers, beardless according to the regulations, become *poilus* in 1914-18). Heroes of the Jungle War in Burma grew beards which, however, disappeared when they returned to more normal conditions. In the German army, where the right to grow a beard was a matter of rank, I have no doubt that discipline broke down in the conditions that prevailed during the retreat on the eastern front. The Americans alone, perhaps, managed to preserve their clean-shaven standards throughout the war, though their addiction to electric razors (clippers, properly speaking) caused many a crisis in their British and European camps and billets.

The Tarzan motif

The type of moustache first popularised by Douglas Fairbanks still appears to be the standard design at Hollywood, and has its devotees in a world where the movies have long been replacing Kings and Courts as mirrors of fashion. The idea, spread by Maupassant, Kipling and others, that women prefer a bristly buss, still has its adherents. Dr. E. J. Dingwall (to whom I am greatly indebted for much assistance) informs me that he has also a great deal of information on the *Tarzan Motif*, which will in due course be made known to the public in another illuminating book on Woman. He proposes to discuss among other things the cult of hairy chests. As to this I was informed that advertisements had appeared in an American magazine setting forth the virtues of a *chest-wig* for those who were insufficiently Tarzanic. But enquiry from *Esquire*—the magazine named—produced the reply that no such advertisement had appeared, with the comment that the idea seemed fantastic, not to say impracticable ; a fact which was (of course) the reason for my morbid curiosity.

A few bearded sects are still reported occasionally (they include one among the Yorkshire colliers), and a new vogue of centenary beards has recently arisen. The beard as a memorial was, I believe, first proposed by a correspondent in the *Irish Times* of May 1, 1911, as a tribute to the memory of Edward VII. It now appears in South Africa, among the descendants of the *Voortrekkers* —as a memorial and once more as a political emblem (of white supremacy and Boer nationalism). Young men in Ironton, Ohio, are growing whiskers to celebrate the hundredth anniversary of their town, even as I write—perhaps they were inspired by the American businessmen (*Life*, April 14, 1947) who did the same thing to celebrate the centenary of their firm.

Loretta Young, in a creditable effort to say something new about England, assured Americans not long since that she had met a British news-hound who grew a beard because it was impossible to buy razor blades. It was astonishing to notice the sensitivity of the London press to this story. The bearded reporter proved to exist, for his colleagues ran him to earth in Southampton, where it is remarkable that he was allowed to explain his beard and not lynched (without a hearing) on a charge of spreading derogatory reports about the state of the Empire. He should have replied (and perhaps he did) that he was only following the advice of the ultra-patriotic *Evening Standard*,[1] which devoted its leading article on August 9, 1947, to an appeal for the return of beards worthy of the descendants of Drake and Raleigh—*the outlet which every man needs for his individualism in times of austerity and control.* This article was but an echo of an artful plea put forward in the *Hairdressers' Weekly Journal* before the war. The safety razor, which did so much to kill the beard, killed much of the barber's trade with it. Hence a wily barber suggested that his colleagues should urge their clients to wear beards again so that they would

[1] I note also an article in *The Star* (October 14, 1948) explaining that West End stores were looking for *kindly-faced men with rosy cheeks* to play Santa Claus (commercial brand), and that real beards were essential. The modern critical child could stomach the racket, but not false whiskers, apparently.

come for trimmings.   *You will at least,* he said, *see your clients twice or three times a week.*

Figaro as Machiavelli

The same note was struck (by the same person surely, and with the same Machiavellian motive) in other articles—e.g. one in the *Hairdressers' Weekly Journal* dated July 4, 1936 :

The *Imperial* and the heavy eyebrows give the wearer a fierce and dominating appearance that can only be found now in the film world.

And again, in the *Rules and Technical Handbook* of the London Academy of Gentlemen's Hairdressing, we read that *No one can go away from the fact that the effect of a beard is manly and distinguished. You cannot help remarking that most people who have a beard are of high standing or distinction.*   A Dublin wit, John D. Sheridan, had an article on *Beards and Bare Faces* in the *Irish Independent,*[1] and though it contained no special pleading for the return of the beard I cannot help thinking that the renewed interest in the subject (I have myself had two articles on it accepted since I began this book) is perhaps comparable to the steady propaganda which preceded the Victorian Renaissance.   One of Mr. Sheridan's valuable observations is the fact that most men, though they now remove their beards, still like to think of them as *strong,* and boast of the trouble they cause.   He regards them as *bare-faced liars.*   I notice that John Brophy, in *The Human Face,* expressed the view that most men at some time try to grow a beard, just to prove that they can do it.   I tried myself twice, with contemptible results.   Fortunately my object was not to test my virility, but merely to avoid the tedium of shaving (during two periods of my life when there seemed to be no imperative need not to look a fool, so far as I could help it).   So the poverty of my chin did not worry me.

The Holy See and the Victorian beard

The Victorian beards brought a last flicker of the old ecclesiastical controversy.   In December, 1860, an Anglican bishop (Rochester) attacked the growing menace, which had evidently

[1] Reprinted in condensed form in *The Irish Digest* for July, 1948.

affected the chins of curates in his diocese. This was the occasion for a spirited defence of the beard in a letter to *The Times* of January 2, 1861, signed W.M. The writer delighted in the fact that the curates concerned were not as compliant as Henry I had been when confronted by Bishop Serlo. Evidently this Bishop lacked the high-pressure violence of his great predecessor, Ernulphus. Beards—often of great prolixity—appeared on many clerical faces from that time, especially those of non-conformists and Low Churchmen (the lower the church, the longer the beard). Nevertheless, a Dutchman, who went to hear the great Spurgeon preach, wrote to him expressing his disapproval of the preacher's beard and moustache, which marked him as carnal and worldly-minded. Bishops continued to resist the innovation, and the first prelate of the Church of England to appear in a full beard was the evangelical John Ryle, first Anglican Bishop of Liverpool —in the very year (1880) from which the decline of the beard among laymen can be traced. Rome resisted similar attempts at innovation, though Wernz and Vidal recall that it was necessary for Pius IX to confirm the old practice *ex mandato speciali*. (In his time an attempt to restore the beard was even made by a bishop, at a Vatican Council in 1870). A Council of the Catholic Fathers at Westminster (1873) and a Plenary Council at Baltimore (1876) applied the Papal ruling to England and America respectively. But as late as January 10, 1920[1] it was necessary for the Church to uphold the rule and the authority of a bishop in enforcing it against Bohemian clergy who wanted to grow beards. It seems to have been a recurring vice among the transmontane barbarians, for Thurston in the *Catholic Encyclopedia* mentions a similar scandal in 1865, when *an attempt made by some of the clergy of Bavaria . . . to introduce the wearing of beards was rebuked by the Holy See*. This was when beards were the *dernier cri* in current fashion, and Fathers *novitatis vel potius levitatis spiritu perducti* fell into an error which it is easier to explain than to excuse.[2]

[1] This was the case of Wratislava, *ubi negatur per codicem datam esse clericis sæcularibus libertatem gestandi barbam.* (*Jus Canonicum*, Wernz and Vidal, Tom II, page 113.)

[2] See Barbier de Montault II, XX, 8.

I have a presentiment that this book must end some time, and that it should be soon. The more is the pity, for there lies before me a vast heap of unused material, enough to make another volume.

The last of the Barber-Surgeons

It is not long since I sat in a barber's chair—*a barber's chair that fits all*, as Procter said in *The Barber's Shop*, coyly suppressing the rest of the sentence. And so sitting (upon my pin-buttocks) I discoursed with the elderly gentleman who was ministering to my needs, speaking of this book, as an amateur who shyly probes a professional for advice. I was surprised when my barber friend informed me that he had himself been employed as a lather-boy, when about six or seven years of age, by a man whom he believed to have been the last of the barber-surgeons. The place was Drayton Park, Holloway, the year, about 1890.[1]

Finding that men still lived who could recall the great *chirurgiens-barbiers d'antan*, who let blood and drew teeth, I wrote to the *Hairdresser's Weekly Journal* inviting further reminiscences. As a result I am now perhaps the only common repository of such information ; and the secrets of my confessional include an affidavit regarding one of the last barber-surgeons of Denmark, also the recollections of a hairdresser whose father was apprenticed to a barber-surgeon at Leipzig in 1878. This enterprising German not only practised barbery and bone-setting, blood letting, dentistry and chiropody, but kept bees for stinging rheumatic patients into health.

But I must leave bee-doctors, also the beards of Havelock Ellis and Dr. Freud (ah, how much I could have said *en revanche* under pretext of analysis). And I must lay aside my notes for a long sermon on a text from Pagenstecher : *Dividimus autem Barbam in Nigram, Rubram & Albam.* Perhaps you will never learn why Judas is represented with a red beard.[2] My vast catalogue of

[1] The reader will perceive that I did not follow the principles of Archelaus, who, when asked how he would be shaved, replied *silently*. He must have missed a good deal. (See Plutarch *De Garrulitate,* where he has other stories relating to barbery.)

[2] See Appendix I.

Bearded Women must also remain unpublished.[1]   You must look for yourself in the rare pages of Burchardus, or the vast tomes of Migne for the story of Galla, the daughter of Symnachus, that holy woman who *elegit magis* (said Gregory the Great) *spiritalibus nuptiis copulari Deo,* and grew a beard—the result predicted by her medical advisors—as a direct result of her sanctity.   There are, however, a few observations on the subject of bearded women that I shall permit myself by way of conclusion, because I began this book with a riddle and hope to end it with an answer.

False beards of the Argive widows

Jacques Ferrand in his *Erotomania* remarks that Hippocrates seems to attribute to passionate love the power of transforming women into men, as was the case of Phæthusa, in the city of Abdera ; for she pined for one Pytheus, and grew a long beard like Galla.   And the same befell Namysia, wife to one Gorgippus. Hence it is not remarkable that many primitive peoples believe the women of olden times to have been bearded, as my friend Mr. Verrier Elwin has recently shown in his *Myths of Middle India*, of which he has kindly sent me proofs.   Doubtless these women of old loved with a love that was more than love. The false beards worn by the women of Argos on their nuptial beds, which mystified Ernest Crawley when he was writing *The Mystic Rose*, may be simply explained upon the same assumption—and a certain Monsieur Quitard once justified them in a learned article.[2]   Having avenged their first husbands with such valour, fighting under the poetess Telesilla against the Spartans, the widows who first acquired this right might well be assumed to love their second husbands with a devotion worthy of men— *beard-worthy*, the highest honour. We, said M. Quitard, only offered ribbons (feminine ornaments) to our heroes, but they (the Argives) gave beards to their heroines.

Now observe your Goddesses of Love. Friga, the Teutonic

[1] See Appendix A.

[2] Reproduced in full by Larousse under *Barbe,* in the *Dictionnaire du XIX Siècle.* The story is alluded to by Herodotus (VI, 77) and (in more detail) by Plutarch (*De Mulierum Virtutibus*).

Venus, was an hermaphrodite, and Verstegen shows us that this goddess wore a great beard, like the Venus of Amathos. *Signum etiam eius est Cypri*, says Macrobius (Sat. III, 8), there is indeed a statue of her in Cyprus, *barbatum corpore sed veste muliebri*. She was worshipped by men clad as women and women in the garments of men. (Telesilla was annually remembered in like manner.) Theophrastus tells the same story, and the Byzantine writer, Joannes Lydus, has a similar account in his *De Mensibus* of a bearded Aphrodite worshipped by the Pamphylians. This bearded goddess is identified by Fraser with Astarte ; and in *The Golden Bough*[1] he gives the authority of Philochorus for the opinion that this original Hermaphrodite represented the moon.

The Moon lives on horseflesh

At last we have the answer to the Rolleston Riddle. For in the same volume of *The Golden Bough* (page 149) you will find a dialogue between the Huzuls of the Carpathians and the moon, in which it is made clear that THE MOON LIVES ON HORSE-FLESH. Now turn to Jacob Grimm's *Teutonic Mythology* and you will find it distinctly stated that witches (who are well-known as worshippers of the moon) eat horseflesh, and that a horse-bone is used as a pipe by trolls who live under hills.[2] And what better survival of the bearded Venus can you wish to find than the witch cult ?

> You should be women,
> And yet your beards forbid me to interpret
> That you are so.

If anyone could doubt the impeccable authority of *Macbeth* I will refer him to *The Witch Cult in Central Europe* and *The God of the Witches*, by our leading witch-huntress, Margaret Murray, who has made it clear that witches and witch-gods are bearded.

The Riddle Solved

Ergo, the connection between hippophagy and pogonotrophy exists, but is transmitted only on the distaff side. The ancient

[1] Third edition (1914) Vol. VI, 259 n.3.
[2] English translation of 1888, Vol. IV, pages 1302 and 1619.

Goddess of Love, the Moon herself—not the cold Diana but that same Babylonian Ashtaroth, of whom Yaweh himself was jealous—has been worshipped through all ages by women. *Her priestesses were bearded* (at least, like the Queens of Egypt, upon ceremonial occasions) but *her priests were eunuchs* ; and it was to her, you will remember, the *Dea Syria*, that *men sacrificed their beards* at Hierapolis. Also it was to this Usurper of the Beard that, in all ages past, and almost universally (wherever the strong and docile brute was known) the horse was sacrificed. What can he symbolise but Man ?

In a distant island it was once the custom that when the king died he was placed upon a chariot in such a way that his head (and doubtless his beard also) dragged in the dirt. Behind the chariot walked a woman, who threw dust upon his head. There may be something in it. . . . Significantly this island was none other than Serendip. As they say at the movies, this is where we came in.

APPENDIX A

BEARDED WOMEN

FOR those interested in Bearded Women I recommend the Index-Catalogue of the Library of the Surgeon General's Office, United States Army. Under *Hair, Abnormalities of*, they will find many titles : Buerlinus (J.) *De foeminis ex suppressione mensium barbatis* (Altdorfina, 1664); Hoyerus (G. L.) *De fæmina barbata* in the *Acta physico-medica Academiæ*, etc. (Nuremberg, 1737, IV. 378-380); Laurence (J. L.) *A short account of the bearded and hairy female* (*Lancet*, 1857, II, 48); and two articles entitled *Case of a bearded woman*—one by Duhring (L. A.) in the New York *Archives of Dermatology* (1877, III, 193-200), the other in the *St. Louis Magazine* (1877, XIV, 584-587). See also Schurig's *Spermatologia* (Frankfort, 1720) and the *Dissertatio de fæminis barbatis* of J. G. Joch (Jena, 1702).

Notable cases are mentioned by Bulwer, who assures us that there was a mountain in Ethiopia where women grew long beards. The bearded woman grenadier, who fought in the army of Charles XII, is mentioned by Père Oudin among others. A number of authentic cases are given by Gould and Pyle (*Anomalies and Curiosities of Medicine*) and further ones will be found in C. J. S. Thompson's *Mystery and Lore of Monsters*. Among other authors already quoted in these pages, Ulmus, Fangé and Procter have useful information, showing the royal patronage often offered to bearded ladies. Two were the guests of the Sultan in 1881 ; and the bearded Helena Antonia, according to Ulmus (p. 307) was a special favourite of Margarita of Austria, later Queen of Spain. The *Acta Sanctorum* (February Tom. III) records the case of a Spanish girl, pursued by a debauched young man, who prayed that her face might be transformed. She was granted a beard, and the young man did not recognise her.

Margaret of Parma, Regent of the Netherlands, was among the most distinguished bearded ladies of history. Those who earned a good living by exhibitions included Josephine Boisdechene, who married twice ; Augustina Barbara (mentioned in Granger III, 153) of whom John Evelyn wrote that *she plaied well on yᵉ harpsichord* ; and Julia Patrana, who was embalmed and exhibited even after her death.

This great respect paid to bearded women is doubtless a relic of the belief (recorded by Alexander of Alexandria) that bearded women were specially gifted, notably as the vehicles of divine oracles. Hence the beard which was grown (according to Herodotus, I, 175 and VIII, 104) by the priestess of Athene among the Pedasians, when any evil threatened their community.

APPENDIX B

BEAVERS

THE French word *bavarder*, to babble, *bavard*, a babbler, and *bavardage*, are from the word *bave*, which gives us also *baver*, to dribble. All these words—babble, dribble, and *baver*, were evolved by onomatoplasm, like the various synonyms of babble—cackle, gabble, tattle, prattle, chatter, jabber and blather. Clearly the origin is similar to that of the word *barbarian*—the *ba-ba* or *bla-bla* of an unknown tongue sounding very much like the noises made by a child. The Latin *bibere* (giving us *bib*, *imbibe* and—via the French—*beverage*) may have a similar origin in the imitation of sound. Hence the cant use of the word *beaver* has much to recommend it, apart from the fact that a beard, like the original beaver, makes a face invisible—though it is not so conveniently shifted as (e.g.) the beaver worn by the ghost in *Hamlet*. Partridge (*Dictionary of Slang*, 1937) mentions *beaver* for a beard or bearded man as *a passing term and pastime of the 1920's*; but Frank Richardson in *Whiskers and Soda* (1910) could already refer to *beavers, as bearded men are technically termed.*

APPENDIX C

THE CAPUCHIN BEARD

ACCORDING to an illuminating footnote in the *Pogonologie* of J. A. Dulaure, beards have sometimes proved inconvenient to their wearers when dancing or impersonating women in plays, which I can well believe. He gives examples from the experiences of the Capuchins, and alleges that those of Montpellier, in the year 1731, acted a tragedy in the dining hall of their monastery, when those who played the parts of women were under the necessity of concealing their beards beneath a parchment covering, painted the colour of flesh. At Lyons, also, where the Capuchins performed for three consecutive days in *Les Fourberies de Scapin*, in 1757, pink taffeta bags were used by those who had occasion to conceal their beards, of whom one showed great grace and suppleness in a Hungarian dance. M. Dulaure says that similar devices were used by the Capuchins of Grenoble and Vienne, and his object in recording them was not (he assures us) to mock the beards of these religious men, but to deplore the frivolity that had caused them to be concealed.

The beards of the Capuchins were nevertheless a source of much criticism which malice, or (it may well have been) *envy* directed against them. Monsieur Dulaure recalls the titles of various tracts written against the beards of those unfortunate friars, during the first part of the eighteenth century, together with the adventure which befell some of the order at Ascoli, when they were put to sleep by a large dose of opium in their food, administered by the cook (a lay-brother) who shaved them one and all while they lay drugged, and so left them ; from which deprivation the brothers took to themselves such shame that they felt no more inclination to stir abroad than David's ambassadors in a similar situation, but kept to the house till they had nourished a new crop of dignity.

Barbe de capucin is a name for chicory, and according to Larousse (article on *Barbe* in the *Dictionnaire du XIX Siecle*) a reference to it in a vaudeville script was censored during the brief and precarious rule of Charles X, the censor writing in the margin *Choose another salad*. The delicate point appears to have been the *capucinades* of the French Court, a *capucinade* being a tedious discourse.

As a comment on the clerical tradition respecting the upper lip, and the necessity for avoiding the defilement of the sacrament, Barbier de Moutault remarks that *les Capucins se rasent complètement la partie qui avoisine la lèvre supérieure.*

APPENDIX D

CZAR NICHOLAS I AND THE BEARD

AUBRIL claimed that Nicholas I renewed the edicts of Peter the Great against beards in general. I can find no confirmation of this except an alleged proclamation of Laszczynski, Governor of Warsaw, of which an English translation appeared in the *Knickerbocker* for 1850 (XXXV, 498), an undated document culled from *The Tribune* (also undated) which had reproduced it from *La Voix du Peuple* (undated). . . . This proclamation stated that the Czar had ordered the Russian and Polish nobles to shave, apparently because beards were considered incompatible with the wearing of uniform, a privilege recently conferred on the nobility. *I call upon the Military Prefects* (runs the alleged proclamation) *to take prompt and efficacious measures to the end that the detestable usage of wearing beards may be repressed, and that the inhabitants abandon this indecent and subversive innovation.* To call a beard an *innovation* seems odd, even after sixty years of efforts to suppress beards. But until the Iron Curtain lifts I fear it may be impossible to verify this document and discover its date.

DEDICATION OF HAIR

OF the office of baptism, according to the Greek rite, Simeon, Bishop of Thessalonica, tells us that after the holy unction the hair of the person's head is shorn in the form of a cross, and this for divers reasons among which he says that it is a sign to mark *that all vain and superfluous thoughts are from that time to be cut off. For this reason* (says he) *monks are entirely shorn.* But why their beards should escape, as they invariably do among the Eastern Christians, Simeon of Thessalonica does not explain. As to what is done with the hair, we have the familiar story of dedication, for it is offered, writes Simeon, by the baptised person to Christ, *as a sort of first fruits,* as the sacrifice of his body ; the hair being, as it were, the exhalation of the whole body. *The chief priest therefore does not carelessly throw it away, but lays it apart in a sacred place.*

For this ceremony there are appropriate prayers, of which English translations will be found on pages 218-220 of *The Rites and Ceremonies of the Greek Church in Russia,* by John Glen King, D.D., a work published in London, in 1772. The Deacon, in his opening prayer, refers to the creation of man, by God, who *on the superior part of the body didst place the head, in which many senses are so disposed as not to hinder each other's operation ; and didst cover his head with hair, to guard it from the changes and intemperate of the air.* The Deacon then offers on behalf of his client *his first fruits, the tonsure of his head,* which he cuts with a pair of scissors, and, having wrapped up the clippings in a small piece of wax, he throws it into the font.

This appears to conflict with the statement that the clippings are laid apart in a sacred place, but we may assume that the sacred locks are not left in the font for the charwoman to clear away ; and Du Cange cites an authority who says that the trophy is given to the child's God-father who (according to some) stamps the wax with the image of Our Lord and keeps it as a manner of gage or tally, in security for the good behaviour of his god-son. This practice, like that of the ceremonial first shaving of the adolescent, had at one time its counterpart in Western practice, as may be seen in the *Oratio ad Capillaturam* of St. Gregory (*vide* Du Cange, *Dissertations sur l'Histoire de Saint Louys* ; Diss. XXII *Des Adoptions d'honneur en fils*). This dedication of a child's hair—or the beard of an adolescent—was not always a gift to God, as we have already observed. It might be a token merely of human adoption, as in the case of Clovis, if we follow the account which reads *ut in tondenda barba Clodovei patrinus ejus efficeretur Alaricus,* quoted by Du Cange, under *Barbam tangere.* The case of that Byzantine Emperor Constantine IV (whose beard was so notable that he earned the agnomen of *Pogonatus*) lies on the border line; for he sent his children's hair to the Pope as a sign, we are told, that he wished them to recognise the supremacy of the Roman See—a very nice point for a scholastic debate on the venerability of the Vatican, its age and origin.

APPENDIX F

POGONOLOGY

I HAVE not added to the length of this book with a bibliography, which would be of enormous length, but have indicated in tracing the history of the beard the chronology of the more important literature relating to it, with some notes on the various writers.

To these names a vast number could be added. Larousse (v. *Barbe* in the *Dictionnaire du XIX Siècle*) appends a bibliography which includes several works which I have not read. A number of works on Continental Barber-Surgeons will be found under the names of Heinrich Berger, Carl Bruhns, D. Burchiello, Hyacinthe Coulon and G. A. Wehrli, among others. There are also many references in Buckle's *Common Place Book* ; but when this was published with the *Miscellaneous and Posthumous Works* (1872) the prudery of the editor or publisher caused many promising items to be omitted, though for some reason they were allowed to remain in the index. (These included some references to close-stools, which I found deleted when writing *Cleanliness and Godliness*, and a reference to *Beards : Arabic Superstition*, about which the present owner of Buckle's MSS. may one day enlighten us). A bibliography of beards by W. D. Macray in *Notes and Queries* (11th S. XI, 262) also gives several titles not mentioned here, including some Bodleian MSS.

Many books completely eluded my search. These included a modern American work, *Concerning Beards*, by Edwin Valentine Mitchell, of which no copy appears to be available in the British Isles, Isadore Dyer's *Science of Shaving* (1727) Eugen Dulac's *Physiologie de la Barbe et des Moustaches* (1842) Georg Gaspar Kirchmaier's work, *de Gloria et Maiestate Barbæ*, and an *Apology for the Beard* by *Artium Magister* (1862). But the saddest omission was the work of my own true predecessor, Dr. Adrien Phillippe, whose *Histoire Philosophique, Politique et Religieuse de la Barbe chez les principaux peuples de la terre* (Paris 1845) is available in the Bibliothèque Nationale, but nowhere in England. Aubril describes this book as extremely rare, because almost all the copies were destroyed by the author himself ; and even Aubril must have written from memory, as he gives an incorrect date and place of publication, mis-spelling the author's name. If I ever revise this book for another edition I must certainly try to visit Paris and consult Dr. Phillippe.

Rhythmical Essays on the Beard Question by W. Carter was a title that interested me (mid-nineteenth century ?) but has also proved untraceable so far. Schelle's *Geschichte des maenlichen Barts* is merely a translation of Fangé's work. Many other titles will be found in other sections of this appendix, of works dealing with specialised aspects of pogonotrophy, and Fangé's list of authors should also be consulted by the serious student. The celebrated Swiss doctor, Théodore Tronchin, is said to have written a brochure on beards, under the pseudonym of

Esculape, but I have not succeeded in verifying this. *De Barba Disputatio* (already mentioned) by Gothofredus Barthius contains little that is not to be found in other works mentioned in this book.

Other works on Church History where clerical beards are discussed are Routh's *Reliquiæ Sacræ* and Duchesne's *Histoire Ancienne de l'Eglise*. Among modern books, G. A. Foan's *Art and Craft of Hairdressing* has an interesting chapter on beards, and there is also *The Hair and Scalp*, with a chapter on *Hirsuties*, by A. Saville. Frank Richardson's frequent references to beards (*circa* 1905-1911) are tedious and historically inaccurate, though he produced one good quatrain on whiskers. The *Western Stamp Collector* of Albany, Oregon, reports a collection of stamps showing bearded heads, in the possession of Walter L. Gates, whose superb beard inspired the idea.

APPENDIX G

SAXON BEARDS

IT must be admitted that some Anglo-Saxon illustrations do *not* appear to bear out the view—commonly accepted—that the Saxons were bearded at least until about a generation before the Norman Conquest. A ninth century MS. of the *Psychomania* of Prudentius is illustrated by drawings which show more shaven than bearded faces ; and about the same proportion of each will be found in an illustrated Anglo-Saxon calendar of about A.D. 1050 (Cottonian Library, Julius, A. IV). These drawings, which depict the activities of the twelve months, might superficially be taken as confirmation of the usual opinion —e.g., that expressed in the *Encyclopæda Britannica* (article on Beards), where the moustache and forked beard are assumed to have been originally characteristic of the Anglo-Saxons, with the comment that *the beard had passed out of fashion before the Norman Conquest.*

There are, however, two difficulties about fitting these old illustrations into such a story. Firstly, there is the general absence of even a *moustache* in these Anglo-Saxon drawings. The moustache was commonly acknowledged, on the clearest authority of all the written evidence, to have been characteristically Saxon. As we have seen, even those who deny that Saxons in 1066 commonly wore beards acknowledge that they certainly wore moustaches, and were by these distinguished from most of the Normans. Secondly, if we accept the testimony of such drawings, those which illustrate Prudentius show a predominance of beardless and moustache-less Saxons about the time that Alfred the Great was drawing up laws to protect the beard ; and we have seen that a *shorn man* in Alfred's Dooms clearly and exclusively describes the priest and the monk.

Alfred died in A.D. 900, and though the precise date of the *Psychomania* MS. at the British Museum (Cotton. Cleopat. C. VIII) is not known, these illustrations are likely to have been executed before rather than after the beard laws were promulgated. They certainly do not present a picture of men desperately anxious to preserve their beards or their moustaches, and they offer what is really a much greater problem than the evidence of Bayeux, because these are not foreign representations but examples of our own indigenous art.

I have contented myself with answering the case as it is usually presented on the evidence of the so-called tapestry. Had Freeman and others concentrated instead on early Saxon art they could have presented a much better case than they did, for which I have in fact no answer, except that we are faced by the apparently irreconciliable testimonies of irrefutable authorities. But the evidence of early Saxon art, if it proves anything at all, proves far more than most of the pandits have been prepared to accept, being as disconcerting to the opinions of Freeman and others as it is to my own conjectures.

As I have shown in the case of the *Marquis Otto*, in Randle Holme's description of the *British Beard* and elsewhere, the word *beard* could refer simply to a moustache. But Matthew Paris so explicitly compares the Saxon beards with those of the Orient that this explanation of the passages quoted in Chapter IV is hardly satisfactory.

APPENDIX   H

SUNDAY SHAVING

As early as 1317 the Pope complained to the French King regarding this practice, as Odoricus Reynaldus informs us in his continuation of Baronius. A Council of Paris, in 1429, forbade barbers to work on Sundays or days sacred to the Virgin or the Apostles—a prohibition repeated in more general terms, to cover all menial employment and the opening of shops at such times. The State was no less zealous, and Charles VI, when renewing the charter of the French *Chirurgiens-Barbiers*, forbade them to work at certain festivals except in urgent cases of surgery. The French barber was forbidden, by a statute of Henry III, to open shop or display his sign on Sundays or other holy days—a regulation confirmed by Henry IV, who extended its application.

Feeling was evidently strong in New England on the same subject, and Richardson Wright in the *New York Herald Tribune* Weekly Book Review recalls that four Pennsylvania barbers were fined for Sunday shaving in 1702, similar action being taken in Boston.

APPENDIX I

THE BEARD OF JUDAS

A CERTAIN Pierre l'Eguillard wrote a book in praise of red beards, under the title *Enopogonérythrée*, published at Caen in 1580. A special significance has always attached to red hair ever since the Egyptians (according to Manetho) used to burn a red-haired man occasionally by way of sacrifice. Mohamet's preference for red beards has already been mentioned, but among the Jews they have been ill-esteemed ever since the descendants of Jacob began to malign the unfortunate Esau. This may be the origin of the Judas legend of which Pagenstecher wrote *forsan ab ipso Apostolo Juda, quem rubram barbam habuisse vulgus cantat, unde hodie adhuc dicitur* :

> Roth Barte nie gut wart
> Roth Bart Schelmen art.

This he connects with *Judas der Ertz Schelm* (the subject of a tract by Abraham à S. Clara). Charlemagne even had to make it a punishable offence to call a man *Red Beard*.

The name Ahenobarbus indicates that no such prejudice existed among the Romans. (The family ancestor had his beard turned red by the Dioscuri, when they miraculously revealed to him the victory at Lake Regillus.) How Barbarossa lived down the tradition I have no idea. It was among the abuse hurled by the French at the English in the Hundred Years War that they were red-bearded (see page 135) and as late as 1601 the Flemish engraver Jean de Glen (*Des habits, moeurs*, etc.) said that the English usually had red hair and liked this colour. I cannot recollect any outstanding English cases, except William Rufus and King John, who was said to have a Judas beard. That of Hudibras was orange, mixed with grey. At least one distinguished Frenchman (François de Harlay, Bishop of Rouen) wore a red-gold beard of great length, which caused his brother-bishop Alphonse d'Elbène to speculate as to which was longer—his beard or some of his funeral sermons. (This Bishop of Rouen nevertheless recorded his objection to moustaches—and to long hair—in a synodical decree of 1618.) Canel cites a rare work of 1633 in which this bearded bishop seems to be mentioned (*mais je ne vis jamais une telle barbe*, said the writer, who claimed that the monks spent two hours a day *à la peigner et attifer*).

The *Jewish Encyclopedia* (v. Hair) says that red-haired persons are held to be passionate and treacherous, relating the idea again to Judas. I do not know whether the traditional representation of Cain with a yellow beard is also of Jewish origin, but this is the meaning of the Cain-coloured beard in the *Merry Wives* (I. 4.23). A much more favourable view was taken by Petrus of Riga, who said that yellow beards were grown by those Israelites who did not worship the Golden Calf—evidently not a large number. Blonde beards were certainly

esteemed in the Græco-Roman world, and much praised by Theocritus. Bearded
men in the Middle Ages and after were often synthetic blondes, just as many
Moslems (other than Turks and Persians) used henna to dye their beards red.
When the Sultan of Zanzibar visited England in 1875 there were many red
beards among his retinue.

The dyeing of beards has an ancient history, which includes the story variously
attributed to Philip of Macedon and to a king of Sparta (Ulmus says Archi-
damus, but does not indicate which of that name). In the Macedonian version
Philip tells Antipater that he does not consider a man who is insincere in his hair
to be trustworthy in his undertakings—*in capillis infidum, in rebus gerendis fide
dignum esse non puto.* For dyes and their application to the beard (religious or
fashionable) I refer the reader to Cheyne and Black's *Encyclopædia Biblica* (Vol. II,
1938-41) ; to the account of Indian Customs in Flavius Arrianus (the voyage of
Nearkhos in the so-called eighth book of the *Anabasis*) ; and to Bulwer, who
quotes Bacon and others respecting the habits of the Turks (they were said to dye
their beards black—which would seem unnecessary—with *a powder made of a
mineral called Alcohole*). Bulwer also discusses dyeing of the beard in England,
especially by old rakes with grey hair. The habit is referred to in *The Alchemist,*
also in *The Silent Woman* and in *Ram Alley* (V, 415) where red is mentioned as a
fasionable colour, in spite of the age-long prejudice. When beards returned in
nineteenth century France, dyeing returned with them, according to Rowland ;
but superstitions with regard to colour do not appear to have been revived.

APPENDIX J

WOMEN AND BEARDS (Male)

THE opinion of Beatrice in *Much Ado* is confirmed by that of Rosaline in Marston's *Antonio and Melida*. She says she will marry when men abandon jealousy, forsake tobacco and cease to wear their beards so rudely long :

Oh, to have a husband with a mouth continually smoking, with a bush of furze on the ridge of his chin, ready still to flop into his foaming chaps ; ah, 'tis more than intolerable.

The Bali Islanders, according to Fangé, used to depilate their faces to please their women ; and in Juvenal's time even the incipient beard of the shaven male disgusted some Roman women, hence :

Sunt quas eunuchi imbelles, ac mollia semper
Oscula delectent . . .

Darwin is quoted by Hilaire Hiler (*An Introduction to the Study of Costume*) as having said that man lost his coat of hair because men and women chose as mates those who were least hairy. But Hiler also mentions the description by Ctesias of the Indian Pygmæi that *they had hair and beards so long as to serve for vesture*. Among such people the opposite principle of selection must surely operate, as may be seen in the case of the Hairy Ainos, where hair is so greatly admired by the women that they tattoo moustaches on their own faces—or did when A. H. Savage Landor wrote his book about these people. (They are our own cousins, as their hair especially indicates, or so Mr. Duckworth affirms in his *Morphology and Anthropology*.) *Tattooing one's wife*, wrote Landor of these false moustahces, *seems to be one of the pleasures of the honeymoon*.

The Aino women do not appear to be so successful as those Australian aboriginies, of whom we learn in *The Golden Bough* (London 1917, Vol. I, 152-154) that they induce beard growth by pricking the chin with a magic stick or stone, the virtue of which consists in its representation of a rat with long whiskers. The female Aino never had occasion to use the *kike-ush-bashui* or moustache-lifter, an instrument shaped like a paper-knife and employed by her husband when drinking (both for its obvious purpose and for pointing gratefully at the person who stood the round). The Ainos (or *Ainus*, if you prefer), disdaining their kinship with Europeans, prefer to claim their descent from bears.